DIABETES

ARLEEN MARCIA TUCHMAN

Diabetes

A HISTORY OF RACE AND DISEASE

Yale

UNIVERSITY PRESS

NEW HAVEN & LONDON

Yale University Press books may be purchased in quantity for educational, business,
or promotional use. For information, please e-mail sales.press@yale.edu (U.S. office)
or sales@yaleup.co.uk (U.K. office).

Set in Scala and Scala Sans type by Newgen North America.
Printed in the United States of America.

Library of Congress Control Number: 2020934121
ISBN 978-0-300-22899-1 (hardcover : alk. paper)

A catalogue record for this book is available from the British Library.

This paper meets the requirements of ANSI/NISO Z39.48-1992 (Permanence of Paper).

10 9 8 7 6 5 4 3 2 1

To my father, Sam Tuchman

1920–2013

CONTENTS

INTRODUCTION
Diabetes Types and Racial Stereotypes

September 1992

I had never had so much fun with my dad. He and his friend were visiting me in Nashville. We were all at the Opryland Hotel, and he was laughing, almost giddy. I was loving it. His friend, however, was getting increasingly nervous. Something's not right, she kept saying. Sure enough, during dinner he started having trouble controlling his tongue and his speech. When the medics arrived and measured his blood sugar, it was 30 milligrams per deciliters. "We don't understand why he's still conscious," they said as they offered him a tube of glucose and told me to get him a piece of pie.

April 1997

My father was still living in Florida when I got the call from my aunt. "You have to come down. Your father is in the hospital and the doctors don't think he will make it. His neighbors found him passed out on the bathroom floor. He must have been there for at least twenty-four hours. I'm so sorry."

September 2003

After moving to Nashville to be closer to his only grandchild, my father had taken a job at Sears. He was at work when I got the call. "Your dad is awake, but he is unresponsive. We're calling an ambulance. Meet us at the hospital." When I arrived, the doctor came out of my dad's room to tell me that I needed to be prepared to say goodbye. He didn't think my dad was going to survive the night.

December 2009

My dad ended up in the emergency room twice within two weeks. Because of a significant change in his electrocardiogram, the hospital admitted him, ordered an angiogram, and discovered a major blockage in a cardiac artery. A scheduled stent operation was aborted, however, when the surgeons realized he had blockages in three arteries. The next step, a planned quadruple bypass, was canceled when the neurologist insisted that my dad's nervous system wasn't calm enough to tolerate surgery. A few days later, my dad decided that he had no interest in such an invasive procedure at his age. He was eighty-nine years old.

May 18, 2013

My son became a Bar Mitzvah. My dad sang the second Aliyah.

May 31, 2013

My dad passed away peacefully in his sleep. He was one month shy of his ninety-third birthday.

I DID NOT LEARN WHAT IT MEANT to have a close relative with diabetes until 2002, when my elderly father moved to Nashville, where I live. Until then, I had no clue about the frequent scares and the frequent, seemingly miraculous recoveries. My father had been diagnosed in 1983, when he was sixty-three years old and still living in Brooklyn. His physician in New York initially assumed he had type 2 diabetes because of his age and the nature of his symptoms: he had been complaining of constant thirst and frequent urination. At the time, his diagnosis made sense. A short, round man, my dad reached five feet, three inches on a good day and weighed about 150 pounds, which qualified as "overweight" on the body mass index scale. A more informed physician might have realized that something was amiss when my dad's weight dropped to about 115 pounds within a year, but it wasn't until my parents retired to Florida in 1985 that an endocrinologist realized that my dad's pancreas was not producing any insulin. My father received a new diagnosis: late onset type 1 diabetes, or LADA.[1] Between 1985 and 2013, when my father passed away, he injected insulin four times a day.

My father's misdiagnosis and rediagnosis would not have happened a hundred years earlier for the simple reason that no one at the time thought of diabetes as consisting of different types of diseases.[2] To be sure, physicians, health journalists, diabetes patients, and family members were all aware that age greatly influenced the progression of the disease. In the days before insulin, diabetes advanced rapidly among the young, leading to significant weight loss, ketoacidosis, and death within a few short years. For those who were middle-aged or elderly, the body's deterioration took place at a slower pace, making it possible to live for several years, although often with significant health problems. People referred to these two forms as acute versus chronic, or severe versus mild, but they did not think of them as differing physiologically and pathologically.

The discovery of insulin in 1921–1922 minimized the differences between the two forms, because those whose bodies did not produce insulin could now inject a hormone that ameliorated the most severe aspects of the acute form. Still, by midcentury there was a growing sentiment that the two types were different enough in their age of onset, seriousness of symptoms, and degree of fatness to warrant a sharper distinction, and the terms "juvenile diabetes" and "adult-onset diabetes" came into more frequent use. By 1979, diabetes specialists considered such differences important enough that they officially divided diabetes into what they called insulin-dependent diabetes mellitus (IDDM) and non-insulin-dependent diabetes mellitus (NIDDM). By 1995, these two were known as type 1 and type 2.[3] Today, as I write, there is considerable discussion about whether this classification continues to make sense.

The medical community actually recognizes more than two types of diabetes. After types 1 and 2, the third most common form is gestational diabetes, in which diabetic symptoms appear during pregnancy and then usually abate after birth, leaving mothers at risk of developing type 2 diabetes later in life. There are also less common forms, including maturity onset diabetes of the young (MODY), neonatal diabetes mellitus (NDM), and latent autoimmune diabetes of adulthood (LADA). What they all have in common is high blood sugar, but beyond that, they are considered to be quite different. For example, type 2, which afflicts roughly 90 percent of all people with diabetes in the United States—and in the world—is believed to develop when the body's tissues become insensitive or resistant to insulin. Type 1, in contrast, appears to be an autoimmune disease that develops when the body attacks the insulin-producing beta-cells of the pancreas, thereby destroying the body's ability to produce any insulin.[4]

Research conducted in the last several years, however, suggests that it may be misleading to draw a sharp line between insulin resistance and beta-cell dysfunction, and that it may make more sense both scientifically and clinically to think of diabetes as "a spectrum of disorders" with various degrees of insulin resistance and beta-cell dysfunction.[5] In other words, the proliferation of diabetes types in the medical literature since 1979 may stem from the medical community's continued struggle to understand what causes sugar to build up in the bloodstream. The belief in the past that something united all the different forms of diabetes may not have been totally wrong.

When I began working on this book, I thought that I would be writing the first history of type 2 diabetes. I intended to complement what we knew from several excellent studies of the history of diabetes, some of which had focused on insulin's discovery and the startling stories, following the hormone's distribution, of individuals literally rising from their deathbeds, and of parents rejoicing that they would not have to bury their children. I was especially inspired by the work of the physician-historian Chris Feudtner, who had turned his attention to the challenges that insulin-dependent diabetes patients faced after the initial excitement of the pathbreaking treatment wore off and complications associated with the disease began to emerge. He showed how those dependent on insulin learned quickly that the hormone was not a cure, but rather a tool for helping them manage their disease. In this way, his history of diabetes was less about "miracles" and more about insulin's role in transforming an acute disease into a chronic disease, which still left individuals struggling to stave off the common complications of blindness, limb amputations, kidney failure, and premature death.[6]

But several years into my research I had an "aha" moment when I realized that it would be anachronistic to write a history of type 2 diabetes. How could I write that history when the idea that diabetes consisted of discrete types emerged only gradually and was not officially recognized until the late 1970s? And what would it mean to distinguish between different types when insulin's discovery meant that those who had suffered from the acute form now had a chronic disease similar, although certainly not identical,

to the chronic form that others had always had? This is not to deny differences between those whose bodies produce no insulin and those whose
bodies produce some, but the goal of trying to tell the history of type 2 diabetes lost its appeal. Instead, I wondered what it meant for diabetes to have
undergone a division into types. Why had this split happened? What was
at stake in insisting on their differences? And what meanings have been
ascribed to the different forms?

These questions became more compelling for me when, at an early stage
of my research, I discovered evidence that there was a racial element to the
meaning of diabetes. For example, a hundred years ago a diabetes diagnosis
for my father, a middle-class Jew whose family had emigrated from Poland,
would almost have been expected: at that time, diabetes was so closely associated with Jews that it was referred to as the *Judenkrankheit*—or "Jewish
disease"—based on stereotypes about Jews as a people.[7]

* * *

Diabetes is a cultural history of a disease whose meaning has changed
markedly over the past 150 years. These changes reflect not only scientific
advances emerging from the laboratory and the clinic, but also shifting
meanings that professional and popular writers ascribed to diabetes as they
struggled to explain its emergence as a leading cause of death.[8] In focusing
on the cultural history of the disease, my primary purpose is to excavate
the ways that diabetes, in all its forms, has been a locus for the expression
of anxieties about economic, social, and political changes over the past century, many of which explicitly involved issues of race.

Consider how the racial profile of diabetes changed over a hundred-year
span. In 1898, a physician reported in the *Johns Hopkins Hospital Bulletin* that diabetes was "a rare disease in the colored race." Some twenty-five
years later, Elliott P. Joslin, arguably the leading diabetes specialist of his
day, informed readers of the *Journal of the American Medical Association*
that diabetes was "two and a half times as common among Jews." Jump
ahead roughly forty years, and Max Miller, an expert on diabetes in Native
American tribes, wrote that "both male and female Pima Indians had an ex-
traordinary frequency of 'diabetes'—higher than that reported in any other
population studied." By the early 1980s, a physician practicing in southern

California was insisting that "Mexican Americans are a diabetic race." And as I write this, in 2019, someone who turns to the National Institutes of Health to learn about the populations most at risk for developing diabetes will read: "African American, Alaska Native, American Indian, Asian American, Hispanic/Latino, Native Hawaiian, or Pacific Islander."[9]

As the image of populations at risk for diabetes shifted, so too did understandings of race. At the turn of the twentieth century, most Americans remained certain that race was an established fact and that the divisions between races were fundamentally biological, although beyond that there was little consensus about whether biological meant unchangeable or even which populations properly made up a race. The challenges to "race-thinking" that began with anthropologists in the 1930s and that exploded in the post–World War II period are part of a story well told in many excellent scholarly works. The result was an attempt to abandon fixed racial typologies and to reimagine race as populations defined by differences in the frequencies of certain genes or traits. Population genetics remains at the core of scientific understandings of race today, with evolutionary geneticists often preferring the language of "genetic ancestry groups." This phrase addresses genetic differences between people, and the variation in gene frequencies among human populations. Evolutionary geneticists, however, also acknowledge that the correlation between ancestry groups and the racial categories employed by the United States census is inexact at best, and so raises questions about what "race" actually means.[10]

Contentious battles are fought today over whether race is a helpful category when it comes to understanding health disparities. Those who argue that it is do not deny that current racial categories are only an approximation of an individual's ancestry, but they still contend that further knowledge of race-specific genetic susceptibilities will ultimately improve health outcomes by permitting greater specificity in treatment protocols. Those who oppose using race view it as a social convention that has little to do with ancestry (or a population's genetic makeup) and everything to do with how a society chooses to distinguish among the people in its midst. Their claim is that the focus on race ignores not only genetic diversity within groups but also other factors—such as poverty—that might better explain differences in prevalence rates. Their fundamental concern is that racial stereotyping risks constraining diagnostic and treatment options in ways that can do harm.[11]

Some who reject the use of race as a substitute for ancestry, including me, still view it as a powerful lens through which to understand health and disease. From this perspective, race has a direct effect on someone's health, but genetic differences, which may or may not exist, are not the primary reason for health disparities. Rather, health disparities reflect far more the racism that populations experience because of the meanings ascribed to different skin colors and other physical attributes. Racial discrimination can lead to inadequate access to quality health care, as well as exacerbate the social conditions of poor health, such as high levels of unemployment, inadequate housing, and underfunded neighborhood schools. It can also generate ill health by producing pathological responses to the stress of living in a society in which white skin color is endowed with privileges denied to others. Racism, in other words, can make people sick. In this way, racism—not race—becomes a fundamental cause of differential disease rates, making it impossible to draw a sharp line between what is biological and what is social.[12]

Previous works have explored the central role of race and racism in the history of disease. Syphilis, tuberculosis, smallpox, plague, malaria, HIV/AIDS, sickle cell anemia, and heart disease are just some of the diseases whose histories have revealed the subtle and not so subtle ways that race and racist attitudes have shaped the spread of disease, the experiences of those who fall ill, and the theories that medical, public health, and civic leaders put forth to account for the unequal distribution of disease.[13] Three studies in the past fifteen years have looked in particular at startling shifts over the course of the twentieth century in the populations imagined to be most at risk for cancer, schizophrenia, and fetal-alcohol syndrome. In each case, the disease was transformed from one associated with middle-class whites to one believed to afflict mostly racial minorities. And in the process, descriptions of those who suffered from the disease became far more judgmental.[14]

Diabetes builds on these studies as it charts a similar racial transformation of a disease. The story, however, is complicated, because diabetes went through not one but multiple such transformations over the more than one

hundred years covered in this book. Beginning in the late nineteenth century and extending to the present, professional and popular writers alike
consistently evoked race to explain the uneven distribution of diabetes,
but the populations considered most at risk have been, at various times,
Jews, whites, Native Americans, African Americans, Mexican Americans,
and Asian Americans. Race—and class to some extent—has thus been a
persistent presence in writings on diabetes, even as the racial group considered most vulnerable changed with time and even as definitions of race
proved highly unstable. It is striking that at times when more than one race
was considered at risk of developing diabetes, race did not have a single
meaning. For example, in the 1980s, when a government task force on
health disparities singled out five races for their high rates of the disease, it
emphasized genetics for only two populations; for the others it pointed to
behavior, stress, and acculturation.

In addition to race, professional and popular writers also noted the strong
link between diabetes and obesity. Joslin even labeled diabetes "a penalty
of obesity" back in 1921, and few questioned his assertion. Yet diabetes did
not become almost synonymous with obesity until the 1990s, when multiple publications began generating alarm about the impending arrival of
an "obesity epidemic," even coining the term "diabesity." Before then—and
certainly well into the 1970s—medical researchers considered obesity to be
just one factor among many responsible for driving up diabetes rates.[15] Also
on their list were heredity, nervous strain, emotional shock, and infections,
to name just a few. Researchers certainly mentioned obesity frequently, but
they rarely used obesity to explain why some populations had higher rates
of diabetes than others. To answer that question, they turned most often
to race.

The centrality of race to the history of diabetes explains why I have organized each chapter around a population considered at one time to have
had the highest prevalence of the disease. The book is thus loosely chrono-
logical, beginning with Jews, who were widely believed around the turn of
the twentieth century to have a diabetes mortality rate between two and six
times greater than that of the rest of the population, and ending with Native
Americans, African Americans, and Mexican Americans, who today are the
groups believed to be most at risk of becoming diabetic. I also occasionally

disrupt this chronology to chart more fully the rise and fall of a given population's close association with the disease.

In exposing the fraught relationship between disease and race, I am not arguing that race should be abandoned as an analytical category. A disproportionate number of people live in poverty, are denied opportunities, and confront racism because of their skin color, and each of these factors increases one's chances of becoming ill. Race is, thus, intimately connected to health outcomes. As such, it occupies a place at the nexus of social conditions and biology.[16] I am also not claiming that differential morbidity and mortality rates have been fabricated or are only culturally determined. In the past, Jews may have suffered disproportionately from diabetes, and today statistically significant studies show that the rate of diabetes is higher among American Indians, African Americans, and Hispanic Americans than among whites as a whole. The critical question is: how have those rates been explained? The answer I offer is that among the many risk factors, which include age, gender, and economic status, none has figured as prominently in explanations of observed health disparities as race. This focus has led to a shift of resources away from efforts to address inequalities in income, education, employment, and social capital, as well as blame being placed on those suffering from the disease.

"I Have Diabetes. Am I to Blame?" This opinion piece, published in the *New York Times* on October 12, 2016, was penned by a woman who described herself as young, black, fat, and struggling with type 2 diabetes.[17] Simply posing the question in such a prominent forum is a reminder that, in our culture, disease has carried social, political, and racial meanings that have in turn reinforced tropes, misled researchers and clinicians, and misdirected resources. My father had his faults, but no one blamed him for his diabetes.

DIABETES

1

Judenkrankheit, a Jewish Malady

When the Jew is thirsty, he has his sugar tested; when the Christian is thirsty, he drinks.

> Albert A. Epstein, 1919

The reason the Jew has more diabetes is not that he is a Jew, but that he is a fat Jew.

> E. P. Joslin, 1924

THE YEAR WAS 1870. JOSEF SEEGEN had been seeing patients at the Carlsbad baths in Bohemia since the summer of 1854, tending primarily to individuals who suffered from diabetes. Over the years, he had become convinced that drinking and bathing in the spa's mineral waters were helping his patients assimilate carbohydrates and thereby reduce the glucose that passed into their urine. What he could not figure out was why over 25 percent of the more than two hundred patients he had seen in the previous fifteen years were Jewish. "This percentage is immense," he declared, even if Jews tended to visit spas more frequently than Christians. In a book he published on diabetes in 1893, he commented that 10 percent would have been unusual enough, given that Jews constituted just over 2 percent of the overall population in Europe. That they comprised one-quarter of his patients suggested that something unusual was going on.[1]

Seegen's publication was just the beginning. As clinicians and medical researchers all over Europe noted that the number of diabetes cases increased as deaths from infectious diseases declined, they confirmed his finding that Jews suffered disproportionately from the disease. These studies also revealed that mortality rates were every bit as troubling as morbidity rates. Jews seemed to be dying of diabetes at a rate two to six times greater than the rest of the population. In the German-language literature, diabetes even came to be known as the *Judenkrankheit,* or "Jewish disease."[2]

Such views made their way across the Atlantic. "There is no race so subject to diabetes as the Jews," proclaimed one New York City physician in 1904. William Osler, perhaps the most famous American clinician of the early twentieth century, noted that "Hebrews seem especially prone to it." A physician with the U.S. Public Health Service concurred, insisting that the tripling of the diabetes mortality rate between 1888 and 1912 in New York City could be explained only by the rapid growth of the city's Jewish population. And roughly two hundred miles away, in Boston, a Jewish physician concluded from his study of the city's death certificates that the rate of diabetes deaths among Jews was two-and-a-half times greater than among "their neighbors." By 1916, Elliott P. Joslin, the foremost diabetes specialist in the nation, could write with confidence in his highly acclaimed textbook that "the frequency with which diabetes occurs in the Jewish race is proverbial."[3] The association between Jews and diabetes would not be seriously challenged until the 1930s, and would not disappear until well after World War II.

What was going on? Might Jews have suffered disproportionately from diabetes around the turn of the century? Perhaps. Jewish immigrants who had fled poverty and hunger in Eastern Europe tended to eat better in their new land, and this may have increased their chances of putting on a lot of weight and thus of developing the disease. Even the poor, who during lean times ate little more than herring, dark bread, and some carrots and beets, usually had plenty of potatoes. One immigrant remembered eating "Sunday, potatoes, Monday, potatoes, Tuesday and Wednesday, potatoes, Thursday and Friday, potatoes, and on the Sabbath you get a potato kugel." Clearly the chronic starvation that had marked the lives of Jews in Eastern Europe had ended. Moreover, as immigrants slowly assimilated to their new lives in America, their ability to provide for themselves and their families improved. Fish and meat were no longer confined to the Sabbath meal; butter, schmaltz (animal fat), preserves, and strudel also became regular fare. To be able to eat—and eat a lot—became not only a sign of success, but also a great joy. "It was lovely here—so much food," recalled one woman who settled in Pittsburgh. "Cake for breakfast!" commented another, adding that "the very idea of serving cake for breakfast struck me as an extravagant fancy."[4]

Of course, plentiful food does not necessarily lead to increased rates of diabetes. Nor does being fat. Most overweight individuals do not have diabetes. But being overweight can increase one's risk of developing the disease, and a daily fare that included ample portions of butter and schmaltz, and that led Jews to gain weight, could have increased their chances of becoming diabetic. So, too, might their experiences as recent immigrants. Studies of migration and disease have provided ample evidence that immigrants, especially those who have escaped lives of hardship and hunger, can develop high rates of diabetes after moving to a new environment. Why this is so remains unclear. Until recently, researchers had focused most on the consequences of a sudden introduction to a "Western lifestyle," with its abundance of dense-energy foods and low levels of physical exercise. In the past decade or so, however, some scholars have begun to examine how the various stresses immigrants face as they adapt to a new home might increase insulin resistance not only by affecting dietary choice (cravings for "comfort food"), but also by triggering inflammatory responses in the body.[5] This suggests that in the early decades of the twentieth century, Jews might have suffered high rates of diabetes in part because of their immigrant status.

Yet as suggestive as these possibilities might be, there are ample reasons to be wary of assertions in the early twentieth century linking Jews and diabetes. For one, most writers who mentioned this link rarely provided statistics to back up their claims. They simply repeated what everyone else was saying. And those who did offer up numbers and patterns offered statistics that were often unreliable. Not only did physicians usually draw on select populations, whether from their own private practice, the patient population of a specific hospital, or those seeking relief at expensive spas, but it was not always clear how to determine whether someone was Jewish—especially when calculating mortality rather than morbidity rates. One

Jewish physician complained that New York City's death certificates had no information about the religious affiliation of the deceased, although that did not prevent him from counting as Jewish anyone buried in a Jewish cemetery or whose personal name, parent's name, or place of birth suggested that they were "of undoubted Jewish origin." Physicians at the time even commented on the tenuous nature of the data available to them. Albert A. Epstein, a Jewish physician who practiced in New York City, was so skeptical of the evidence linking Jews and diabetes that he claimed that statistics showing the Jews' predisposition to the disease only taught us how easy it is to "prove anything by statistics not sufficiently analyzed."[6]

To add to this confusion, the exact nature of diabetes remained a mystery. By the final decades of the nineteenth century, the medical community may have known that the pancreas was the damaged organ and that its islets of Langerhans, the site of insulin's production, had the greatest impact on the disease, but no one was sure what caused the islets to malfunction. (This remains unclear even today.) Even the discovery of insulin in 1921–1922, which radically transformed the management of the disease, did little to clarify its fundamental cause. Instead doctors pointed to a wide range of possibilities, including heredity, obesity, dietary excesses, a strenuous life, nervousness, infection, viruses, mental shock, and co-morbidities including arteriosclerosis, syphilis, acromegaly, gout, and Bright's disease (today called nephritis, or inflammation of the kidneys). One author even blamed diabetes on processed foods, condemning in particular "the patent roller-made flour, which is deprived of all the coarser part of the flour." As an exasperated physician summed up the conundrum in 1919: "Unlike many other morbid states, the immediate cause of this disease is unknown."[7]

Medical practitioners were clearly feeling frustrated in their efforts to bring a level of certainty to the diagnosis and treatment of diabetes. If only diabetes could be understood as well as the infectious diseases! Buoyed by recent discoveries of the bacterial and viral causes of many infectious diseases, by the beauty and simplicity of the model "one germ, one disease," and by the development of effective treatments such as diphtheria antitoxin, physicians, patients, and popularizers alike wondered whether noninfectious diseases might also stem from a single cause. By the late 1920s this impulse would lead to increased interest in genes, which were imagined as the "cause" of non-infectious diseases in the same way that "germs" caused infectious diseases. In fact, the idea that diabetes was transmitted as a single recessive Mendelian trait was first suggested in the 1920s, although at that time nearly every discussion of the etiology of diabetes began with the caveat that its cause was "still debatable."[8]

Even more challenging, especially for those intent on improving the care they offered their patients, was the lack of standardized tests for determining whether someone had diabetes. Nineteenth-century physicians may have had chemical tests to detect the presence of sugar in the urine without relying on their taste buds (as their predecessors had done), but the lack of uniformity in testing meant that results from different examinations could not be properly compared. Besides, glycosuria (sugar in the urine) was not always thought to signify diabetes: physicians believed that a high sugar diet, an overly active thyroid, liver disease, or even a normal pregnancy could all cause it. One solution to this lack of certainty was to treat any patient who had sugar in the urine as though he or she had diabetes mellitus, at least, as Joslin suggested, "until the contrary is proven."[9] But clearly anyone who followed the diabetes specialist's lead would find more diabetes in the populations they examined than someone who worked with a more restrictive definition.

Fortunately for those who preferred not to treat all their patients with glycosuria as diabetic until proven healthy, blood glucose tests became available in the early twentieth century. Yet even then there was considerable room for interpretation. There was no agreement, for example, on the concentration of blood sugar that should result in a diagnosis of diabetes. Nor did clinicians and researchers agree on the time of day to administer the blood test, how long a person had to fast before taking the test, how much glucose to administer during the test, or how quickly the individual's blood sugar level had to return to normal for the person to be given a clean bill of health.[10] What meaning, then, could be ascribed to a claim that Jews suffered disproportionately from diabetes, when "diabetes" was not clearly defined?

The definition of "Jew" was equally ambiguous. Even putting aside the debates that took place in the early decades of the twentieth century over whether Jews constituted a distinct race, the Jewish population in the United States was heterogeneous. Did claims that "Jews" had high rates of diabetes include Sephardim, who had emigrated from Spain and Portugal as early as the seventeenth century? Or did it refer only to Ashkenazi Jews, who had made their home in Europe following the diaspora? And if only the Ashkenazis, did that group include German Jews, who had started their migration to the United States in the 1830s and had achieved a level of wealth and accomplishment by the end of the nineteenth century? Or did it refer to the millions of Eastern European Jews, primarily from Russia, who had begun to arrive in large numbers in the 1880s and who frequently began their new lives in poverty? Only a few who commented on the high rate of diabetes among Jews made any distinctions among these groups, and among those who did, there was rarely agreement. To some, Russian Jews suffered most because of the particularly "cruel persecution" to which they had been subjected, while others claimed that German Jews' greater wealth and "characteristic modes of living," which included greater "mental exertion," made them more susceptible to the disease.[11]

In short, we cannot know for certain whether "Jews" did, in fact, suffer disproportionately from "diabetes" in the decades around the turn of the twentieth century. Which Jews? Based on which statistics? Working with which definition of the disease? It is impossible to know whether they were overrepresented in the patient populations of those physicians who published statistical studies, or whether, as implied by Epstein's joke about a thirsty Jew checking his sugar levels rather than taking a drink, Jews went to physicians more often than other populations when they were not feeling well. It is thus impossible to answer the question of *whether* Jews had a higher rate of the disease. But we can explore *why,* despite the highly ambiguous nature of the data—an ambiguity acknowledged at the time—virtually no one questioned the fundamental link between Jews and diabetes during the first three decades of the century. Not even Epstein, who, despite drawing attention to the unreliability of the statistical evidence, conceded the likelihood that Jews were, in fact, more predisposed to diabetes. Better safe than sorry, he reasoned, as he recommended that Jews take proper precautions to prevent the onset of the disease.[12]

Diabetes as a "Jewish Peril"

The seemingly high rate of diabetes among Jews in the United States first attracted attention in the last decades of the nineteenth century, as diabetes rates in general appeared to be rising rapidly. Recognizing that improvements in public health and nutrition meant that more people were living into adulthood and developing a wide range of chronic diseases, health professionals noted two ways in which diabetes stood out. First, although many more people died from heart disease and cancer, the mortality rate for diabetes was increasing more rapidly than for these other ailments. According to one diabetes specialist, its rate had jumped 150 percent between 1850 and 1880.[13] And second, Jews seemed to be affected disproportionately. In examining the relationship between the two, these writers ended up constructing racial narratives about the disease.

Some of these narratives were decidedly antagonistic toward Jews. J. G. Wilson, a surgeon with the U.S. Public Health Service, was particularly disdainful. In a study he conducted on "Jewish psychopathology" just a year after he wrote about diabetes, he referred to Jews as "a highly inbred and psychopathically inclined race." Wilson made this claim while he was stationed at Ellis Island, the U.S. port of entry for most Eastern European Jews. His sense of discomfort with this group, whose clothing, language, and mannerisms seemed so alien to him, was clear in two ways: the speed with which he moved from correlation to causation, assuming that the simultaneous increase in both the mortality rate from diabetes and the Jewish population meant that Jews were responsible; and his insistence that Jews had such a high rate of this disease because of "some hereditary defect" exacerbated by "the practice of inbreeding." Wilson's decision to refer to the Jewish practice of consanguineous marriages—which was being hotly debated at the time by Jews and non-Jews alike—as "inbreeding" not only fed anxiety about the close-knit nature of Jews, but also tainted the diagnosis of diabetes with hints of incest.[14]

Wilson was writing at a time of intense anxiety over the seemingly endless flow of immigrants from Eastern Europe to the United States that had begun in the 1880s. In 1911, just a year before Wilson published his study of diabetes in New York City, a congressional committee known as the Dillingham Commission had produced a lengthy report recommending that immigration be curtailed. As part of its investigative work, the committee had prepared an analysis of the racial makeup of the existing immigrant population, a clear indication that race was to be a critical factor in deciding who among the "tired," the "poor," and those "yearning to breathe free" would be allowed to continue to enter the country. Working with standard anthropological classifications, the members of the commission began by dividing the immigrant populations into five major races—Caucasian (white), Malayan (brown), Mongolian (yellow), American Indian (red), and Ethiopian (black)—before separating them further into subgroups, alternatively referred to as "peoples," "nations," or, confusing matters further, "races." In the end, and by employing a combination of biological, linguistic, and cultural characteristics, the Dillingham Commission identified roughly six hundred "branches or divisions of the human family" throughout the world, forty-five of which could be found in the United States.[15] Jews, also referred to as Hebrews, were among them, along with Celtics, Alpines, Teutonics, Mediterraneans, Slavonics, and many others, but it remained unclear exactly who was related to whom and how. One of the questions that received considerable attention was whether Jews should be considered white.

This was not an academic question. The five major races were understood to exist in a hierarchy, with whites representing the most "civilized" of the groups and blacks and American Indians the most "savage." According to the 1790 naturalization law, only "free white persons" could apply for citizenship, and in the early years of the American republic this included Jewish immigrants, who hailed primarily from Germany. But later in the century, the influx of millions of Eastern European Jews, with their strange language, clothing, and overall appearance, cast doubt on this classification. A group of radical nativists jumped into the fray, going to great lengths to cast the latest influx of Jews as "thoroughbred Asiatics." As strange as that may seem today, the question of whether Jews were fundamentally "oriental" or "occidental" dates back at least to the Middle Ages, when Christian writers often depicted them as turbaned and oriental as a way of highlighting their otherness. According to radical nativists, Jews still bore the imprint of their years wandering in the desert when they were little more than a nomadic tribe. Describing them alternately as primitive, tribal, and "Mongoloid," some claimed that they had descended from the Khazars, a Turkic people who allegedly converted to Judaism in the eighth century. Whatever the specific allegations, casting Jews as "oriental" raised the hope—at least for the nativists—that Jewish immigrants seeking entry might be denied under the terms of the 1882 Chinese Exclusion Act, which barred Chinese laborers from entering the United States.[16]

The members of the Dillingham Commission did not join the radical nativists in questioning whether Jews were white. But they evidently struggled with the *degree* of Jews' whiteness, revealing their embrace of early twentieth-century beliefs that some groups were whiter than others. This was apparent in their criticism of the Bureau of Immigration's previous classification of Jews as "Slavonic" and thus as "Aryan," and their reclassification of them as "Semitic," which placed them lower on the race ladder. Given the widespread belief that Semitic peoples stemmed originally from Africa, this change raised further questions about Jews' whiteness. Indeed, although never a popular belief, some considered Jews to be "essentially Negro in habits, physical peculiarities and tendencies," possessing both "Mongoloid" and "Negroid" traits. The motivations behind this change became evident when the commission concluded its work in 1911 and recommended that the government enact a restrictive immigration law. It took another decade, but the commission's report finally bore fruit: in 1921, and again in 1924, with the passage of the Johnson-Reed Act, the government put in place restrictive immigration laws that reduced the number of Jews entering the United States from a record high of 120,000 in 1921 to just 10,000 three years later. As the eugenicist Charles Davenport, who had advised the Dillingham Commission, wrote to a friend shortly after the legislation passed: "Our ancestors drove Baptists from Massachusetts Bay into Rhode Island, but we have no place to drive the Jews to. Also they burned the witches but it seems to be against the mores to burn any considerable part of our population. Meanwhile we have somewhat diminished the immigration of these people."[17]

A decade before Davenport penned these words, J. G. Wilson, the surgeon with the U.S. Public Health Service, had voiced related concerns. The same year the Dillingham Commission published its final report, and one year before he blamed rising diabetes rates on the influx of Jewish immigrants, Wilson had published an article in *Popular Science Monthly* on "The Crossing of the Races." This was Wilson's opportunity to articulate the criteria he believed the government should employ as it crafted its immigration policy, and his message was clear: there are good immigrants and bad ones, and Jews belonged to the bad group. Notably, Wilson did not base this determination on biological race, despite the title of his article. Unlike his peers who spread widespread panic about the effects of race mixing on the vigor of wholesome American stock, Wilson believed that "racial amalgamation" had long been a part of human history and should be embraced, at least as long as it took place "between different branches of the white races." In fact, he believed that some racial crosses, such as between Teutons, Britons, and Celts, had produced positive results, and he could well imagine future intermarriages between "real Americans" and select immigrants that would be similarly beneficial. What worried him was not the biological mixing of the races, but their moral mixing. He wanted the government to restrict entry to those immigrants who would have a positive impact on "our *habits* of *thought,* upon *our morals,* and upon *our institutions,*" in short, on "our spiritual selves."[18]

Wilson claimed that history provided the best clue to an immigrant group's moral mettle, so he proceeded to offer a brief lesson about each of several populations, reading their past to see what it revealed about the group's character and whether they would be capable of adopting "those Anglo-Saxon habits of thought which we must insist upon as necessary to good citizenship in a great republic." His conclusion was that Italians, Magyars, Poles, and other Slavs had all demonstrated their ability "to adopt the ways of western civilization." Jews, on the other hand—he referred to them as "the other type of immigrant"—had failed the test. In his interpretation of their history, Jews had been welcomed in many different lands from biblical times to the present, and each time they had begun by being treated as equals. Invariably, however, they had drawn others' wrath by insisting on "certain special privileges" and keeping to themselves. This "clannishness," Wilson insisted, reinforced by Jews' refusal "to intermarry with those of other religions," worked against ensuring that immigrants adopt, rather than obliterate, "our inherited Anglo-Saxon ideals."[19] Diabetes, Wilson may well have thought, was a just punishment for Jews' insistence that they "breed" only among themselves.

The hostility that Wilson evinced in his discussion of Jews and diabetes was, however, the exception rather than the rule. Far more common in the diabetes literature was subtle trafficking in negative stereotypes. Thus one physician attributed Jews' high rate of diabetes to the love of the "Hebrew race" for "high living," adding that "they are given to parties, they congregate together and have frequent and irregular meals." William Osler wrote of Jews' particularly "neurotic temperament." A journalist weighed in, blaming Jews' "racial tendency to corpulence." And Haven Emerson, professor of preventive medicine at Columbia's College of Physicians and Surgeons, and a previous commissioner of health for the city of New York, put the onus on Jews for spreading what he called "this great luxury disease." In doing so, he drew on not only widespread fears of the drastic changes shaking the foundation of American society in the interwar years, but also negative images of the Jew as the embodiment of much that was wrong with modernity.[20]

Emerson honed his argument in an article entitled "Sweetness Is Death," published in 1924 in *The Survey,* the leading journal of the social work profession. In the first two-thirds of his article, Emerson did not even mention Jews. Instead he drew in his reader by presenting disturbing statistics about the fifteen-fold rise in the annual death rate from diabetes between 1866 and 1923, and by targeting the social, economic, and cultural changes that were making the trend difficult to reverse. Emerson mentioned, for example, the way the new "motorized and mechanistic existence" reduced the need for physical labor and thereby reduced the number of calories a person burned. But what truly disturbed him were challenges to the moral fiber of the nation. These included the growing "self-indulgence," the increase in "lazy comforts," the "sugar coating" of meals, the desire for little more than "the satisfaction of . . . caprice." Indeed, if anything, Emerson's diatribe in the first pages of his article was against "the idle rich" and their embrace of conspicuous consumption, not Jews per se. Diabetes rates were going up, he ranted, because Americans had become "the grossest feeders among the nations . . . bulging with the money bags of the world, fairly oozing with wealth, eating every day much more than any of our allies or opponents of the war . . . and, as it were, dying of overeating."[21]

"Sweetness Is Death" is clearly about more than diabetes. It is also Emerson's denunciation of so many of the changes taking place in the years following the Great War. Labeling diabetes "a great luxury disease," he expressed deep anxiety about the transformation of fundamental aspects of American life: the economic prosperity that stemmed from the mass production of consumer goods, including clothing, radios, cars, and magazines; the rise of print culture and advertising, which encouraged citizens to support the new consumer culture; and a credit economy that allowed working-class and middle-class individuals to participate in new leisure activities, whether they had the means or not. New cultural activities also took shape during the "roaring twenties," with the proliferation of dance halls, movie theaters, and jazz clubs, offering venues where traditional gender roles and staid sexual mores could be flouted publicly. To Emerson, diabetes was symbolic of all that he loathed; "a disease of wealth and feeding and fatness," it provided physical evidence of what was, in essence, moral turpitude. And nowhere, he added, is this "better shown than in the story of the races."[22]

This was Emerson's segue to his discussion of diabetes's prevalence among Jews. In support of his argument that diabetes and wealth went hand in hand, he claimed that tuberculosis, "a disease always fostered by poverty, low standards of living and food shortage," barely affected Jews, whereas diabetes ran so rampant among them that it was "commonly known in Europe as the '*Judenkrankheit.*'" Yet Emerson's explanation for this proclivity did not fit the picture he had just painted, for he described Jews as "merchants, storekeepers, [and] needle workers," who were "abundantly though cheaply fed." In other words, by his own account they were not the "idle rich." Still, by defining Jews as the most at risk of developing "this luxury disease," and by linking the disease to "wealth and feeding and fatness," Emerson reinforced an image of the rich and fat Jew, hoarding his money and indulging himself while the rest of the world struggled with hunger and deprivation.[23]

This image was finding particular resonance in the early decades of the century, when the "fat Jew" became a potent symbol, in one historian's words, of "the potential for disease and decay" associated with modernity.[24] The fears to which Emerson gave voice in his essay—that self-indulgence and hedonism were replacing self-discipline and asceticism as the social values to which one should aspire, and that the "American way of life" was rapidly coming to an end—reflected the changing meaning of fat from a marker of affluence and influence to a symbol of gluttony and decadence.

In this context, the fat—and diabetic—body of the Jew became one important site where these anxieties played out.

It is possible that Emerson painted this picture unintentionally. Indeed, he specifically added that "it is not money in the bank, nor being a Jew . . . that determines the excess of diabetes deaths."[25] At least in theory, he seemed to be writing, anyone who had "the means to grow fat," and who then chose "self-indulgence" over "self-control," ran the risk of developing the disease. But by attacking the character of those who had diabetes, while naming Jews as the "race" with the highest rate, he rendered them guilty by association.

A clear link between fat, Jews, and diabetes is also evident in the writings of Joslin. As the leading diabetes specialist in the United States in the first half of the twentieth century, and a physician of considerable international fame, Joslin may have shaped the conversation about Jews and diabetes more than any other individual of his day. Author of the widely read textbook *The Treatment of Diabetes Mellitus,* which first appeared in 1916 and went through ten editions before his death in 1962, Joslin specialized in diabetes care decades before medical specialization became popular. Why he chose this specialty is unclear, although his experiences with his mother and his aunt, both of whom developed the disease when they reached middle age, may have influenced him. By 1916, when the textbook's first edition came out, he had examined a thousand individuals in his clinic. According to one physician, this was "the largest number of diabetic cases in the literature observed by one man."[26]

Like other physicians, Joslin noted early on that the high rate of diabetes among Jews was "proverbial," but he did not weigh in on whether race had anything to do with it until 1924, when he declared unequivocally that "diabetes [is] not a congenital stigma of the Jewish race." Were that the case, he reasoned, "it should be manifested from youth to old age." But that is not what he observed in the Jewish patients he had treated in his clinic over the previous quarter of a century. Comparing them with the rest of his patients, he found that the rate was unusually high only when they entered the fourth and fifth decades of their lives, a time, he claimed, when Jews packed on the pounds. In fact, Joslin found that 85 percent of his Jewish diabetes patients were overweight in comparison to just 70 percent of Gentiles. "The Jew," he concluded, "in my opinion, is not prone to diabetes because he is a Jew, but rather because he is fat."[27]

Why Joslin chose to speak out in 1924 against a link between Jews, race, and diabetes can only be surmised. Perhaps he was troubled by the anti-immigration sentiment that had resulted in the recent passing of the Johnson-Reed Act. He may also have been watching with apprehension the rising anti-Semitism at home and abroad and felt that he should speak out. Yet like Emerson, and despite his best intentions, Joslin continued to play into negative stereotypes—this time of the fat Jew—effectively replacing "the stigma of a congenital tendency" with the stigma of obesity.[28]

Just three years earlier, Joslin had labeled diabetes "a penalty of obesity," encouraging his colleagues to think of the fat diabetic as akin to the alcoholic. Neither, he insisted, deserved pity. Indeed, he recommended shaming them into making a change. "It is all nonsense," he declared, "to use polite terms for being 'just fat.' It is generally prudent and always far more effective to say to the patient: 'You are too fat,' than cautiously to remark: 'You are a trifle obese.' Fat diathesis!," he exclaimed, using a word common at the time that referred to a constitutional predisposition. "Granted there is one person in a thousand who has some inherent peculiarity of the metabolism which has led to obesity, [but] there are 999 for whom being fat implies too much food or too little exercise, or both combined."[29]

Again, as with Emerson, Joslin was not targeting Jews alone. Indeed, he even claimed that his Jewish patients were beginning to understand the importance of losing weight, realizing sooner than most that in the near future "one may be almost ashamed to have diabetes." But the admiration he may have felt for those who heeded his message did not prevent him from employing language that propelled the image of "the fat Jew" as a health threat to the nation. This is vividly evident when Joslin tried to convince his colleagues that diabetes could be eradicated if it were approached with the same logic and energy that had been employed to eradicate infectious diseases. "To stamp out a pestilence," he explained, "one studies and attacks it where its ravages are worse. Yellow fever was investigated and prevention found in Cuba, not in the United States. The pathway is equally plain in diabetes. First, this disease is known to be fifteen times as frequent among adults; second, this disease is ten to twenty times as common among the fat; third, this disease is two and a half times as common among Jews and slightly more so among Jewish females. Any campaign to eradicate diabetes, therefore, should yield maximal returns if directed toward its prevention and discovery in adult, fat females, and particularly in Jews."[30]

This passage is remarkable in many ways, beginning with the jingoism in Joslin's language as he suggests that diabetes, like yellow fever, may have foreign roots. Whether he intended it or not, this assertion would have resonated with individuals like Wilson who blamed Eastern European Jews for rising rates of diabetes in the United States. Comparing diabetes to a "pestilence," situating it in the body of Jews, and encouraging his colleagues to "stamp it out" also brings to mind the radical measures favored by eugenicists (although, as we will see in Chapter 2, Joslin explicitly rejected any talk of sterilizing people who had diabetes). As he railed against the "pestilence," he gradually narrowed his target population, beginning with fat adults and ending with fat Jewish females, despite stating clearly that Jewish women had only a "slightly" higher rate than Jewish men. In this way, Joslin helped to shape the meaning of fat, which was not only becoming increasingly stigmatized in the interwar years, but also increasingly feminized. Obesity was also being linked to the immigrant body, and especially to Jews.[31] If you were Jewish, diabetic, fat, and female, you had four strikes against you.

Neither Emerson nor Joslin, I am convinced, set out to paint a negative picture of Jews. Nevertheless, their writings reflected and advanced common stereotypes that displaced onto Jews many of the anxieties associated with modernity. Emerson did this while remaining unclear as to whether he considered diabetes a racial disease; Joslin did so while explicitly rejecting that assertion. But whether blaming race or behavior and lifestyle, both cast Jews as a population that burdened the health of the nation. Two years after Emerson published "Sweetness Is Death," the *New York Times* ran an article with the ambiguous title, "Diabetes as Jewish Peril."[32] Whether diabetes was perilous to Jews or Jews were the peril remained unclear.

Not all writings on Jews and diabetes trafficked in racial stereotypes. To the contrary, the vast majority simply repeated the claim that Jews had an unusually high rate of the disease, suggesting that the link between Jews and diabetes made so much sense that few saw any reason to question it. Certainly, the idea that race-specific diseases existed was neither novel nor

contested at the time; medical writers often attributed perceived disparities in the prevalence of specific diseases to the character of an entire race.
Thus, in the nineteenth century, cholera was said to afflict the Irish disproportionately because of their immorality, evidenced by the filth and poverty
in which they lived. Later in the century, syphilis was said to run rampant
among blacks because they lacked the ability to control their "instincts, pas-
sions and appetites."[33] Thus, it would not have seemed unusual to include
negative comments about the alleged character of Jews in explanations of
why they suffered disproportionately from diabetes. Indeed, if you had to
match the imagined characteristics of a population with the imagined characteristics of a disease, you could not have done better around the turn of
the century than to pair Jews and diabetes. Both had come to symbolize
what many considered the worst aspects of modern life.

But physicians at the time saw diabetes as more than a consequence of
consumerism run amok. After all, consumerism did not define all of modern life; societies that were deemed the most "modern" were also believed to
be the most "civilized." Yet civilization also came with health risks, producing stresses and strains that resulted in increased rates of diabetes as well
as other so-called diseases of civilization, such as cardiovascular ailments
and cancer. According to the Swedish physician Emil Kleen, whose work
circulated widely in the United States, diabetes flourished where "culture"
abounded and where "civilized humanity" could be found; it thus tended to
afflict those who demonstrated "greater intellectual exertion, keener emotions, higher nervous development, more earnest struggle for existence,
more urgent demands, [and] a more intense culture." Frederick Shattuck,
Jackson Professor of Clinical Medicine at Harvard University, also asserted
that diabetes was most prevalent in "civilized regions," and "especially
among brain workers." William Osler concurred. To him, diabetes was a
"disease of the higher classes," far more common among those who possessed great wealth, itself a marker of class standing.[34]

Few questioned Jews' inclusion in this "civilized" elite. The nineteenth-
century physician Josiah Clark Nott claimed that they were "in intellect . . .
ranked among the first of the human family." Leroy Beaulieu, a French
economist whose work *Israel among the Nations* received international atten-

tion, commented that he did "not know a more intellectual race." Even the German eugenicists Erwin Baur, Eugen Fischer, and Fritz Lenz—whose co-authored textbook *Human Heredity* influenced Hitler's racial theories as well as early human genetics instruction in the United States—praised the Jews for their unusual "intelligence and alertness," their exceptional "mental activity," the "disproportionally large number of great musicians" in their midst, and "their feeling for humanity at large." To them, Jews were not as advanced as Teutons, who belonged to the Nordic race; they were instead "oriental" with some admixture from the Near East. But still, these eugenicists declared, after "the Teutonic, the Jewish spirit is the chief motive force of modern western civilisation."[35]

Jews and diabetes both occupied ambivalent places in discourses about modernity. As symbols of success taken to excess, and of an advanced society without restraint, they fit together like a hand in a glove. No wonder diabetes came to be known as the *Judenkrankheit*.

Jews as the "Most Nervous of Civilized Peoples"

Anti-Semitic sentiments are evident in many of the explanations for the alleged high rate of diabetes among Jews. But such sentiments alone cannot account for the widespread belief that Jews suffered disproportionately from diabetes, if only because many Jews agreed that the disease posed a particular problem for people of Jewish descent. Anyone, for example, who turned to the twelve-volume *Jewish Encyclopedia* in the early twentieth century to learn about diabetes would have read: "Statistics prove conclusively that the disease occurs among Jews from two to six times as frequently as it does among non Jews." Published in the United States between 1901 and 1906, the *Jewish Encyclopedia* was cast in the spirit of the French *Encyclopédie*, that is, it was intended to counter prejudice by sharing knowledge about Jews obtained through the use of modern scholarly methods. In this way, the *Encyclopedia*'s founders believed, Jewish people would become familiar to others, and suspicion of those who appeared foreign would melt away. The *Encyclopedia* was thus filled with biographical entries, descriptions of holidays and traditional foods, religious observances and terms, cultural

practices, and historical events. It also included articles on scientific, medical, and anthropological topics that directly challenged any assertions that
Jews were an inferior race.[36] The article on diabetes mellitus fit this mold.

The two authors of the entry on "Diabetes Mellitus," Joseph Jacobs and
Maurice Fishberg, were well known in medical and anthropological circles.
Jacobs, an Australian-born historian, folklorist, statistician, and journalist,
had built a reputation for himself as an expert in Jewish history and in the
use of scientific methods to study modern Jewish problems. Although he
had made England his home, he spent several years in New York helping
to oversee and produce the *Jewish Encyclopedia*. His co-author, Fishberg,
a Russian-born, American-educated physician and anthropologist, was the
medical examiner at United Hebrew Charities, an organization that took
shape in the last decades of the nineteenth century to provide assistance to
the poor. A leading expert on the physical anthropology and diseases of the
Jews, Fishberg never missed an opportunity to advocate for the continued
immigration of his people. Agreeing, for example, that "the immigration of
sober, healthy and industrious people to the United States is desirable," he
amassed evidence demonstrating the good hygienic habits and comparatively low mortality rate of Russian Jews living in the tenements of New
York City's East Side. This proved, he contended, that "the Russian Jew is
as desirable as any other class of foreigners and better than many."[37] When
Fishberg wrote entries for the *Jewish Encyclopedia*, he had a similar goal
in mind.

It is not surprising, then, that the central message of the article on diabetes by Jacobs and Fishberg was that it "is not a racial disease of the Jews." For
support, they cited studies that showed that the rate of diabetes was high in
other groups, such as "the educated classes of natives in India and Ceylon";
that French Jews did not appear to have a higher rate than their non-Jewish
neighbors; and that the various communities of Jews in the United States
had different rates. (According to Jacobs and Fishberg, German and Hun-
garian Jews suffered far more than Russian Jews, among whom the rate
"is certainly no more—perhaps it is even less—frequent than among other
races.") Yet despite their acknowledgment of differences among American
Jews, and despite insisting that race had nothing to do with differential
rates, they still lumped all Jews together when they offered a reason for "the

frequency of the disease among Jews." The only "reasonable" explanation, they informed their readers, was the Jews' "extreme nervousness, the Jews being known as the most nervous of civilized peoples."[38]

Thus, even as Jacobs and Fishberg denied racial traits, they ascribed nervousness to Jews, drawing on a widespread belief that diabetes and the nervous system were intimately connected. This belief drew on experimental studies showing that the stimulation of nerves, which enervated the internal organs, resulted in a release of adrenalin, which then caused the liver to break down glycogen and produce a mild glycosuria. Almost every discussion of diabetes's etiology at the time included some reference to the nerves—whether nervous strain, nervous temperament, nervous derangements, nervous tension, or the nerve-shattering aspects of city life. Indeed, Jacobs and Fishberg believed there was "no room for doubt" that "sudden emotional excitement, grief, terror, worry, and anxiety" triggered the onset of the disease.[39]

Jacobs and Fishberg were also drawing on a robust literature that cast Jews as a particularly nervous people. Most fully developed in the writings of the nineteenth-century French neurologist Jean-Martin Charcot, the image of "Jewish nervousness" became, in one historian's words, part of "the standard *fin-de-siècle* rhetoric." Physicians throughout Europe commented on it, agreeing that "the Jews have a hysterical and especially nervous disposition to an overwhelming degree." Jacobs and Fishberg endorsed this image in another article they wrote for the *Jewish Encyclopedia* on "Nervous Diseases," in which they informed readers that "Jews are more subject to diseases of the nervous system than the other races and peoples among which they dwell."[40]

There was, as a result, nothing new about the connection that Jacobs and Fishberg were making between diabetes, nerves, and Jews. But where some non-Jews viewed Jews' proclivity toward nervous diseases as a sign that they were a particularly pathological race, Jewish physicians and anthropologists offered alternative explanations for the labile nature of Jews' nervous system. One explanation drew on geography: Jews' nervousness arose because they had for centuries been concentrated in cities, where the pace of life was fast, streets and living quarters were crowded, community ties were weaker, and the business deals inherent in urban living necessitated a quick wit and competitive drive. Cities were enervating to all their inhabitants, but Jews suffered to a greater degree from urban life for two reasons. First, they occupied some of the most demanding jobs, whether as merchants, businessmen, financiers, or cultural elites, assuming responsibilities far beyond menial tasks. And second, other populations had the benefit of being periodically invigorated by an influx of immigrants from rural areas, who brought in "pure, fresh, healthy country blood." Jews, in contrast, lacked this "rejuvenation," with the consequence, in Fishberg's words, "that the evil effects of the strained, nerve-shattering city life have been deeply rooted on their [Jews'] bodies and minds, and this in turn has been transmitted to their offspring."[41]

In addition to geography, history provided an explanation for Jews' "nervous taint." Indeed, when Josef Seegen first noted Jews' unusually high rate of diabetes, he blamed it on their "labile nervous system," which he attributed to "the long history of suffering, which the Jewish people have had to endure over thousands of years." Jewish commentators ran with this explanation. Hermann Oppenheim, for example, whose *Textbook of Nervous Diseases for Physicians and Students* became a standard in his field, and which was translated from German into English in 1911, blamed the high rates of "neuroses and psychoses" among Jews on the fact that they had been "persecuted and oppressed, mostly only tolerated among the nations, living in peace for short times only, and then again tormented." The Philadelphia physician Solomon Solis-Cohen, who maintained—in contrast to Jacobs and Fishberg—that Russian Jews had the highest diabetes rate of all the Jews, blamed it on the particularly "cruel persecution" they had experienced. As he explained, "the consequent emotional disturbances must have affected profoundly their autonomic nerve system; and autonomic-endocrine imbalance is . . . a potent factor in the pathogenesis of diabetes." And to Albert Epstein, a specialist in nephrology at Mount Sinai, who spoke in 1919 to the National Conference of Jewish Charities about diabetes, everything could be explained by "the conditions under which the Jews have lived for many centuries, particularly during the middle ages, [which] have been such as would shatter the most resistant nervous system. We know," he added, "what baneful influences suffering and misfortune can exercise on the mental and physical being of man. The recent war affords many sad examples of that. How much more profound must that influence be on a people who for many generations, year in and year out, from the cradle to the grave, have endured oppression, privation, and every possible mental distress!"[42]

It is easy to understand why Jews would favor an explanation that turned nervousness, and by extension diabetes, into a symbol of Jews' oppression rather than a source of shame. Diabetes was not an outward expression of the "disease and decay" deep in the body and soul of Jews; rather it signified the centuries, even millennia, of hateful and oppressive practices that Jews had had to endure. Yet an argument that attributed high rates of diabetes to centuries of discrimination also ran the risk of suggesting that the disease was, in some sense, racial. Indeed, in one part of his talk, Epstein described how the physical consequences of such discrimination had produced "a profound and indelible impression" on the bodies of Jews, one that had been "transmitted from generation to generation."[43] Nevertheless, he insisted that he was not talking about a racial trait, but rather an acquired one.

In drawing this distinction, Epstein was gesturing toward the work of the eighteenth-century French naturalist and evolutionist Jean-Baptiste Lamarck. Best known for his theory of the inheritance of acquired characteristics—and his explanation for how the giraffe ended up with a long neck— Lamarck had postulated that organisms exposed to new environmental pressures responded with new habits, which led them to use some body parts and to cease using others. The changes in these body parts were then transmitted to future generations. Ridiculed by his contemporaries for suggesting that organisms *willed* their body parts to change—which he never did—Lamarck ended up appealing to turn-of-the-century evolutionists troubled by Darwin's theory of natural selection and its image of "nature, red in tooth and claw." The inheritance of acquired characteristics seemed, in contrast, to provide a more humane picture of organisms surviving harsh environmental pressures by developing new and creative ways to respond.[44]

Epstein's decision to cast Jews' experience with diabetes as an example of an acquired trait would likely have appealed to his audience. Indeed, Lamarck's popularity among Jews was so profound that the German racial hygienist Fritz Lenz drew attention to it, insisting that "the fondness of the Jews for Lamarckism" rested in their "wish that there should be no

unbridgeable racial distinctions." Distinguishing between racial and acquired traits—which was widespread in the first decades of the twentieth
century and was variously referred to as primary versus secondary racial
traits, static versus fluctuating racial traits, or "racial proclivities" versus
"temperamental characteristics"—allowed Jewish anthropologists to separate those traits "transmitted by heredity from generation to generation,
irrespective of the environment" from those that were a product of time
and experience. This is what allowed Fishberg to write that "the nerve-
shattering" effects of city living have "been transmitted" to the offspring of
Jews, while still denying that this constituted a racial trait. It also provided
the logic behind Solis-Cohen's linking of "cruel persecution," "autonomic-
endocrine imbalance," and "the pathogenesis of diabetes."[45]

To Epstein, the fact that there was no mention of diabetes or its symptoms in the Bible or the Talmud, despite the "rich . . . discussion of medical
subjects" in those texts, meant that the disease could not be racial, since
racial traits had to have existed "from time immemorial." Lest someone
suggest that diabetes did not turn up in old Jewish texts because the disease
did not yet exist, he insisted that ancient Chinese texts included a description of the disease. Thus there was only one conclusion: ancient Hebrews
did not suffer from diabetes; their proclivity for the disease could only have
developed over time; and this was probably a result of persecution having
rendered them a "high-strung and nervous people." Diabetes, he told his
audience, was "acquired not racial." It may have been biological and heritable, but it was not a permanent marker of the Jewish race.[46]

Jewish writers' willingness to embrace an image of Jews as a nervous and
diabetic people stemmed in part from the nonracialized stories they were
able to construct to explain this characteristic of their people. But it also reflected the positive connotation affixed to the label "nervous," which marked
Jews as highly advanced on the evolutionary scale. To quote the French
economist Leroy Beaulieu, whose words Maurice Fishberg frequently cited,
Jews were "the most nervous and in so far the most modern of men." No
wonder Jews suffered from a disease that flourished where "wealth and culture" abounded, "civilized humanity" could be found, and the stresses of
life were paramount. Importantly, Jews were also believed to be most at risk
of developing angina, which was alleged to occur "usually in the sensitive,

nervous type, as the Jew, or in the tense, efficient American, rather than in the dull, happy negro or the calm, accepting Chinaman." "What can we do to prevent diabetes?" asked Frederick C. Shattuck in 1904. "Very little," he responded. "Human life in civilized regions unavoidably tends to become more complex, the struggle for existence fiercer, competition of all kinds, but especially among brain workers, more keen; and we must recognize nerve overstrain as one of the predisposing causes of diabetes."[47] In short, diabetes may have marked Jews as a sickly race, but it also symbolized their place among the cultured elite. It was the price they paid for having devoted themselves to a life of intellectual pursuits, mental exertion, and nonphysical activities and entertainments.

Diabetes was considered a "Jewish" disease in the early twentieth century because science, medicine, and culture all worked together to produce a slate of explanations for the disease's high prevalence among Jews. For some, diabetes revealed the Jews' gluttony and neuroses; for others it marked the centuries of suffering that Jews had endured; for yet others it was a sign of Jews' highly civilized state. But all agreed that in one way or another Jews made up a distinct race. That belief, which had seemed the sturdiest of all, would not last.

When Jews Became "White Folk"

In the interwar years, the idea that races were fixed in time and place, and that the social order was similarly set in stone, came under intense scrutiny. Anthropologists painted pictures of human populations as historically on the move, migrating across continents as they explored new lands, conquering—or being conquered by—the peoples they encountered. The idea that the "blood" of different races had, as a result, long ago lost its purity was reinforced by the picture of African Americans, Jews, Italians, Irish, French Canadians, and others all mingling in the burgeoning urban centers, where, as a result of industrialization, emancipation, and immigration, groups of individuals who had rarely encountered one another were now living and working in close proximity. A social order predicated on biological differences could accommodate an idea of racial admixture only with difficulty. As anthropologists like Melville J. Herskovits insisted that

the ancestry of the American "Negro" population was part African, part Indian, and part Caucasian, and sociologists like Maurice H. Krout similarly
contended that the "white race . . . is as thoroughly blended as is any other
race," a frightened and powerful segment of white society fought back. Trying with great difficulty to preserve what might be left of the "purity" of the
"American race," they enacted restrictive immigration and antimiscegenation laws.[48]

Those fighting to protect this racial "purity" continually encountered
challenges from an increasing array of individuals. These included biolo-
gists, whose new understanding of the mechanics of inheritance led them
to question the legitimacy of racial categories; sociologists, like W. E. B.
Du Bois, who attacked the scientific foundations of racism in a public debate in 1929 with one of the nation's leading eugenicists, Theodore Lothrop
Stoddard; anthropologists, who tackled ideas of both racial purity and racial
fixity; and many others.[49] Although not the majority in any of their disci-
plines, they made their voices heard.

Among the loudest was the anthropologist Franz Boas, an émigré from
Germany who headed up the Anthropology Department at Columbia
University between 1899 and 1942. His insistence that races were best
understood as products of culture rather than as biological entities helped
to transform anthropology from a science whose fundamental goal had
been to classify and ultimately rank the races to a science that studied,
in one scholar's words, both "the adaptation and change of peoples over
time." One of Boas's most frequently cited studies, which he published in
1912, demonstrated that among seventeen thousand immigrant children
in the United States, the head shape of Sicilian and Jewish children born
in the United States differed in a statistically significant way from that of
their parents. Boas did not interpret this as proof that evolution was taking place; instead he saw it as evidence that the human skull had enough
plasticity to adapt directly to environmental influences. Stoddard may have
dismissed this study as little more than "the desperate attempt of a Jew to
pass himself off as 'white,'" but there was no question that by challenging the scientific validity of cranial measurements Boas was attacking
what had long been considered an unchanging and thus ideal marker of
racial difference. For if the size and shape of the skull, or any other physi-

cal characteristics, were responsive enough to environmental influences to change in a generation, what exactly had race scientists been measuring? As the anthropologist J. H. Fleure observed, if Boas's conclusions were true, they "would destroy the foundations of anthropological research for race history."[50]

Boas and other critics did not put race to rest. Indeed, even they continued to employ language that made it sound as though races were real. But there could be no question that the "racial alchemy" of the United States was changing significantly. Nowhere was this more pronounced than in the shifting criteria for who counted as "white." As historians have shown, one of the outcomes of the Johnson-Reed Act was the gradual disappearance of the different shades of white that had mattered so much to the Dillingham Commission, and their replacement by a monolithic white population, increasingly referred to as "Caucasian." This did not mean that perceived differences between populations that hailed from different nations disappeared after 1924. They did not. By organizing peoples according to their national origins in the *Dictionary of Peoples,* and by establishing quotas based on those national origins, the federal government had even imparted new meaning to those differences. But whatever might have continued to separate Jews, Italians, Irish, Teutons, and French Canadians from one another was rarely talked about as racial. Some of these populations may have been less desirable than others, but they were all white and thus potentially assimilable, capable of becoming American citizens. That put all of them in a different category, for example, than Asian immigrants, whom the Johnson-Reed Act defined as nonwhite and completely banned.[51]

That Jews would become white had by no means been a given. After all, according to a study President Herbert Hoover commissioned, the purpose of the Johnson-Reed Act had been to increase "the Nordic racial types of northwestern Europe," who "resemble[d] more closely the prevailing stock in our country," and limit "the Mediterranean and Alpine types of southern and southeastern Europe." Yet declining numbers of Jews and other "undesirable types" ended up giving birth to a new imperative, which was to assimilate the proportionally smaller number of non-Nordic immigrants, if for no other reason than to drive a wedge deeper between whites and nonwhites. There is a certain irony here: legislation that drastically reduced the number of Jews who were allowed to enter the United States also opened the door to their inclusion among the "white" elite.[52] This did not take place overnight, and it may even have taken somewhat longer for Jews than for other non-Nordic populations, but reactions to the virulent anti-Semitism that exploded in Europe in the 1930s hastened the Jews' reconfiguration as Caucasians. Evidence of their successful assimilation became particularly apparent in the postwar years, as Jews received benefits like the GI Bill and government-backed mortgages, which allowed them to join the white flight out to the suburbs. Many Americans may still have viewed Jews as different by virtue of their religion, customs, and culture, but it became less likely that they would think of these differences as biological.

As the image of Jews as a distinct race faded, talk of diabetes as a Jewish disease also diminished. Nevertheless, it was not unusual well into the 1950s to read that Jews had a high prevalence of the disease. Indeed, in 1941, the Jewish medical journal *Harofé Haivri* published a special issue covering a symposium that had taken place on "Diabetes among Jews." Joslin, who provided the introduction to the issue, considered it "eminently proper for the Hebrew Medical Journal to issue a number on diabetes. All authors attest to the frequency of this disease in the Jewish race." Indeed, to one of the symposium's participants, the Philadelphia physician Gershon Ginzburg, the greater prevalence of diabetes among Jews remained "an undeniable fact."[53]

Joslin continued to link diabetes to Jews in subsequent editions of his *Treatment of Diabetes Mellitus*. William Osler's *The Principles and Practice of Medicine* included the same message in the sixteenth edition in 1947 that had appeared in the first edition in 1892: "Hebrews seem especially prone to [diabetes]." And as late as 1954 readers of the *Nebraska Medical Journal* were still learning that when it came to diabetes, "Jewish persons are unusually suspect."[54]

Still, a close look at these and other publications reveals that important changes were under way. For one, those who worked the hardest to sustain this message made up an older group of researchers. Among the participants in the 1941 symposium, for example, most were in their sixties. Joslin, the oldest of them, was seventy-two. They also provided precious little new material, drawing instead on studies they had conducted decades earlier. In doing so, they ignored studies that had begun to go beyond the simple message that race played no role in Jews' experience with diabetes to doubting whether the rate of diabetes among Jews was particularly high.

Jacob Schwartz, for example, a physician at Beth-El and Brooklyn Women's Hospitals in Brooklyn, New York, reported in 1934 that only 2.9 percent of the 4,398 Jewish patients he had seen in his practice had diabetes. This rate, he pointed out, was directly comparable to what Joslin had found in the general population. Louis Zisserman, who practiced medicine at the Jewish Hospital in Philadelphia, also found no difference in the diabetes mortality rate among Jews and non-Jews when he examined the hospital's records for the years 1930 to 1938. "This is in direct contradistinction to the figures generally published," he announced. And Harold Blotner, a Boston physician who gave army selectees their final medical examination at the Boston Armed Forces Induction Station before they left for service in World War II, went even further in 1946 when he questioned whether the diabetes rate among Jews had ever been disproportionately high.[55]

Blotner's doubts stemmed from his analysis of the medical examinations of almost seventy thousand selectees, which showed that Jews, who made up 6 percent of a control group of 7,350 men, made up 5.8 percent of those who had diabetes. This was exactly what one might expect if Jews did not have a special proclivity for the disease. Blotner noted as well that Jews were overrepresented in the group of individuals who already knew they had the disease (9.1 percent) and underrepresented among those whose diabetes was first discovered during his medical examination (4.1 percent). This suggested to him that the high rate of diabetes that had been found among Jews in the past had probably reflected their greater awareness of their disease—and not a higher incidence—and that this stemmed from the fact that "they live in urban areas chiefly and appear to visit the doctor quite readily for various complaints." In short, more urine tests had meant that more cases of the disease had been found.[56]

The 1930s and 1940s were decades of transition. Evidence was accumulating that suggested the need to rewrite the story of Jews and diabetes, while professional and popular authors alike continued to repeat the refrain that Jews were particularly susceptible to the disease. The two different points of view simply existed side by side. Only in the 1950s did the tide turn in favor of those who insisted that Jews were no more susceptible to diabetes than other groups. Backing them up were studies emerging from the newly established state of Israel.

As early as 1951, just three years after Israel's founding, a study appeared based on statistics gathered from the food-rationing authorities in the country's three largest cities: Tel Aviv, Haifa, and Jerusalem. A synopsis of the study, published in the *Journal of the American Medical Association,* pointed out that "the number of persons suffering from diabetes mellitus in Israel is, on the average, no higher than in other civilized countries." As the summary made clear: "Nothing confirms the opinion that the tendency of Jews to contract the disease is two to four times higher than in other races, as is often stated in textbooks."[57] Subsequent studies in the following decade reached the same conclusion. To Hermann Steinitz, who focused his analysis on Tel Aviv, "the opinion that diabetes is much more frequent among Jews than among other peoples . . . is not based on exact statistics." To A. M. Cohen, one of the founders of the Israel Diabetes Association, a comparison of diabetes rates among Ashkenazi, Sephardi, Yemenite, and Kurdish Jews in Israel "repudiates the statement accepted in the literature that diabetes is more common among the Jewish race." Cohen had found that none of the four groups he had studied had a rate higher than those for non-Jews in other parts of the world, although he had uncovered some significant differences among the four groups. Most striking was the extremely low diabetes rate among very recent immigrants from Yemen and Iraq, which at 0.06 percent was among the lowest in the world. In contrast, the descendants of Yemenite and Kurdish Jews who had emigrated to Israel decades earlier—Cohen referred to them as "old or 'settled'" immigrants—had rates comparable to that of Ashkenazi and Sephardic Jews. For Cohen the reason for this difference was simple: the new arrivals had previously had "little or no contact with . . . the Western mode of life and food habits." The increase in their diabetes rate was, thus, nothing more than a "result of a change in the environmental conditions."[58] Neither genes nor race played any role.

When the Jewish cardiologist Dennis Krikler decided in 1970 to survey the medical literature to determine "the present state of knowledge" regarding "diseases of Jews," his short paragraph on diabetes mellitus stated simply that "impressions" that Jews suffer disproportionately from diabetes have "not been borne out." By this time, few were left who would have disagreed. Indeed, the sources that Steinitz, Cohen, Krikler, and others cited when criticizing a literature that linked Jews and diabetes were, for the most part, decades old. To be sure, the assertion that diabetes afflicts Jews disproportionately has never totally disappeared. As recently as 2002, for example, an online article on "Jewish Diabetes" repeated the claim that there was a "higher incidence of diabetes among Jews."[59] But such statements have been rare since the 1960s. I have found that most people today are surprised to hear that Jews were once believed to be particularly vulnerable to the disease.

* * *

There may be a temptation to credit new empirical studies with taking down the once widespread belief that Jews suffered disproportionately from diabetes. And no doubt they played a role. The studies that emerged from Israel in particular received considerable attention in the professional and popular press. But it would be a mistake to give empirical studies all—or even most—of the credit. After all, clinical investigations in the 1930s and 1940s had already challenged the reigning wisdom about Jews and diabetes. Yet professional and popular writers alike paid little attention to those findings, continuing instead to draw on an older literature that purported to have evidence of the Jews' proclivity to the disease. Thus, the better question may be: why did these empirical studies become more believable in the postwar years?

This question is all the more intriguing because the empirical studies produced in the postwar years did not demonstrate unequivocally that diabetes rates among Jews were low. Blotner skewed his findings, for example, by using the birthplace of the parents of his study subjects as the criterion by which to determine his subjects' nationality. This means he classified anyone whose parents had been born in the United States—whether of Jewish, Italian, Irish, or Canadian French descent—as "Old American." As it turned out, "Old Americans" had by far the lowest rate of diabetes: although they made up 45 percent of the control group, they made up only 13.3 percent of the cases.[60] His message was clear: the longer one lived in the United States, the less chance one had of developing diabetes. Blotner never explained his rationale for classifying his subjects in this way, but as a Jew he may have hoped to paint a picture that touted the benefits of assimilation.

Tellingly, in a study Blotner published three years earlier based on the medical examinations of 45,650 inductees, he had reported a high rate of diabetes among Jews, but still interpreted his finding in a way that favored assimilation: he claimed the rate was higher among Jews who lived in isolation, where their old "habits and customs" could prevail, and lower among those who lived in "mixed communities."[61]

The results of empirical studies, then, go only so far in explaining why the link between Jews and diabetes was finally broken in the postwar years. Equally significant were changing understandings of race. The labeling of diabetes as a *Judenkrankheit* had made sense when Jews were believed to make up a distinct population biologically. The heyday of this practice, the last decade of the nineteenth and the first three decades of the twentieth century, coincided with a time when few challenged this claim, not even Jews who may have tended to define race differently than many of their non-Jewish peers, but who did not yet challenge the concept of race itself. As Jews became "white," however, and especially as scientific racism came increasingly under attack in the postwar years, fewer and fewer articles claimed that a proclivity to diabetes had anything to do with Jews' unique biology. Instead, Jews' experience with diabetes became part of discussions about the higher susceptibility of middle-class whites to the disease.

Research exploring the link between Jews and particular diseases did not disappear. As early as the 1930s, scientists recognized that Tay-Sachs disease occurred with unusual frequency among Jews, but they also noted that while it favored Ashkenazi Jews, its rate among Sephardic Jews was no different than in the rest of the population.[62] In subsequent decades, studies of French Canadians from Eastern Quebec, Cajuns from Southern Louisiana, and the Pennsylvania Dutch also revealed a high prevalence of Tay-Sachs, breaking the unique link between Ashkenazi Jews and the disease. Thus, few considered the presence of this disease in a population a racial trait; instead it was thought to be a genetic mutation that had established itself in a reproductively isolated population. This focus on genetic frequencies and particular populations was a far cry from the practice early in the twentieth century of arguing for a clear connection between an entire population's characteristics and the prevalence of a disease.

But while the strong link between Jews and diabetes began to weaken in the 1930s, the connections between race, diabetes, and civilization persisted until after World War II. Popular and professional sources continued to insist that diabetes and other diseases of civilization proliferated among middle- and upper-class whites while being virtually absent among so-called primitive populations. Diabetes thus continued to symbolize the "civilized" nature of those who suffered most from the disease, even as its rapid rise among society's "best" raised fears of a civilization in decline. Given these tensions, diabetes became fertile ground for anxieties about the destructive nature of consumer capitalism.

2

Whiteness, Self-Restraint, and Citizenship

All kinds of [diabetes] patients have been treated, the courageous and the cowardly, the enterprising and the slothful.

John R. Williams, 1921

Diabetics . . . make a good deal better citizens than the average.

Hannah Lees, 1936

IN 1936 THE JOURNALIST HANNAH LEES published an article in *Collier's*, a literary and political weekly magazine, titled "Two Million Tightrope Walkers." Her goal was to draw attention to the increasing number of people in the United States estimated to have diabetes. The image Lees evoked—of two million people trying to balance on a thin rope, with any misstep risking a fall into dire medical problems and eventual death—conveyed the seriousness of what professional and popular writers alike were beginning to consider a potential public health nightmare. Recent statistics revealed that diabetes had become the ninth leading cause of death in the country, a significant jump from the twenty-seventh place it had held in 1890. "Diabetes Mortality Up 58% in 30 Years," announced the *New York Times* in 1933. Morbidity rates were also skyrocketing. In 1934, the Metropolitan Life Insurance Company estimated that almost half a million people already had diabetes, and that if nothing were to change, another 2,500,000 people would develop the disease before they died.[1]

Such large numbers fostered competing claims about what could be driving up rates, since no one believed that the influx of Jewish immigrants to the United States could alone account for diabetes's astronomical rise. Amid discussions of the relative contributions of family history, obesity, diet, stress, and viruses, diabetes became entangled in debates over the threat that consumer capitalism posed to older virtues of modesty, frugality, and self-discipline. As a disease associated with overindulgence, diabetes symbolized—as we have already seen in Haven Emerson's diatribe—a life lacking in self-restraint. Yet at the same time, the strategies deemed necessary to manage the disease, including constant self-monitoring, began to assume significance beyond their role in staving off kidney failure, blindness, and gangrene. They also came to signify the practices that would help Americans free themselves from the opprobrium of having become, during the interwar years, "the grossest feeders among the nations."[2]

The anxieties evident in writings about diabetes reveal the authors' concerns with more than the medical aspects of the disease; they also indicate deep divisions over which values mattered most during a time of massive social, economic, political, and demographic change. Such differences of opinion surfaced clearly in the aftermath of insulin's discovery, when those who hailed the hormone as a miracle drug proved unable to silence fears that individuals with diabetes might now think they could eat whatever they wanted, indulging their appetites with impunity. The eugenically minded further lamented that insulin was keeping the "unfit" alive into their reproductive years, allowing them to contribute "defective genes" to the gene pool. This led some to recommend that anyone who had diabetes be forbidden from marrying. Others countered that those who controlled their disease modeled self-discipline and would likely make ideal parents. Central to these battles, especially in the interwar years, were questions about how to define and protect what it meant to be white.[3]

I have already mentioned the gradual erasure in the years following the Johnson-Reed Act of the different shades of whiteness that had once been part of the country's racial imagination, and how they had been replaced in the interwar years by a monolithic "Caucasian race." But the boundaries that divided "Caucasians" from everyone else remained porous, leading to numerous attempts to clarify who belonged to this group and who did not.

The passage of a flurry of antimiscegenation laws in the interwar years is one example of such boundary work. The 1924 Virginia Racial Integrity Act, for example, defined whites as having "no trace whatsoever of any blood other than Caucasian," and forbade marriage between anyone in this group and nonwhites. But perceived threats to an imaginary whiteness came not just from fears of admixture—"taints" from without—but also from concerns that the number of eugenically "unfit" whites was increasing.[4] Writings on diabetes during this era reflected these fears. Nowhere is this clearer than in distinctions between "good" diabetes patients and "bad" ones.

To the physician J. R. Williams, diabetes patients included "the courageous and the cowardly, the enterprising and the slothful." Haven Emerson divided them into those who practiced "self-control" and those who took the "easy way out of the consequences of dietary sins." Lees took this distinction one step further and insisted that "diabetics . . . make a good deal better citizens than the average. They are never wasters and drunkards," she elaborated, "because they have to learn early in their disease to be controlled and self-reliant. They have greater intelligence than the average and they develop it by constant use. . . . Of course there undoubtedly have been diabetics with weak characters but they didn't live very long to tell the tale."[5]

Lees was claiming that individuals with diabetes, whose bodies were unable to regulate blood-sugar levels, were better qualified to participate in civil society than the average person whose blood-sugar metabolism worked just fine. And her reason rested on the daily routine necessary to manage diabetes, which instilled the self-discipline and self-reliance hailed by many to be a necessary component of responsible citizenry. In this scenario, diabetes made a person better by requiring constant monitoring and a life of restraint.

Diabetes was not the only chronic disease in the early twentieth-century United States to inspire teachings on the virtues of living abstemiously and practicing self-control. Advice literature related to cancer, diseases of the heart, and tuberculosis—the three greatest killers at the time—also reveal assumptions and instructions similar to those in the diabetes literature: an emphasis on individual responsibility rather than social conditions; strict moral codes as a means of preventing disease; recommendations for the close surveillance of bodies; and a sense that growing numbers of individuals were potentially at risk of becoming ill.[6] Still, diabetes stood out in degree, if not in kind, because of the widespread belief that in comparison to other chronic diseases, successful treatment rested primarily in the hands of patients. Thus where the importance of early detection dominated the cancer advice literature, manuals for living with diabetes concentrated on proper rules for daily living and strategies for practicing self-control. Those who mastered these rules and strategies—who learned to restrain themselves, live modestly, and reject gluttony—became in the process "better citizens than the average."

In the 1930s, when Lees's article appeared, *Collier's* had over two million subscribers.[7] Although the demographics of its readership cannot be known definitively, it is likely that the vast majority of subscribers were white and middle class. Certainly, the images that filled the pages of *Collier's* suggest that this is the population the editors set out to attract. Taking up almost half of the front page of Lees's article, for example, was an image of a white physician warning an elegantly dressed white couple of the dire circumstances that would befall them should they fail to curb their appetites (Figure 2.1). This was the population, the editors of *Collier's* evidently believed, that had the most to gain from reading what Lees had to share.

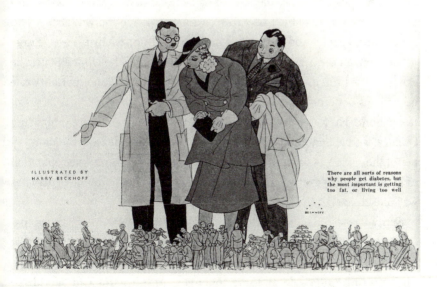

Fig. 2.1. The illustrated first page of "Two Million Tightrope Walkers," an article by Hannah Lees published in *Collier's* on May 15, 1936. *Collier's Magazine* is a registered trademark of JTE Multimedia, LLC 435 Devon Park Drive, Bldg. 500, Wayne, PA, 19087.

The editors had good reason to believe this was the population to target. In the interwar years, medical writers were still claiming that diabetes "rises with wealth," afflicting those "in the most comfortable situated
classes" more than any other group. They even described diabetes as a
"clean" disease of whites, in contrast to "dirty" diseases, such as tuberculosis and syphilis, that plagued the poor and especially the so-called red,
black, and brown races.[8] A diagnosis of diabetes was thus consistent with
cultural understandings of what it meant to be middle class and white. Still,
as the distinction between "good" and "bad" diabetes patients made clear,
not all whites were considered equal. Some were "cowardly," "slothful," and
"weak," while others made model citizens. During these interwar years,
then, such distinctions became part of broader conversations about race,
class, and citizenship, helping to promote a set of model behaviors that allegedly defined what it meant to be white and American.[9]

A Cultural Shift from "Frugality" to "Luxury"

The characterization of diabetes as a symbol of uncontrolled consumption dates back at least to the late nineteenth century, when diabetes rates
began to soar. It may have been uncommon to divide individuals with diabetes into "good" and "bad," but already in 1890, when Charles Purdy
penned one of the first major textbooks on diabetes in the United States, he
wasted little time in blaming the 150 percent increase in the mortality rate
of diabetes between 1850 and 1880 on "the decided change in the habits of
the nation." He found it deeply troubling that Americans were embracing
"luxury" and abandoning the "frugality" that had long defined the moral fiber of the nation. As a result, the United States was earning "the reputation
of being the most extravagant nation in the world." The high rate of diabetes
was one clear sign to him of that extravagance.[10]

Purdy wrote little about the specific social and economic changes that
concerned him, other than to lament the "inflation of the currency" that
took place during the war, which presumably had increased the purchasing power of the people. But one could well imagine this Chicago physician reacting more generally to the developments transforming his city.
Industrialization, mechanization, new modes of transportation and com-

munication, the rise of banks, and the availability of credit were all altering the lives of Americans, creating an urban environment at odds with the rural and small-town communities that had been home to 95 percent of the population at the beginning of the century. Gone was the homogeneity of what the historian Robert Wiebe has called the "island communities" of the antebellum period, where townspeople recognized themselves in their neighbors and knew one another by name, face, or reputation.[11] Instead, a rapidly growing working class, fueled by the influx of immigrants from both rural America and Eastern and Southern Europe, coexisted and sometimes mingled with an increasing number of emancipated African Americans, along with Native Americans fleeing the poverty of the reservations to which they had been forcibly removed.

There was a hustle and bustle to urban life as people traveled to work, perhaps catching a quick ride on one of the new cable cars instead of making their way slowly on foot. At the end of the day, they might stop into one of the new department stores, where they could choose from a dizzying array of low-priced luxury items, such as silk, porcelain, and tea. Or they might spend an evening pursuing pleasure in the new music clubs and dance halls. The excitement this generated among the millions of people who frequented the new stores and other venues of entertainment was, however, cause for dismay among others. Purdy, who saw little more than an abandonment of values he held dear, gave voice to anxieties shared by many others who were, in the words of one historian, experiencing "dislocation and bewilderment" as a result of these changes.[12]

Such feelings of dislocation continued to escalate as American cities grew in size and number, radically altering how people lived, worked, and played. By the "roaring twenties," the first decade in which more Americans lived in urban than in rural areas, tensions were exploding between, at the greatest extremes, those who looked backward—to an imagined past when American families embraced middle-class values grounded in the Protestant work ethic—and those who sought to push the boundaries of what was considered acceptable. This was, after all, the decade of jazz clubs, dance halls, movie theaters, automobiles, art deco, and the Harlem Renaissance. But it was also a time of intense backlash against these "experiments," evident in Prohibition, the Scopes Monkey trial, the passage of a national restrictive immigration act, and the Supreme Court's upholding of a legal challenge to the coercive sterilization laws that state legislatures had been enacting since the turn of the century. Antimiscegenation laws also grew in number, with a revived Ku Klux Klan stepping in to make sure that they were obeyed. Everywhere one looked, the state appeared to be growing long arms, expanding its administrative apparatus in order to better manage the increasing complexities of modern life and, in the process, reaching deeper into the private lives of citizens. But the "search for order," as Wiebe has described the drive of Progressive-era reformers who sought to forge a new nation after the Civil War, relied not only on coercive measures enacted through legislative bodies and the courts. It also required that the nation's citizens take responsibility for disciplining bodies, minds, and actions—their own, those of their families, and in the case of medicine and public health, those of patients and the public writ large.[13]

Public health materials in the first decades of the twentieth century were replete with instructions on how to achieve health by practicing self-governance. Whether they were targeting high infant and maternal mortality rates, tuberculosis, venereal disease, cancer, or diabetes, health educators encouraged individuals to change their personal habits voluntarily, an approach that seemed most consistent with the principles of the democratic nation they were trying to build.[14] People would be motivated by promises of good health, a long life, and a chance to demonstrate that they understood and could act on modern, scientific approaches to solving society's problems. Those who monitored themselves and their families were, at the same time, signaling that they possessed the traits needed to be appropriate stewards of the new nation.

Against this backdrop, those with diabetes began to be divided into two groups. Similar to a distinction between the "deserving" and "undeserving" poor, the "heroic" disabled veteran eager to rehabilitate and the "pariah" willing to live off a government pension, and the "good" mother of the nation's future citizens and the "immoral" one, a division between "good" and "bad" diabetes patients indicated the weight being placed on individual responsibility at a time of heightened anxiety about the future of the nation.[15] Purdy may have associated the disease of diabetes with an abandonment of frugality, but those with diabetes were now being differentiated—

and no one played a greater role in promulgating this differentiation than Elliott P. Joslin.

Joslin's Prescription: Perfect Control

The son of a successful shoe manufacturer and the heiress to a fortune acquired in the leather tanning trade, Elliott Joslin enjoyed a "gentleman's upbringing" among New England's social elite. He was born in 1869 in Oxford, Massachusetts, grew up in the Congregationalist church, and was educated at Yale College and then Harvard Medical School, where he received his M.D. in 1895 and later joined the faculty. Combining his own financial resources with the considerable wealth of his wife, Elizabeth Denny Joslin, he purchased a three-hundred-acre farm in his hometown of Oxford as well as a residence on Bay State Road in the Back Bay of Boston. From this residence, which was just down the road from the Charles River and some of the city's most elegant mansions, Joslin set up his office and began specializing in diabetes, long before medical specialization had become the norm in the American medical profession.[16]

Joslin's reputation derived in large part from his authorship of the textbook *Treatment of Diabetes Mellitus*. He also wrote a companion text, *A Diabetic Manual for the Mutual Use of Doctor and Patient,* in which he translated dense medical knowledge into information useful to both general practitioners and their patients. Like the textbook, this went through ten editions in his lifetime. He also published 240 articles, spoke at medical conferences and congresses, and produced radio programs intended to educate the public on medical matters. As early as 1921, one of his colleagues commented that "when we think of diabetes, we think Joslin."[17]

Joslin's approach to diabetes care, although not universally shared, earned widespread respect. Although some doctors were inclined to allow some laxity in patients' control over their daily activities, for Joslin, strict control over all aspects of life was essential, with no detail too minor to monitor. The section of his textbook entitled "What Every Diabetic Patient Should Know" offers a small taste of what his advice looked like. Along with general information about the need to move one's bowels daily, get ample sleep and adequate exercise, chew one's food slowly, clean one's teeth, eat less rather than more, avoid anxiety, and test one's urine before breakfast, Joslin offered instructions on how to determine what foods to eat. Take, for example, vegetables. After dividing all of them into groups based on the percentage of carbohydrates they contained, he explained: "Even if the 10 per cent., 15 per cent., and 20 per cent. vegetables are allowed, vegetables from the 5 per cent. group should be taken as well. Usually it is allowable to substitute for a given quantity of 5 per cent. vegetables one-half as much from the 10 per cent. group, one-quarter as much from the 15 per cent., or one-sixth as much from the 20 per cent. Exchange vegetables for fruit only under advice."[18]

Not surprisingly, many people with diabetes found it difficult to follow such advice. One twenty-year-old man insisted that "to diet as doctors expect us to is not only uncomfortable but impossible." Although he did his best to "weigh and measure" everything he consumed, he occasionally splurged and ate "three marshmellow sundaes." Some individuals also struggled financially. To become an expert on the content of foodstuffs and allowable substitutions, to prepare the appropriate foods, and to measure and weigh everything consumed required both time and money. One young man remembered that his mother had weighed every bit of food he had eaten for seven years. Small wonder that those who had enough resources often hired private-duty nurses to care for them or for their loved ones.[19]

Joslin was not completely blind to the expenses involved in the care he prescribed—in fact, he occasionally forgave a bill or helped secure a free hospital bed for a patient in need—but this awareness did not temper his expectations of patient compliance. Perhaps he required full obedience because of his belief that diabetes usually afflicted those with ample means; financial concerns would not have posed a roadblock for them. But Joslin also valued an orderly life in and of itself. A frugal man who ate sparingly, he once bragged that he had kept a steady weight throughout his adult years, neither losing nor gaining a single pound.[20] He also worked hard, spending long days examining patients and long evening hours writing up meticulous notes, filling out patients' charts, and catching up on correspondence.

Joslin held all of his patients to the same exacting standard to which he held himself, considering them responsible if they failed to keep their urine free of sugar, lapsed into a diabetic coma, developed gangrene, or put on too much weight. In fact, he once claimed that "to get fat shows a lack of moral character."[21] Visible signs of the disease's progression were, in other words, indications not simply of the individual's failure to follow the doctor's orders, but also of a *moral* failure. Not that Joslin absolved doctors of all responsibility for keeping their patients on track. Casting them as both medical advisers and moral guardians, he once encouraged a group of physicians to make sure that their "warning and admonition" to the diabetes patient to watch his diet, check his urine, and examine his feet "penetrate . . . deeply the souls of your cases." In that way, should a complication set in, "the unhappy patient will feel compelled to say: 'Doctor, you warned me. . . . You are not to blame for my condition.'"[22]

Joslin also imagined that at least some diabetes patients would become "apostles of food hygiene," taking the teachings of their physicians to relatives and friends as they spread the gospel of clean habits of living. He spelled this out most clearly in an article he published in 1921 in which he labeled diabetes "a penalty of obesity" and contrasted those who became fat and should be "ashamed" with a different type of patient, one who "know[s] the disease, and can be counted on and should be encouraged to disseminate information about its prevention."[23]

To help his reader visualize this type of person, Joslin introduced Louisa Drumm, a seventy-nine-year-old woman who had come to his office on March 30, 1920. She had diabetes and received instruction during her visit on how to test her own urine. She died shortly thereafter from pneumonia, but in the short time between her visit to Joslin and her death, she had "examined the urines of ten others in her boarding house, and in so doing discovered the presence of diabetes in a boy." The boy ended up in Joslin's office and although we never learn what came of him, Joslin credits Drumm with saving this child's life. He even ends his article with a quotation from the "Parable of the Good Samaritan": "Can one not appropriately say to younger patients: 'Go thou and do likewise'?"[24]

In this way, Joslin created caricatures of diabetes patients, with the "bad" selfishly indulging their excessive appetites and becoming fat, and the "good" monitoring not only themselves but also relatives, friends, and neighbors. Joslin's understanding of personal responsibility thus extended to the care and monitoring of others, although one's obligations amounted largely to surveilling their habits and offering encouraging or admonishing words. Ultimately, then, if physicians and "apostles" did their part and an individual's condition nevertheless grew worse, blame could be placed only on the choices the individual made, as though each and every person had the same obstacles and challenges to overcome.

Joslin, as we have seen, was not alone in juxtaposing two types of diabetes patients whose differences had everything to do with their alleged moral nature. To "the courageous and the cowardly," and "the enterprising and the slothful," J. R. Williams added "the attentive and interested, and the indifferent." He went on: "These types are mentioned because the character of the individual has much to do with the outcome [of the disease]. To successfully contend with diabetes a patient must not only be wisely advised, but he must also possess courage and a willingness to learn and assist, to create new dietary habits and eliminate old ones."[25]

One might be tempted to think that these two "types" had something to do with the distinction we make today between type 1 and type 2 (or what was once called juvenile and adult) diabetes. But doing so would be a mistake. As already mentioned, the medical community at the time believed overwhelmingly in the "unity of diabetes." To be sure, physicians recognized that those who developed the disease at a young age usually manifested severe symptoms more rapidly than if the disease first appeared later in life. For these young patients, a diagnosis of diabetes often meant that they would be dead within a few short years. William Osler even referred to "*acute* and *chronic* forms," but he maintained that "there is no essential difference between them, except that in the former the patients are younger, the course more rapid, and the emaciation more marked." Others took this idea a step further, cautioning that a division between acute and chronic forms served only "practical purposes," since "these two types may pass indifferently from one to the other in the same subject at any time during the course of the disease."[26] Diabetes would not, in fact, be officially divided into different diseases until the late 1970s, when most physicians had abandoned any belief in the unity of the disease.

The distinction between "good" and "bad" patients during this earlier era, then, had nothing to do with physiological differences and everything to do with "character." Character was, moreover, most often judged by the individual's performance of the kind of self-governance advised by the doctor. In the pre-insulin days, the doctor's orders focused almost exclusively on adherence to a specific diet, even though there was little consensus on what that diet should entail. Were fats okay? What about protein? Carbohydrates? Fruits? Did types of food matter, or did one just need to watch total calories? How many daily calories, moreover, was ideal? The most popular of the pre-insulin diets, Frederick Allen's "starvation diet," limited calories to five hundred per day. Advocates of this treatment method, which included Joslin, believed that they were extending the lives of their patients by months if not years, although critics were not convinced. Yet despite such disagreements—indeed, despite basic therapeutic ineffectiveness—patients were still held responsible if they "failed" to keep their blood sugars in check.[27]

When insulin was discovered in 1921–1922, it changed forever the way diabetes was imagined, experienced, and treated. The discovery took place at the University of Toronto, where John J. R. Macleod, Frederick G. Banting, Charles H. Best, and James B. Collip carried out the scientific work leading to the isolation of this pancreatic hormone. Medical researchers had first learned about the importance of the pancreas in the pathophysiology of diabetes in 1889, when Oskar Minkowski and Joseph von Mering at the University of Strasbourg had removed the pancreas from a dog and realized that they had unintentionally created a diabetic condition. Subsequent research, by these scientists and others, drew attention to clusters of cells scattered throughout the pancreas, known as the islets of Langerhans and believed to be the site of an "internal secretion." Macleod and his team were the first to isolate this secretion, which they subsequently named insulin.[28]

Preliminary tests of insulin produced remarkable results, especially for individuals whose bodies were incapable of producing any of the hormone. In one particularly famous case, adherence to Allen's diet had left fifteen-year-old Elizabeth Hughes—daughter of Charles Evans Hughes, U.S. secretary of state and later chief justice of the U.S. Supreme Court—weighing under fifty pounds, barely able to walk, and near death.[29] Within five weeks of her first insulin injections, she had gained ten pounds and expressed her joy that she could now expect "a normal, healthy existence." After six years of insulin therapy, she married a young lawyer, Thomas Gossett, and went on to have three children and eight grandchildren. Such stories of sudden recovery led to newspaper articles with titles like "Diabetes, Dreaded Disease, Yields to New Gland Cure" and "Insulin, Science's New Cure for Diabetes." One *New York Times* article shared the experience of a sixteen-year-old boy who had lapsed into a diabetic coma only to be brought back to life by the administration of insulin. According to the journalist, this marked "the first case on record in the annals of medicine in this city where a patient has been rescued from death when a diabetic coma had set in."[30]

Such stories fed excitement about the promises of scientific medicine to radically transform the experience of disease. First infectious diseases, and now diseases of "disturbed metabolism," were proving to be no match for the laboratory. Given that insulin basically ended diabetes's death sentence—especially for those with the acute form—these accolades were well deserved. What these pronouncements ignored, however, was the reality that insulin was not a cure and that life for those with diabetes and their families continued to be marked by daily struggles. In the words of physician and medical historian Chris Feudtner, insulin transformed an acute disease into a chronic condition.[31]

Insulin did nothing to erase the distinction between different types of patients, however. On the contrary, for those already inclined to read diabetes as a sign of society's overconsumption of goods—and to see calorie limits and monitoring of daily activities as an antidote to that overindulgence—insulin was a threat. In the words of Haven Emerson, the hormone led too often to the abandonment of the "self-control and self-restraint" that distinguished "man . . . from the brute." An article in *Time* magazine similarly warned that insulin could not "protect one against the ravages of self-indulgence. Curbed cravings cannot now be satisfied with impunity." The Metropolitan Life Insurance Company also jumped into the fray. In an article in their monthly magazine in January 1930 with the catchy title, "Rip Van Winkles," the company accused "the million diabetics" in the country of being asleep, "lulled into a false sense of security" by insulin and thinking that they could now take whatever "liberties" they wanted with their diet. Should they do so, the company warned, they would soon see how, "with crushing swiftness," diabetes would kill.[32]

Insulin may have been a "miracle" drug, but by promoting the message that "tight" control of blood glucose levels could postpone—if not eliminate—the long-term health complications of the disease, it also sharpened the line between those labeled good and bad.[33] In theory, everyone now had the tools to keep his or her disease in check. In the post-insulin era, high blood-glucose levels could have only one meaning: the individual who had diabetes had failed to make good choices and live a model life.

Insulin and the False Promise of Independence

The model life for someone with diabetes had long been defined by a commitment to restraint and moderation. What insulin made possible was also a life free of dependence on others. At least, this was the promise. This is evident in a set of before-and-after photographs that appeared in 1923 in the *Journal of the American Medical Association* (Figure 2.2).[34] The before photograph portrays a barely clothed and emaciated young child in the

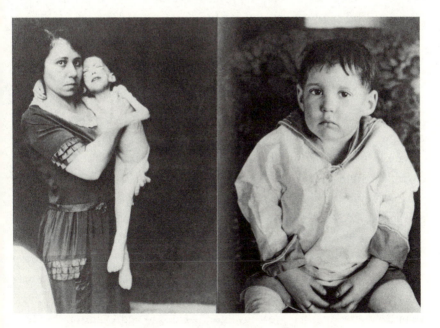

Fig. 2.2. Dr. Ralph Major's patient, before and after insulin treatment. The photograph appeared in Ralph H. Major, "The Treatment of Diabetes Mellitus with Insulin," *Journal of the American Medical Association* 80, no. 122 (June 2, 1923): 1597–1600. Courtesy of the Clendening History of Medicine Library, University of Kansas Medical Center. Wellcome Collection CC BY.

arms of his mother. The viewer can see much of the child's body. He seems to be in considerable pain, his face contorted, his eyes squinting. His ribs are protruding and his arms and legs are so thin that one can easily imagine them snapping under his own weight. Only his mother's grip appears to be keeping this child from falling apart. The "after" photograph zooms in so one sees only the child's head and shoulders. The mother is gone. The boy is now clothed in what looks like a sailor's uniform. He is staring at the photographer, his eyes big and alert, his cheeks deliciously chubby, his face filled out and healthy looking.

Yet even a moment's reflection reveals the illusory nature of this independence. After all, the boy is very young, and so will remain dependent on his mother—or another adult—for years to come. This would have been true of any young child, but especially one who would need help managing his disease. For despite the understandable excitement that accompanied the discovery of insulin, and even though those with diabetes no longer had to live in as much fear of extremely high blood sugar levels and ketoacidosis, they now had new worries: first, that insulin might lead to a sudden drop in blood sugar, sending them into hypoglycemic shock; and second, that they may develop long-term complications—such as blindness, kidney failure, and amputations—that had long afflicted those living for decades with the mild form of the disease. Thus many people who had diabetes remained dependent in multiple ways: on parents, if they were children; often on caregivers in later years; and for those whose bodies produced either little or no insulin, on the hormone and all the paraphernalia (needles, strips, syringes, scales) needed to manage their disease.

By framing insulin as a means of acquiring independence, and, more importantly, by pathologizing dependence, these photographs denied the realities of patients' lives and the conflicting feelings they and their caregivers often experienced when they learned that they would need to inject the drug for the rest of their lives. Mina Miller Edison, the second wife of Thomas Alva Edison, responded with dread when Frederick Allen, who had been attending the great inventor, decided to add insulin to her husband's treatment plan. "I am sick over the idea," she wrote to their son on July 12, 1931, "but it seems that it had to be done. Dr. Allen is very nice but I do wish that other means had been tried before resorting to insulin."[35]

What Mina did not acknowledge in this comment is that other means had been tried. Edison had been diagnosed with diabetes eight years earlier at the age of seventy-seven. Since that time he had been managing his disease solely through diet, fasting occasionally for four days at a time to get his sugar to a tolerable level, although frequently ending the fast with a binge when, Minna complained, he would consume "more than he ha[d] in ages."[36] Nevertheless, this toggling between fasting and binging had worked well enough until early 1931, when Edison's health began to fail. By July he was spending most of his time in bed, too exhausted to complete the work he had begun at the request of his friend, Henry Ford, to find an alternative rubber source for automobile tires. Only at this point did Allen start his patient on insulin, yet by then it was too late. By October, Edison was dead.

One may very well ask why Allen had not started his patient on insulin sooner. Neither Edison's nor his doctor's reasons are known, but Mina's letters reveal her horror at the thought of the new routine, which she considered both "a nightmare" and "an ordeal." She felt this way even though they had hired a private nurse to give the injections and monitor Edison's progress. For Mina, insulin was not a miracle drug that would allow her husband to return to a life of independence. Had that been her image, she may very well have welcomed—perhaps even suggested—that her husband begin this treatment regimen earlier. To her, insulin signified that her husband had become an invalid, dependent on the ministrations of others and on the new drug.

Mina Miller Edison's reaction to insulin stands in stark contrast to that of Elizabeth Hughes, likely because they were dealing with different forms of the disease. Hughes, who had the acute form of diabetes, did not have the option of managing her disease with diet alone; her body produced no insulin. Nevertheless, individuals who had to inject insulin to survive occasionally voiced sentiments similar to those found in Mina's letters. Twenty-year-old James Albertson, who shared his experience with diabetes in an article he penned in 1938 for *American Mercury*, claimed that being dependent on insulin was "very much like being a cripple with a crutch." Several decades later, Ralph Bunche, U.S. diplomat and winner of the 1950 Nobel Peace Prize for his role in brokering peace in the Middle East, voiced similar apprehensions. Refusing to take insulin, despite experiencing extreme exhaustion, a declining appetite, and the rapid loss of thirty-five pounds, he shared his concern that he would become "enslaved" by it. When he heard of Sheikh Abdullah of Kashmir's near death from acute diabetes in 1967, it made him think of his own infirmities. By that point, Bunche was struggling with severe loss of vision and was feeling as trapped by the disease as by the hormone. "I feel sorry for him," Bunche remarked. "He is a great figure of a man but diabetes can take him down. It is insidious in that it seems to erode one's life away—sapping strength in many ways and keeping one entirely at its mercy. I sometimes feel like a doomed prisoner."[37]

The fears and concerns that Mina Edison, Albertson, and Bunche articulated, while clearly a response to losses in their own and their loved ones' physical abilities, were also shaped by the cultural and political meaning of dependence. In a society that went beyond merely idealizing rugged individualism to making "independence" a key qualification for adulthood and thus, by implication, for citizenship, becoming dependent carried a heavy burden. At various times since the founding of the republic, women, African Americans, the poor, and the disabled had all been denied rights, including citizenship, because of their alleged "dependence," whether that dependence was understood as economic (not owning property or their own labor) or intellectual (being incapable of thinking for themselves). Such denial of rights and privileges is all the more evident if we think not only of "legal" citizenship, which basically confers political rights, but also of "social" citizenship, which includes but is not restricted to the right to employment, education, housing, marriage, and military service.[38] The history of the United States since its founding shows that while legal citizenship has been extended to an increasing number of peoples, social citizenship has not followed in step.

A robust body of scholarship has laid bare how attitudes toward gender, race, and class have informed who receives the privileges of full citizenship and who is either denied those privileges completely or relegated to the status of second-class citizen. Disability scholars have in particular encouraged us to recognize the way that such discriminatory practices have long employed the language of dependence and disability for their justification. Thus, one strategy for denying political rights to African Americans was to group them, in the words of Charles S. Johnson, the first black president of Fisk University, "with cripples, persons with recognized handicaps." Those opposed to women's suffrage also often cited women's "great temperamental disabilities," which allegedly rendered them incapable of thinking rationally. Equally disturbing, when groups fought back to claim rights for themselves, they rarely came to the defense of individuals with disabilities. Instead, their strategy was to insist that they were not disabled—a tactic that, although sometimes effective, also legitimized disability as a reason to discriminate. As a result, people with physical and cognitive impairments suffered two kinds of discrimination: they were (and continue to be) denied rights because of the perception that they are not able to act responsibly in a participatory democracy, and, as other groups pressed for full access by arguing against their own particular disability, they were devalued for being among those perceived as disabled.[39]

In the years following insulin's discovery, individuals with diabetes struggled to understand the meaning of this new drug in their lives. There can be no question that it gave many of them the miracle of a longer, fuller life, allowing them to contemplate a future beyond the average of three years post-diagnosis for those with the acute form, and six years for those with the milder form. It also raised new questions about the nature of diabetes, its effect on one's ability to be a "productive" member of society, and its relationship to other conditions widely viewed as "disabilities."

In this regard, Albertson's story in *American Mercury* deserves a closer look, because central to the young man's narrative is his reconfiguration of the relationship between dependence, independence, and disability.[40] The comparison he made between insulin and a crutch, for example, appeared near the beginning of his article, yet by the end he was telling the reader that he was "unsure" whether, given the chance, he would want to "rid" himself of the disease. He leads his reader through this transition by turning every disadvantage associated with diabetes into a gift. Thus he describes in detail how he has to "thrust" something like a "medium-sized sewing needle" into his upper arm "once, twice, three, and even four times a day," something he had done roughly fifteen thousand times since he received his diagnosis thirteen years earlier, at the age of seven. Yet his purpose is not to garner sympathy but to paint himself as someone with "courage." It is his friends, he tells the reader, who "turn a little pale" when they witness what he must do.

In a similar fashion, Albertson turns his reliance on a diabetic diet into an opportunity for him to practice "will power." The constant threat of low blood sugar becomes a chance for him to learn how to take care of himself, whether by carrying candy in his pocket or knowing how far he is from the nearest drugstore. He even turns a "humiliating" experience—telling a date that he had diabetes and her responding with pity—into an opportunity to demonstrate how he takes control of his life. In this case, he decided that on future dates he would hide his disease and just "order and eat," an action, he realized, that "may be taking several years" off of his life, but that nevertheless shows him to be in charge of his own fate.

Albertson saved the biggest advantages for last. These were the longer life and greater chance for economic success he believed he would enjoy when compared to those who did not have the disease. Because in living a life of moderation he had to refrain from smoking, drinking, and emotional upsets; eat and exercise regularly; and get enough sleep, he was likely, he contended, to "live to be much older than many of my healthy contemporaries." Moreover, without "a healthy body to fall back on," he had more incentive to succeed financially since failure would mean not having enough resources to take care of himself. Put differently, Albertson argued that it was his very dependence on insulin and a special diet that motivated him to achieve the economic "independence" he needed to handle the expenses of managing his disease.

In this way, Albertson reframed the meaning of dependence (whether he did so intentionally or not is unclear). He was not denying that, like a "cripple," he needed his "crutch." But he also insisted that the fact of his dependence had taught him to assert his will, making decisions most days to restrict his diet, take his insulin, and pursue a life of moderation. Even deciding occasionally to ignore his disease and eat and drink like a "normal" person was not a lapse of judgment or a failure of self-control but rather a risk that he had calculated and consciously chose. If the ideal citizen was someone capable of both financial independence and independence of thought, then, James Albertson was suggesting, one could hardly do better than to have diabetes.

It is possible that Albertson had read Lees's article in *Collier's* from two years earlier, in which she had linked diabetes with citizenship. His description of himself certainly fit the positive image she had portrayed. He may, however, also have been trying to counter messages that painted a far less favorable picture of both insulin and the person with the disease. For alongside the excitement about insulin as a "miracle" drug and the picture of "good" diabetes patients were two narratives that preyed on a broad set of social fears. The first, described earlier, focused on the bad choices that individuals made as rampant consumerism destroyed their moral compass. To the extent that diabetes stood symbolically as the price people paid who engaged in "immoral" behaviors, the discovery of a treatment that lessened the pain of that punishment was viewed with mixed feelings. What would prevent people from living a life of overindulgence now?

The second narrative also tapped into a cultural current of the day: eugenics. Some worried that insulin was allowing individuals with diabetes to reproduce, when previously they had been unable to have children, either because they had died before reaching reproductive age or because they had had difficulty conceiving.[41] Either way, "nature" had previously worked to prevent an increase of "defective genes" in the human gene pool. But now, as one eugenicist commented, medicine and public health were doing away with natural selection, which had kept "all races purged of the unfit, the ill-adapted," while allowing "the weakling, the defective" to "arrive at maturity and commingle his blood with that of the strong." The result was that our "present humanitarian methods" were "driving the race toward decadence."[42] Fifteen years after insulin's discovery, Priscilla White, an expert on diabetes and pregnancy, estimated that of the ten thousand births they anticipated each year from diabetic women, 1,250 babies would later develop the disease.[43] Eugenicists took note.

Concerns about Passing on "Defective Genes"

Eugenics, a term coined in 1883 by Charles Darwin's cousin, Sir Francis Galton, means literally the "science of good birth." Galton had set out to apply Darwin's ideas about natural selection to humans, worried that "misguided" humanitarian policies were allowing "unfit" individuals to pass on their defective genes to future generations. The imagined threat to the future of the human race resulted in the passage of laws—earlier in the United States than in any other country—that permitted the coercive sterilization of those deemed eugenically "unfit." The primary targets of this legislation were not individuals with diabetes or other medical conditions, but rather the so-called feebleminded. Allegedly identified by poor performance on IQ tests, the "feebleminded" just as often received this label because of perceived antisocial behaviors, such as illegitimacy, criminality, or unemployment. During the late 1920s and 1930s, a time considered to be the "high water mark of eugenic sterilization in the United States," roughly twenty-five thousand individuals underwent surgery to ensure that they would never reproduce.[44] Individuals who had diabetes were not among them, but whether they should be encouraged, or even allowed, to reproduce was a topic of considerable debate.

In 1927, the same year that Justice Oliver Wendell Holmes defended the Supreme Court's decision to uphold the Virginia state eugenics law with his famous comment that "three generations of imbeciles are enough," Herbert Spencer Jennings, a zoologist and geneticist at Johns Hopkins University, spoke passionately about the need to restrict the proliferation of "defective genes." The occasion was the Twenty-Third Annual Meeting of the National Tuberculosis Association, and the title of Jennings's talk was "Health Progress and Race Progress. Are They Compatible?" What is notable about Jennings's talk is his lack of interest in the fate of the "feebleminded" or what the eugenicist Harry H. Laughlin called "the socially inadequate." Rather, his focus was on individuals with medical conditions who were benefiting from recent advances in chemistry. And his message was that social programs, public health initiatives, and modern medical advances had all become so successful in reducing mortality rates that society was becoming inundated with "the halt [lame], the blind, the weak, [and] the variously deformed and degenerate."[45] Jennings had no wish to see these individuals suffer, but he was equally adamant that individuals sporting such "defective" genes should be kept from propagating. Among those he targeted were people with diabetes.

Jennings was troubled by "that pitiful half-formed thing, a cretin," who could now take a thyroid hormone and become "a normal human being"; the "diabetic," who could now take insulin and live a long life; and the person suffering from "intersexuality or other discordant condition" who could now be rendered "normal" with sex hormones. Chemotherapy, he explained, might be able to restore individuals to "normality," but their genes "remain defective" and are passed on to the next generation, who must also be treated, and so on ad infinitum. In the end, "each must carry with him an arsenal of hypodermic syringes, of vials, of capsules, of tablets. Each must remain within the radius of transportation of the synthetic chemical laboratory on which he depends. This picture is not an attractive one."[46] To Jennings, in fact, it was the apotheosis of dependency.

Despite appearances, Jennings was not criticizing the great medical breakthroughs of his day. He, like many of his peers, viewed these accomplishments as the very symbols of an advanced civilization. But he feared that the ability to use science to bring "the environment under control" was now being employed to reverse the progress of evolution. It was one thing, he insisted, to apply scientific knowledge to the relief of individual suffering, but such compassion must not be extended to the next generation. In what was by far the most animated part of his talk, he insisted that preventing even one person with defective genes from propagating would be "a gain." He went on: "A defective gene—such a thing as produces diabetes, cretinism, feeblemindedness—is a frightful thing; it is the embodiment, the material realization of a demon of evil; a living self-perpetuating creature, invisible, impalpable, that blasts a human being in bud or leaf. Such a thing must be stopped wherever it is recognized. The prevention of propagation of even one congenitally defective individual puts a period to at least one line of operation of this devil. To fail to do at least so much would be a crime."[47]

Demon, evil, creature, devil, crime. Jennings directed this powerful language, and the fear it evoked, to those in health care, trying to convince them to take seriously their responsibility to prevent the propagation of those known to be defective. Yet when it came to specific measures, Jennings came up short—for technical reasons. He believed that the conditions he was targeting were transmitted as Mendelian recessive traits and that meant, given what was known at the time about genetics, it would be nearly impossible to eliminate them.

The difficulty was that recessive traits could not easily be detected. As the rediscovery of Mendel's work in 1900 had made clear, people who appeared normal could still be carriers, their genotype remaining hidden unless they had children with other carriers or with someone who had the same condition or disease. Even then, Mendel's laws dealt in probabilities, not certainties. The children of two carriers had only a one in four chance of inheriting the "defective" gene from both parents and manifesting the disease. The primary tool available at the time for determining patterns of inheritance, the family pedigree, required time and depended on knowledge of a person's medical history, which many individuals lacked. Thus, eugenicists were in a quandary. They could target those who appeared to be manifesting signs of disease, and for conditions that were associated with social deviance, such as "feeblemindedness," that was often done. But a decade before Jennings gave his talk, several scientists had calculated that it would take thousands of years to eliminate an undesirable trait that was transmitted as a recessive gene. Jennings was aware of this, admitting that "progress" had to await a time when genetics would "advance far beyond its present point."[48]

Jennings's admission, however, did little to silence eugenic concerns. The number of people with diabetes was increasing too rapidly; eugenics itself was growing in popularity (by the mid-1930s, eugenic sterilization laws were in place in thirty-one states in the United States); and American physicians were aware of discussions taking place in Europe about whether or not those who had diabetes should be permitted to reproduce.[49]

England, Denmark, and France were all involved in these discussions, but Americans paid most attention to Germany, especially after the Nazi government passed the Law for the Prevention of Genetically Diseased Offspring (Gesetz zur Verhütung erbkranken Nachwuchses) in 1933, just seven months after assuming power. The "Sterilization Law," as it was otherwise known, sanctioned the compulsory sterilization of anyone determined to be suffering from feeblemindedness, schizophrenia, manic-depressive insanity, epilepsy, Huntington's chorea, hereditary blindness and deafness, grave bodily malformations, and chronic alcoholism. Diabetes was not included, but there were German physicians who believed it should have been.[50]

Those in favor of including diabetes shared their American colleagues' concerns that insulin was harming the race by allowing individuals with defective genes to reproduce. Those opposed did not deny this point, although they countered that too little was understood about the exact nature of diabetes inheritance to justify such a drastic measure. Besides, one critic insisted, diabetes had little in common with the conditions already targeted by the Sterilization Law, which usually entailed either a gross physical defect or some kind of intellectual impairment. Diabetes, in contrast, afflicted individuals with "above average intelligence."[51]

Holding people who had diabetes in high regard was one thing; allowing them to reproduce was quite another. Ferdinand Bertram, a diabetes specialist and medical director of Hamburg's General Hospital, recommended making use of the "Marital Health Law," which the German government passed in 1935, and which required anyone wishing to marry to be certified as "fit" by the Genetic Health Courts. Demanding that marriage be denied to all but the mildest cases of diabetes and to any two people who had a family history of the disease, he also insisted on the termination of any pregnancy in which signs of diabetes appeared, for the sake of not only the mother, but also reasons of genetic inheritance.[52]

Back in the United States, Elliott Joslin was following this conversation and growing increasingly alarmed. A frequent visitor to Europe, and especially to Germany where he had spent several months early in his career, Joslin attacked the German government for its "crusade against diabetics" and for considering "exterminat[ing] diabetics upon the ground that advances in diabetic therapeutics had reached an impasse." In two pieces that he penned in the 1930s, he voiced his concern, but he did not condemn eugenics per se. On the contrary, he bragged that "diabetics . . . are being taught more than any other group the value of eugenics."[53] He simply had a different assessment of what made good eugenics when it came to diabetes. Joslin did not go so far as to argue that the disease of diabetes improved the gene pool. But what surfaced in his writings as well as in the writings of others was a sense that people with diabetes possessed laudable traits that should be passed on to the next generation. Those eugenicists who held this view considered the possible transmission of the "diabetes gene" a worthwhile risk.

Were "Diabetics" Superior?

"You cannot indict a whole nation, the major portion of a nation or even 1 percent of a people without causing a reverberation throughout the world." So began Joslin in an article he published on diabetes in 1935 in *Medical Clinics of North America,* a journal devoted to exploring problems that physicians encountered in their daily practices. With Germany as his target, Joslin went on to dismiss as absurd any argument that claimed diabetes could be eliminated if individuals with the disease would simply be sterilized. The problem, as Jennings had clearly articulated eight years earlier, was that diabetic carriers could not be detected. So even if you sterilized everyone who had diabetes, you would still be left with those whose disease remained hidden. Extrapolating from existing estimates of the number of diabetes cases in the United States, Joslin estimated that one in four individuals was a "hereditary diabetic carrier," and clearly "you cannot eliminate one-fourth of a nation." Besides, Joslin added, it would be "unfair" to sterilize the siblings of those who had diabetes, since it was possible that some of them would not have the hereditary trait.[54]

As compelling as this numerical argument might have been, Joslin's criticism of sterilization rested not on statistics but on his insistence that people with diabetes, despite their disease, were highly accomplished individuals whose elimination would entail a great loss for society. To drive home his point, he turned to a "concrete" case involving the daughter of a middle- to upper-class family. Joslin asked his readers to imagine the following scene: "An attractive young woman comes to your office and asks you if she can get married. A moment's conversation suffices to disclose that she is unusually intelligent; she is evidently physically strong, because she is a champion tennis player, often rides to hounds for six hours at a time, has driven an automobile recently 300 miles a day, and repeatedly dances all night. In the midst of city gaieties she has learned stenography and typewriting and, what is more, secured a job."[55]

This amazing young woman, he added, who took insulin twice a day, also watched her diet, so that at a height of 63 inches and a weight of 117 pounds, she was a little underweight and doing extremely well. Importantly, like Louisa Drumm, the apostle he had featured in one of his earlier writings, she understood "her disease." For Joslin this meant that she managed her blood sugar levels successfully, never being "so careless as to develop coma."[56] Diabetes, Joslin was announcing, was a disease that any intelligent person could and should be able to control.

"Now, what would you do under these concrete conditions?" Joslin asked his readers. Would you advise her to marry or to remain single the rest of her life? He responded to this rhetorical question by explaining that he first asked her about her fiancé. Was "he a good boy?" Were they in love? Did their parents approve? Would there be enough money to care for her if she became ill and needed hospitalization? Was money there to provide special hospital care should she become pregnant? Most important, was there a history of diabetes in his family? Satisfied with her answers, Joslin tells his readers that he said "get married and God bless you."[57]

Joslin did not share his patient's exact answers or her name. Indeed, this particular woman may never have existed. Although it is unlikely that she was a total fabrication, she may well have been a composite of several women who had sought his advice over the years. But her authenticity barely matters, for Joslin had not set out to tell this woman's story for the sake of painting an accurate picture of her life with diabetes. Rather, in choosing an intelligent, strong, tennis-playing, horseback riding, young (presumably white) woman for his "concrete" case, he wanted to make sure his readers understood what might be lost if those who had diabetes were denied the right to reproduce. Fully embracing the eugenic language of his day, he told them how his experiences not only with this woman but also with "500 other diabetic girls and 500 other diabetic boys" had led him to "admire the backbone and the brains of the average diabetic and I truly believe on the whole they are superior to the common run of people and therefore their good qualities merit cultivation. . . . I think they are less apt to drink, far less likely to have syphilis or gonorrhea, and distinctly less to have, what is anathema to me, 'nervous prostration and nerves.'"[58]

Joslin was far from alone in admiring the "brains of the average diabetic." As Harold Bowcock of Emory's School of Medicine asserted, "all medical authors state that diabetics as a group, are more intelligent and smarter than other patients." Priscilla White, who gave intelligence tests to 169 diabetic children at the Joslin clinic, found that a third "were of superior intelligence." German critics of the sterilization of diabetes patients made similar claims about this population's superior mental faculties. This message was picked up in the popular press as well. We have already noted Hannah Lees's comment in *Collier's* that diabetics "have greater intelligence than the average and they develop it by constant use." Articles in *Hygeia,* a periodical published by the American Medical Association for the express purpose of enlightening the public "in matters of medical science," shared similar views. In one, a woman described her experience with diabetes, stating boldly that she had "always been considered somewhat above the average in intelligence." And the author of an article in *Parents'* magazine went so far as to recommend that "precocious children" be screened more frequently for signs of the disease because "diabetic children are as a rule very energetic mentally."[59]

Intelligence was the most important "positive" trait that individuals with diabetes could boast as far as eugenicists were concerned, but it also made sense that they would have this trait. After all, those who had diabetes were still imagined as white and middle class, an idea reinforced by statistical studies, therapeutic recommendations, and even images in the media. Drawings that accompanied a *Hygeia* article on "the emotional life" of the "diabetic" are priceless in this regard (Figure 2.3). The author, Ione Leonard, who had the disease, describes the mood swings she experienced before she learned how to train her mind and body and "regulate" her feelings. Such emotional upheavals are portrayed in several images that surround the article, all of them depicting a very well-dressed middle- to upper-class married couple. In a few images the "diabetic" is shown as either in a rage or depressed, although significantly it is the husband, not the wife, who has the disease. Switching the gender roles in this way meant not only that a potentially disturbing image of a "madwoman" could be avoided; it also made it possible to put the wife in the normative role of caretaker, charged with monitoring the emotional excesses of her husband. This normativity was displayed as well in an image of the couple dancing at a ball, he dressed in a tuxedo and she in a gown; and in a scene in their living room, where she is playing the piano while he listens intently. Emotional mood swings, the article seems to be announcing, may threaten this marital bliss, but this is also the population best positioned to master "the 'regulation' of the emotional side of man."[60]

"Brains count," explained Joslin in the manual he prepared for diabetes patients and their doctors, in helping the treatment to be successful. But knowledge was not enough. "This is a disease which tests the character of the patient," he added, "and for success in withstanding it, in addition to

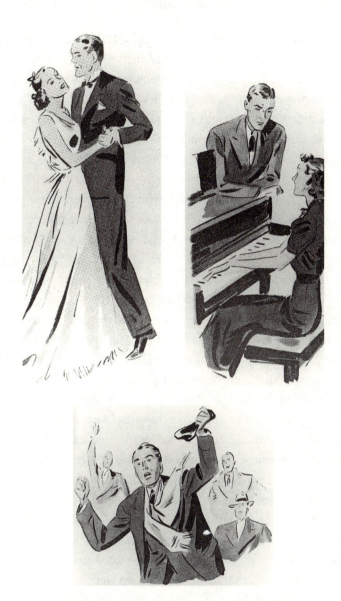

Fig. 2.3. From the opening page of Ione Leonard,
"A Diabetic's Disposition," *Hygeia* 17 (1939): 310.

wisdom, he must possess honesty, self-control and courage."[61] Those were traits, of course, largely believed to be the purview of those who were white and middle class. Thus the eugenically minded faced a conundrum. Committed to eliminating the "unfit," they nevertheless recognized that someone with a defective gene might, on balance, have "better" material to pass on to the next generation than someone who lacked that gene. Fitness, in other words, was relative. Besides, most understood that genetics was basically a game of chance. If diabetes were transmitted as a Mendelian recessive trait, which most believed at the time, the children of someone with diabetes were unlikely to develop the disease unless the spouse was a hidden carrier. Thus those who had the disease simply had to avoid marriage to others who had it or anyone with a history of diabetes in the family.

Even if it remained risky to allow people with diabetes to reproduce, Joslin believed it was a risk worth taking because by marrying and having children, they were increasing the chances that the next generation would have more of the positive traits believed to be at a premium in people like themselves. As early as 1921, Joslin had claimed that "the potential power of the diabetics in this country for good almost offsets the harm that results from their having the disease." Twenty-five years later he was still praising them, fighting anyone who suggested they should not be allowed to marry. If we do "forbid marriage," he asked, "who will be left to halt the falling birth rate if all unsound individuals in the country are forbidden to have children? There are many individuals one meets on the street who are far less desirable to choose for fathers and mothers than diabetics."[62] People with diabetes, he was saying, should not be subjected to restrictive legislation; on the contrary, under the proper circumstances it might very well be good eugenics to actively encourage them to reproduce.

One year after Joslin published his attack on German eugenic practices, Lees's article "Two Million Tightrope Walkers" appeared in *Collier's*. Lees probably had interviewed Joslin or at least read carefully his article in *Medical Clinics of North America*. Not only does she mention him several times, but her essay reads as though she had taken his message, which he had written for his medical colleagues, and repackaged it for the two million subscribers of the magazine. Joslin may not have gone so far as to claim that "diabetics make better citizens than the average," but in many ways

Lees was doing little more than stating boldly what was clearly a subtext in many of the decade's writings on diabetes.

"Diabetics" as "Better Citizens"

What could diabetes have had to do with citizenship? If we think about the right to vote, perhaps not much. But if we think instead about what some scholars have called "biological citizenship" or "biocitizenship," then the answer is a lot. Focusing largely on twentieth-century notions of citizenship, scholars have drawn attention to how political and cultural elites employed bodily differences as a way of distinguishing, in one social theorist's words, "between actual, potential, troublesome and impossible citizens."[63] The use of biological differences to justify the inequitable distribution of resources and power was not, of course, a creation of the twentieth century; nor was there anything new about the imposition of social constraints on how "proper" citizens should behave. One need only think of Victorian codes of conduct to recognize this. What distinguishes twentieth-century projects, however, was the degree of reverence afforded to medical knowledge in defining what was "proper" or "normal," and the power that experts in medicine and public health enjoyed as a result. Thus, in the first half of the twentieth century, alongside the expansion of the administrative apparatus of the state and the growth of industrial capitalism, a number of developments took place: an increasing conviction that the well-being of the nation depended on the mental and physical health of its citizens; the expansion of public health departments, which made it feasible to monitor the behaviors of the population; and greater expectations that citizens would manage their own health. In fact, the willingness and ability to assume responsibility for one's own health became an indicator that one had enough reason and self-governance to perform civic duties.[64]

Evidence abounds that during this era, medicine and public health gained the power to determine which populations would enjoy social and economic privileges and which would be denied them. One study, for example, of Mexican, Chinese, and Japanese immigrants in Los Angeles around the turn of the century has shown how public health officials painted them as dirty immigrants and "'permanently foreign'" no matter how many generations they had lived in the United States. Depicting them as health threats served as justification for policing their daily activities, preventing them from negotiating higher wages, and keeping them from seeking housing and employment anywhere in the cities in which they lived. Chinese Americans suffered a similar fate in San Francisco, where they were painted as unwanted aliens and public health pariahs. As a result, they were subjected to house searches, raids, and quarantines until they adopted "a strategy of bourgeois self-regulation" and transformed themselves into "model citizens," proving not simply that they could assimilate into modern society, but also that they could do it better than others.[65]

Lees's article makes the most sense when it is read in relation to these other studies. Ostensibly about diabetes, the article is also about the set of characteristics believed essential for a democracy to thrive. Blurring the boundaries between the person already diagnosed with the disease; one who has the disease and does not yet know it; and the person who may develop diabetes because of the lifestyle he or she is pursuing, Lees spelled out what was necessary to nurture these traits. The "Two Million Tightrope Walkers" in her title certainly referred to the estimated two million people in the country believed to have diabetes at the time, but it isn't difficult to envision Lees also thinking about the two million subscribers to Collier's, who, at least in the imagination of most professional and popular writings of the day, represented the demographic group most likely to develop the disease.

After a short introduction in which Lees provides some basic facts about the disease, explains the importance of the pancreas, shares a cute story about the discovery of insulin, describes the hormone's influence on the lives of those with diabetes, and mentions the roles of obesity and heredity in predisposing someone to the disease, she asks her readers, "Now supposing you've got diabetes. . . . Diabetes isn't a thing you get over. So what do you do about it?" In answering the question of how that person had to live, she spares no detail. "A diabetic must know the exact food value of any given breakfast, lunch or dinner," she writes, which means that:

> your typical diabetic has to be a dietitian so that he can measure and weigh his foods; a laboratory technician so that he can test for too much sugar in his system; a nurse so that he can give himself shots of insulin, the proper

amount at the proper time and under sterile conditions; and even a doctor, for he has to watch himself constantly for symptoms, symptoms of too
much sugar, and, after he has taken insulin, symptoms of too little sugar,
symptoms of cold or fever or even a sore toe. . . .

He has to learn about maps, too, insulin maps, for unless his case is
pretty mild he has to inject insulin so often . . . that the skin would thicken
up and not absorb the stuff . . . if he always stuck the needle in the same
place. So he has to learn to chart off his body like a navigator.

He has to learn to like his meals without sugar and his fun without hotcha. No riotous living for him. He can't measure his insulin if he hasn't
measured his sleep. He can't eat except measured foods at measured times.
He can't drink much . . . [lest he] might get to feeling too gay or too hungry
and forget all about measuring his food and sleep.[66]

The life Lees spelled out for a person with diabetes was one of constant
measurement, all day, every day, for the rest of one's life. Scales, needles, cal-
ibrated vials, manufactured insulin, urine tests—these technologies made
bodily surveillance possible. And sitting in the driver's seat is the person
with diabetes, the new "patient expert," who is dietician, laboratory techni-
cian, nurse, and doctor all rolled into one. Those with diabetes had to weigh
and measure everything they put in their mouths, looking for the perfect
balance between calories and insulin, and then test their urine or blood to
see if its sugar content fell within the "normal" range. The number they
got—more than how they felt—told them whether they had succeeded or
failed, and since exercise and sleep also affected how rapidly food was me-
tabolized, every aspect of daily life had to be measured as well.

What Lees described here was a strategy for managing diabetes—for
managing life—that built on a relatively new understanding of the disease.[67]
Diabetes had long been known by its symptoms of unquenchable thirst,
excessive urination, and extreme weight loss. In the twentieth century.
what was growing increasingly important, in contrast, was the concentration of blood glucose. While symptoms still mattered, especially for those
who experienced complications such as blindness, amputations, or renal
failure, those symptoms were less signs of diabetes than of the failure to
control it. For those intent on staving off complications, their experience
of the disease was largely symptomless, dominated instead by the daily re-
gimes of monitoring and management. What is remarkable about Lees's

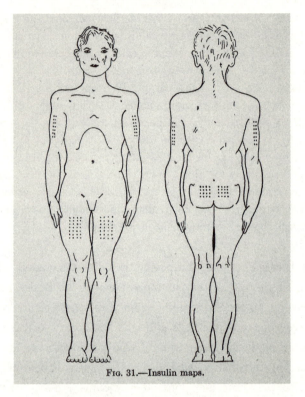

Fig. 31.—Insulin maps.

Fig. 2.4. Insulin maps. Reprinted from Elliott P. Joslin, *A Diabetic Manual for the Mutual Use of Doctor and Patient,* 7th ed. (Philadelphia: Lea & Febiger, 1941), 121. Copyright 1941 by Elliott P. Joslin.

prescription, though, is her insistence that those with diabetes make this monitoring and management visible by thinking of their bodies as spatial and temporal maps. Henceforth, they would chart specific sites of intervention and then read the marks to know where she has been—the thickened skin that prevents the absorption of insulin—and where she needs to go (Figure 2.4). Diabetes is thus brought under control, reduced to a silent disease controlled via measurements and charts.

Lees's challenge, of course, was to convince those with diabetes to sign on to this life of hypervigilance, to agree to chart, measure, and map their daily bodily functions. And this brings us back to the article's intended audience. The picture that accompanied her article, as briefly noted, depicts an erudite-looking physician talking to an extremely well-dressed couple, she of normal weight and in a fashionable hat; he obese, in a dark suit, and wearing a monocle (Figure 2.1). The physician is pointing to a mass of similarly well-dressed people in a crowded restaurant—without facial features and miniaturized so that they appear at the central figures' feet. Most are of ample weight and food is in abundance; we see whole turkeys being delivered on trays, and a table piled high with sweets in the background. The caption reads: "There are all sorts of reasons why people get diabetes, but the most important is getting too fat, or living too well."

The picture and caption reinforce the reigning belief that the population most at risk for developing diabetes is white and middle class, even upper class. It makes sense, moreover, to assume that the man is the one at risk, given his great girth. Indeed, he is looking at the scene with what appears to be trepidation. Perhaps he has just received a diagnosis of diabetes from his physician? But the physician is directing his comments to the wife, not the husband. Is he telling her that it will be her job to keep her husband on his strict regimen and to avoid the life of indulgence on display at their feet? Her countenance is more difficult to read—she is studying the scene, but shows no fear. She even seems aloof. But maybe her reaction is not to anything her doctor may be saying about her husband, but rather about her. Perhaps he is telling her that if she continues to live like the people down below, she too could become diabetic. The message of this article may not, in other words, be aimed alone at those with diabetes (and their loved ones), but also at the magazine's readers, each of whom had the potential to develop the disease. Everyone is walking a tightrope; the wrong choices can send anyone plummeting down. To plummet, moreover, means to lose one's identity, to become one of the faceless, teeming masses of people—like those in the picture—who want nothing more out of life than to indulge their appetites. This is why "diabetics," at least those who succeed in managing their disease, "make better than average citizens." By expertly reining in their impulses, eating moderately, exercising regularly, and regulating their emotions, they had learned to avoid temptation and to live a life of "self-restraint."

One did not, of course, need to be diabetic to follow this regimen. Put differently, Lees was suggesting that all of her readers were potentially diabetic and thus advised to follow suit. They were to become their own dieticians, lab technicians, nurses, doctors, and navigators—observing, monitoring, and evaluating the minutiae of their lives. This was the goal of the "civilizing" mission—everyone had to agree to surveil their own bodies and manage their own risks. To be worthy of full citizenship meant quite literally to embrace the responsibility of governing all aspects of oneself.[68]

*　*　*

So tight a link existed between diabetes and class that when evidence emerged in the 1930s that poverty did not offer protection from the disease, it received little notice: the poor remained invisible in the diabetes literature.

This invisibility is not surprising. Those who studied and cared for poor people worried most about exceedingly high infant and maternal mortality rates, as well as diseases such as pellagra, syphilis, gonorrhea, and especially tuberculosis and other respiratory ailments. In the first decades of the twentieth century, the extent of even these problems remained invisible to vast numbers of Americans who knew little about the hardships of life in the foothills of Appalachia or in the deep South. The Great Depression changed that. Drought, dust storms, crop failures, bank closures, and the eventual collapse of the economy brought the lives of the poor to the front pages of newspapers and magazines. Photojournalists like Dorothea Lange documented the abject poverty of rural America, rendering visible the lack of food, shelter, and sanitation across the country. Public health studies also brought home how such conditions exacerbated health problems that had long plagued the poor. In Kansas, infant and maternal mortality rates jumped 66 percent in 1935 during a three-month period when dust storms swept across the state almost daily. Respiratory infections increased three-fold as well.[69] Small wonder that diabetes attracted little attention.

This situation would slowly change as the country grew more aware of the dangers of chronic diseases for the poor. Some of this awareness stemmed from health researchers' shift in focus from mortality to morbidity as they came to believe that death rates were a poor indicator of the economic cost of chronic diseases on the nation. An important turning point came in 1935–1936, when the government published the results of a nationwide health survey initiated two years earlier by the U.S. Public Health Service (USPHS). The study was part of FDR's New Deal, and it was designed to document how disease and disability trapped individuals in cycles of poverty. For two years, enumerators—hired off the relief roles and trained for the job—went house to house, covering eighty-three cities and twenty-three rural areas spread across nineteen different states. They collected data on age, marital status, sex, race, country of origin, employment status, income, relief status, and the number of inhabitants in the home, and coupled this with information about how illness had affected each individual in the household. Speaking to someone (usually the housewife), they gathered information about approximately 2.8 million people. The first published report of this work came out in 1935–1936. The National Health Survey on Chronic Disease and Disability showed that chronic diseases burdened the poor more than the well-off. This was true whether one looked at disease prevalence, mortality rates, days lost from work or school, or individuals who were permanently disabled. According to one calculation, families on relief suffered 87 percent more chronic illness and 47 percent more acute illness than those with annual incomes in excess of $3,000 (equal to about $54,000 in 2017).[70]

Diabetes was by no means the leading cause of disability. Defining disability as the "inability, because of disease, accident or impairment, to work, attend school, or follow other usual pursuits" for a period of at least seven days, analysts found that minor respiratory diseases and accidents headed the list, followed by diseases of the digestive system and then degenerative diseases. But although rates of diabetes were relatively low, the survey showed that they rose as poverty increased. The same was true of other degenerative diseases: individuals on relief suffered the highest rates of all. According to one report, diabetes was 1.5 times "as frequent among relief families as among those in comfortable circumstances." Another report claimed that diabetes was one of the diseases that offered proof that rates of chronic disease were tied more closely to levels of poverty than were rates of acute diseases. The *New York Times* reproduced these findings in an article titled "Deaths among Poor Exceed Others 100%."[71] By the late 1930s, government reports, journal articles, and newspaper accounts were all providing evidence that questioned the link between diabetes and wealth.

Yet it would take several more decades before diabetes lost its close association with the "comfortable" classes. The images that Hannah Lees, James Albertson, and Ione Leonard had produced in the interwar years all but drowned out reports beginning to suggest that diabetes might be linked more to poverty than to wealth. For those who studied, treated, and wrote about diabetes in this early era, poor whites were invisible. So were people of color. At least at first, empirical evidence could not overturn an image of diabetes so deeply entrenched in cultural assumptions about race, class, and disease.

3
Misunderstanding the African American Experience

[Diabetes] is rare in negroes.
> Thomas B. Futcher, 1897

Diabetes in negroes is not different in any way from the disease as found among white people.
> Eugene J. Leopold, 1931

The unusually high percentage [of diabetes] among colored females as observed here was completely unanticipated by us.
> Christopher McLoughlin, 1951

RECONSTRUCTION MARKED THE NADIR OF HEALTH conditions for African Americans, the vast majority of whom lived in the South. Left to fend for themselves following Emancipation, and often illiterate, penniless, malnourished, and homeless, the newly freed men and women fell ill in vast numbers. Tuberculosis ran rampant, infant and maternal mortality rates skyrocketed, and syphilis spread quickly. Epidemics of cholera, yellow fever, and smallpox claimed the lives of young and old alike. No one, however, either during Reconstruction or in subsequent decades, believed that diabetes was contributing to the high death rate of African Americans. Arthur R. Elliot, a white faculty member of the Post-Graduate Medical School in Chicago, encountered no opposition when he announced at the 1904 meeting of the American Medical Association that he had "never seen a case of diabetes in the negro." A fellow physician added that he had also "never seen a case of diabetes in them," and did not know of any other practitioner who had. Black physicians agreed. Charles Wainwright Birnie, the first African American doctor to practice medicine in Sumter County, South Carolina, remarked in 1910 that "any physician either in private or hospital practice can count on the end of his fingers the number of cases of diabetes he has noted within the Negro race."[1]

Might these claims that diabetes rates were low among African Americans have been accurate when they were made? Perhaps. As already noted, diabetes rates tended to rise when the death rate from infectious diseases and malnutrition fell, allowing individuals to survive to an age when chronic ailments were more likely to develop. This "epidemiological transition" occurred among the country's white populations by the second decade of the twentieth century, even if not all whites benefited equally. African Americans, however, who lived in either poor rural communities or impoverished neighborhoods, which were often ignored when municipal departments invested time and money in public health initiatives, continued to experience high rates of infectious diseases and to suffer distressingly high infant and maternal mortality rates throughout the first half of the twentieth century. Such disparities suggest that poverty and racism may have led to more early deaths, thereby keeping diabetes rates low in black communities.[2]

African Americans' experiences of poverty and hunger, coupled with the physical labor often demanded of them in their jobs, may also have kept diabetes rates low by producing conditions that led to their being underweight and undernourished. A 2007 study of pension files of U.S. Civil War veterans, which compared differential diabetes rates among black and white veterans, found that rates were lower among the black veterans. Since the files contained information on weight and occupation, the researchers were also able to determine that African Americans had lower body weights on average and were more likely to have physically demanding jobs: 93.6 percent of black veterans were engaged in either agricultural or manual labor as compared to 48.6 percent of whites.[3] Although the authors mentioned nothing about poverty, it is not difficult to imagine how insufficient resources could have exacerbated this trend.

Another reason to doubt that diabetes was burdening black communities in the early twentieth century is that most African American physicians, nurses, and community health leaders said little about the disease.
This was certainly the case with the National Negro Health Movement: established by Booker T. Washington in 1915 to improve the health of black
communities, it paid little attention to diabetes or any other chronic condition. Diabetes also appeared infrequently in the pages of the *Journal of the
National Medical Association,* the official publication of the National Medical
Association, which was founded in 1895 because the American Medical Association refused membership to physicians of color. Health professionals focused their attention on what they understood to be the most serious
health risks in their communities. With tuberculosis accounting for 50 to
60 percent of the total death rate for black people in the first decade of the
twentieth century, and with the overall death rate for black children under
the age of five more than double that for white children, diabetes did not
register as a great enough threat.[4]

Still, it is unlikely that diabetes rates were as low as many asserted. As
we have seen, the definition and diagnosis of diabetes were clouded with
ambiguities. What concentration of glucose in the blood or urine warranted
the diagnosis? Which tests were most reliable? Given that practitioners did
not use the same measurement tools, how could comparisons between different races even be made?

Of equal importance, the vast majority of practitioners rarely saw African
Americans in their clinics, hospitals, and private practices, raising the possibility that the allegedly low rate of diabetes among black individuals (similar to the allegedly high rate among Jews) reflected the degree of contact
between physicians and different communities rather than the actual incidence of disease. If frequent visits to doctors may have inflated the rate of
diabetes among Jews (as some claimed), then infrequent visits, especially to
those physicians likely to publish articles on diabetes, may have reinforced
the impression that African Americans suffered little from it. If, moreover,
the small number of white physicians who tended to black patients rarely
tested their patients' urine because diabetes was not "supposed" to afflict
this population, then cases of diabetes would also have gone underreported.

In addition, reliable vital statistics for African Americans living in the South, where roughly 90 percent of all black people in the United States still resided in 1900, were basically nonexistent. When Daniel H. Williams, an African American physician from Chicago, traveled to the region at the turn of the century to learn about the health status of black communities, he found that accurate information was available only in big cities that had boards of health. In rural areas, in contrast, "there were to be found no statistics of any kind bearing on the death rate." To Walter G. Alexander, an African American physician from Orange, New Jersey, the failure of most southern states to establish a registry for births and deaths meant that whatever passed as statistics was simply "erroneous."[5]

Claims of low diabetes rates in black communities must also be read with caution because the question of who, exactly, counted as "Negro" lacked a clear answer. Mary Gover, assistant statistician in the U.S. Public Health Service, provides evidence of this confusion in a report she published in 1927, "Mortality among Negroes in the United States." After describing black people as both "a more homogeneous racial group" than whites because they tended to have native-born parents, and "a heterogeneous group" because of admixtures with whites, she nevertheless concluded that they are "still quite distinct in environment and racial characteristics." This ambiguity was also evident in attempts to quantify the amount of blood that warranted the designation "Negro." In Florida, for example, "Negro" applied to anyone in possession of "one-eighth or more of negro blood," while in some other states, one-sixteenth or one-thirty-second sufficed to legally classify someone as "Negro." Virginia's Racial Integrity Act of 1924 adopted the most extreme criterion, declaring that any person who had a "trace whatsoever of blood other than Caucasian" had to be classified as "colored." The "one drop rule," as it came to be called, not only narrowly defined who would henceforth count as white; it also collapsed all other groups into the single category "colored." To W. E. B. Du Bois, this way of conceptualizing race "utterly vitiated" the validity of studies that purported to explain differential death rates by recourse to race. How, he challenged, could race explain anything if "Negro" included everyone who had a drop of Negro blood, regardless of "their percentage of white or Indian blood"?[6]

Such cautions and concerns underscore the difficulty of determining with any confidence whether diabetes troubled black communities in the early decades of the twentieth century. Even setting aside the ambiguities surrounding the terms "black" and "diabetes," the available evidence does not permit a simple conclusion. For although the prevalence of diabetes among African Americans seems to have paled in comparison with that of infectious diseases, this does not mean that the rate was lower than among whites. And even if it was lower, high rates of tuberculosis, syphilis, and other diseases may have been masking *rising* rates of diabetes. The claim, in other words, that diabetes was rare may have been accurate in the late nineteenth century, but a few decades later that may no longer have been the case.

This, at least, was the contention of a small number of white and black physicians and researchers, who began in the second decade of the century to argue that diabetes rates among African Americans were increasing, and in some cases surpassing those of whites. These claims drew on studies from southern cities like New Orleans, Baltimore, and Atlanta, where white physicians with university appointments came into contact with African Americans in out-patient clinics and public hospitals. They included evidence from studies in northern cities, like those conducted by Louis Dublin, health statistician for the Metropolitan Life Insurance Company, which was one of the largest insurers of black and white wage earners in the first half of the twentieth century. And they incorporated the experiences of a growing number of African American physicians who noticed increasing rates of diabetes among their middle-class clientele. Their reports, however, received very little attention. As late as 1985, readers of the Heckler Report, a government-commissioned study of health disparities, expressed shock when they learned that black people were dying of diabetes at significantly higher rates than were whites. The information they read for the first time was not, however, new. It had been noted and put aside, then noted and put aside, again and again.[7]

To argue that this neglect occurred because other health problems always seemed more pressing is to ignore the social, economic, and political reasons that African Americans continued to suffer so much longer from infectious diseases than whites did. The claim also misses the point that most physicians and public health officials did not label diabetes "less important" than other diseases; they simply did not "see" that the disease was becoming a problem in black communities despite accumulating evidence. Preventing this evidence from entering the medical mainstream were several interlocking cultural images: the sustained image of diabetes as a "disease of civilization," believed to afflict only those with highly sensitive nervous systems; a picture of African Americans as "dull" and "happy" (when not violent) and thus distinctly "uncivilized"; and the erasure of class differences among African Americans, which rendered middle-class black people invisible within American society. Poor blacks were not "advanced" enough to suffer from diabetes, and middle-class blacks "did not exist." Until either the image of diabetes or the image of black people changed, diabetes as an African American health problem would not be seen.[8]

The Idea of Racial Immunity

When a small number of physicians began in the 1920s to draw attention to the problem of diabetes in black communities, they were directly challenging a widespread belief that Africans and their descendants were immune to the disease. The Swedish physician Emil Kleen articulated this view in his book *On Diabetes and Glycosuria,* in the same section in which he had remarked on the high rate of diabetes among those who experienced "the intensity of cultivated life." Like American Indians and Aboriginal Australians, he explained, Africans had an immunity to the disease, a sign that they lacked the "higher nervous development" that produced high rates of diabetes in "civilized" populations. Thomas Futcher, a professor at Johns Hopkins University School of Medicine, shared this view, commenting in a single essay that "mental shock, nervous strain, and worry appear to favor the occurrence of the disease"; that diabetes was "rare in negroes"; and that "African and Mongolian races enjoy considerable immunity in their own countries."[9] Taken together, these claims indicated that immunity to diabetes signified a race's primitive nature.

Racial immunity might seem an unlikely sign of a group's supposed inferiority. After all, immunity signals the absence of a disease, and so suggests health. But no one in the waning years of the nineteenth century was claiming that African Americans were healthier than whites. On the contrary, their overall bad health was taken for granted, although the reasons for it engendered considerable controversy. Some blamed their poor health on the inability of formerly enslaved individuals to handle their newly won freedom. Frederick L. Hoffman's widely read 1896 study, "Race Traits and Tendencies of the American Negro," advanced this view. As the statistician for the Prudential Life Insurance Company, Hoffman had access to mortality tables, and he insisted that an impartial review of the available statistics showed that the race was on the road to extinction. The population's "excessive mortality" from such infectious diseases as syphilis and tuberculosis stemmed, he insisted, from *"the race traits and tendencies"* of black people and not from "the *conditions of life.*"[10] What slavery had kept in check, in other words, was now being given free rein.

Kelly Miller, a black mathematician educated at Howard University and Johns Hopkins University, issued an immediate rebuttal, offering alternative data that showed the black population increasing, not decreasing. He also argued that high morbidity and mortality rates had nothing to do with innate racial traits and everything to do with social factors. The genius of his approach was to turn to studies of London's poor, which revealed health problems similar to those of black people in the United States. Class, not race, he argued, best explained excessive mortality. Miller's arguments had little influence on the white medical community, however, and the question of why blacks' life expectancy remained lower than that of whites continued to be the subject of debate.[11]

To resolve the apparent contradiction between ill health and disease immunity, medical researchers and physicians read African Americans' low rate of diabetes as biological "evidence" that they lacked the sensibilities and sensitivities that made a race like the Jews so prone to the disease. Similar to other scientific studies that alleged to offer proof of the inferiority of the "African race" and its descendants, medical writings often presented black people as occupying a step lower on the evolutionary ladder than whites, which meant that they were considered less developed neurologically. "The higher the organization, the higher the physiological development, the higher the nervous system, the greater the sensation," asserted a physician at the meeting of the Saint Louis Medical Society in 1884, adding that this is why black people, who had "less brain" and a "less developed" nervous system, did not suffer from "a great number of diseases" that afflicted whites."[12] This physician and his colleagues were studying malaria and gonorrhea, but the same logic underpinned writings on diabetes, especially since most considered the disease to be linked to the nervous system through the adrenal gland's role in stimulating the liver to release sugar into the bloodstream. Thus, as Isaac Ivan Lemann, who practiced medicine in New Orleans, informed his audience at the 1920 meeting of the Southern Medical Association: "Nervous strain, intense application to business, mental shock and worry have frequently seemed to play an important role, at least in precipitating the phenomena of the disease [diabetes] or aggravating it. The negro race is to a very great degree free from these influences. The average individual is happy-go-lucky, living from hand to mouth and from day to day, without great responsibilities and without great ambitions which carry with them great cares. . . . The mental and nervous make-up of the negro is in marked contrast to that of the Jews, among whom diabetes is disproportionately frequent."[13]

Delivered at a time of heightened anxieties about the mixing of the races, when states reinforced antimiscegenation laws and the Ku Klux Klan policed boundaries through lynchings and other acts of brutality, these words reveal a deeply troubled racial imagination. Lemann drew here on a widely disseminated caricature of black people as simple-minded, lackadaisical, and carefree. Popularized around the turn of the century in minstrel shows, magazines, and cartoons, the figure of the "black Sambo" denied the experiences of black men (and women) who after Emancipation continued to be traumatized by daily acts of terror.[14] Lemann's erasure of this reality created an image that stood in stark contrast to that of "the nervous Jew," whose nerves were allegedly fraught because of millennia of discrimination. Thus, despite having both experienced long histories of prejudice, discrimination, and brutality, African Americans and Jews were constructed as polar opposites: one primitive, the other civilized; one carefree, the other high-strung; one simple-minded, the other intellectually astute. In this way, the diabetes literature produced, legitimized, and proliferated two sharply drawn, differentiated stereotypes that put the two groups at cross-purposes.

Lemann was not, however, merely playing from an old script; he was also changing the narrative. At the same time that he employed blatant racial stereotypes to explain variations in rates of diabetes, he also questioned whether black people possessed a racial immunity to the disease. To be clear, he left no doubt that "some racial make-up" explained the prevalence of diabetes among Jews; he was also adamant that white and black people differed "not only in physical make-up, but also in mental and moral habits." Thus he did not cast doubt on the notion of biological race itself. Nor did he doubt that diabetes was "a disease of the well-to-do."[15] Still, he insisted that previous studies of diabetes and race had mistakenly compared all white people, whether poor or wealthy, with all black people, almost all of whom lived in poverty. In contrast, Lemann explained, his data came from two institutions that served poor black and poor white patients. And based on his data from the New Orleans' Charity Hospital and the Touro Infirmary Outdoor Clinic, he concluded that class offered a better explanation than race for why diabetes rates differed between groups.

Lemann had first made this claim in 1910. At that time, he had found that although diabetes rates were lower for poor African Americans than for poor whites, the difference was not significant.[16] Now, in 1920, with another decade of data under his belt, he was able not only to confirm his earlier finding that diabetes was not "rare among the negroes," but also to demonstrate that in the intervening years both populations had experienced a similar increase in diabetes rates. The rate for poor whites had jumped 94 percent, while the rate for poor blacks lagged just slightly behind, at 83 percent. To Lemann, this provided evidence that "whatever influences have contributed to the increase of diabetes, noted by Joslin and other observers, have affected white and negro alike and the latter has shown no especial immunity to the operation of their forces."[17]

It is unclear whether Lemann recognized that his emphasis on poverty could be interpreted as challenging some of the tenets of scientific racism. His comments provide ample evidence that he continued to traffic in racial stereotypes, even as he opened the door to the possibility that some racial traits stemmed from the conditions of life rather than from biology. Perhaps his understanding of race was closer to that of Lamarck than Darwin, allowing for a greater role for the environment in establishing racial traits. Lemann's silence on this matter leaves us without an answer. But evidently the implications of his study were all too clear to members of his audience, and they struggled with what they had heard.

"I should like to ask the author of the paper whether there was a great deal of admixture of white blood in the darkies in whom he noticed diabetes." This question came from Mary Freemon, a physician from Jacksonville, Florida, who shared her own observations that the darker a person's skin, the more he could tolerate "shock and accident." Taking for granted the stereotype that whiteness and nervousness went hand-in-hand, she explained that while she had never "seen a black negro who showed any high degree of nervousness, no matter what ailed him," she had noticed that "the more white blood they have, the more nervous they become." Another physician piped up, adding that the only time he had ever diagnosed diabetes in a black person, that person had been "a mulatto." The question, therefore, was whether "white admixture" might explain Lemann's findings. Lemann, however, insisted it could not. On the contrary, he responded, he had found the disease among "pure jet-black negroes," not just those with light skin.[18]

Beyond questioning how Lemann was explaining the diabetes he had found among African Americans, some in the audience challenged Lemann's premise that diabetes was even a problem in this population. One physician contended that New Orleans was not representative. Another, who had spent twenty-five years in private practice in Memphis, Tennessee, and who worked primarily with black patients, remembered only one case of the disease. Nor had he encountered many cases of diabetes when he had attended the large number of black patients who received care at Memphis General Hospital. A physician from Louisville, Kentucky, wondered whether the diabetes cases Lemann had found were "true diabetes" rather than "transient glycosuria." Only one physician sided with Lemann, going on to predict that the rate among black people would increase "when they live as the white people do."[19]

Lemann published his study in 1921 in the *Southern Medical Journal,* thereby reaching individuals who had not attended his talk. But the mixed nature of his message—that black people lacked a racial immunity to diabetes; that white people appeared to suffer more than black people from diabetes, but only if class was ignored; that race might not explain differential diabetes rates between black and white people, but it did explain the high rate of diabetes among Jews—meant that few writers, either professional or popular, knew how to interpret his claims. Hyman Goldstein, a faculty member at the University of Pennsylvania, cited Lemann in an article on "Diabetes in the Negro," in which he presented evidence that diabetes occurred in this population "more often than one is led to believe." His own review of records from several Pennsylvania hospitals confirmed this finding, revealing six female and two male "colored patients." Yet when Goldstein concluded his article, he made no mention of the higher-than-expected frequency of diabetes among African Americans. Instead, he reminded his readers that "diabetes is much less common in the Negro than in the white population."[20] It is as though he had forgotten what he had written in the beginning of his article and had allowed himself to fall back on the accepted wisdom in his field.

Other writers simply seemed unaware of Lemann's work. A 1923 *Time* magazine article, entitled "The War on Diabetes," claimed that diabetes rates were "the lowest in the southern and western states largely because Negroes are less susceptible than whites." Haven Emerson, in his article "Sweetness Is Death," asserted that "it is the Negro, whether in southern states or in northern cities, who gives the lowest diabetes death rates." And the official statistics of the Department of Commerce from the same year reported that the nation's diabetes mortality rate was lower for black people than for whites.[21]

In subsequent decades, as new studies suggested that the rate of diabetes in black communities was increasing, Lemann's publications received more attention. To the pathologist Julian Herman Lewis, writing in 1942, Lemann deserved credit for having been the first to provide "actual statistics" comparing diabetes in white and black populations.[22] But in 1921, Lemann's argument that differential disease rates could better be explained by class than by race did not attract many followers. Part of the problem—as was evident in Lemann's own confusing remarks—was that few white professional or popular writers were ready to abandon the idea of biological race. They were also still wedded to the idea that diabetes afflicted wealthy people. Both of these assumptions shaped the image of diabetes well into the 1940s. But by that time, studies had accumulated suggesting that New Orleans was not an anomaly after all.

New Data and Old Stereotypes

Such evidence began to appear in the late 1920s, and the person most responsible was the statistician Louis Dublin. In 1909, when he first began to work for Met Life, it was one of the four largest life insurance companies in the country. The sociologist Lee Frankel, whom Met Life had recently hired to head up a new welfare division, was responsible for bringing Dublin on board. Frankel wanted to set up a pilot visiting-nurse program and he tasked Dublin with determining the efficacy of the program. The young statistician realized early on that the information the nurses collected could be used for epidemiological studies, and he began by focusing on infectious diseases. Soon, though, he was also looking at chronic diseases, producing his first study of diabetes in 1918.[23]

A decade later, Dublin would insist that diabetes rates were every bit as high among the company's black policyholders as among its white policyholders, but that is not what he saw in the data he analyzed in 1918. Examining almost eight thousand deaths from diabetes that his company had recorded between 1911 and 1916—which he described as "by far the largest aggregation of cases of this disease which have as yet received extended statistical treatment"—he looked for patterns in several demographic categories and found nothing surprising when it came to race: black wage earners appeared to have a lower death rate than whites. Yet although the numbers were right in front of him, Dublin overlooked the fact that the *rate of change* among black individuals over that five-year period had been significantly higher for blacks than for whites (Figure 3.1). Among black women in particular, the rate had jumped 91 percent as compared to just 22.4 percent for white women. Dublin made no comment about this—perhaps because he did not see it—but by 1928 he had become convinced that racial disparities in diabetes rates had disappeared.[24]

Ten years had made a difference not only in diabetes rates, but also in the number of black wage earners insured by Met Life. One of the few major life insurance companies to sell policies to African Americans, Met Life

TABLE III.—MORTALITY FROM DIABETES, CLASSIFIED BY COLOR AND BY SEX. DEATH RATES PER 100,000 PERSONS EXPOSED. SINGLE YEARS IN PERIOD 1911 TO 1916. EXPERIENCE OF METROPOLITAN LIFE INSURANCE COMPANY, INDUSTRIAL DEPARTMENT.

Year.	Persons.	WHITE.		COLORED.	
		Males.	Females.	Males.	Females.
1911 to 1916	14.4	10.8	18.5	9.5	11.4
1916.........	15.9	11.5	20.2	11.6	14.8
1915.........	15.1	10.3	20.0	8.1	14.4
1914.........	14.2	10.5	18.4	10.0	10.4
1913.........	13.9	10.8	17.5	8.9	10.9
1912.........	13.7	10.3	17.7	9.7	9.2
1911.........	13.3	11.3	16.5	8.1	7.7

Fig. 3.1. Diabetes mortality rates by race, 1911–1916. From Louis I. Dublin, "Mortality Statistics of Diabetes among Wage Earners," *Medical Record* 94 (October 12, 1918): 632.

had roughly 2.5 million black policyholders by 1928.[25] Since the company rarely ventured into the South, these numbers reflected the great migration of black people who had left their homes and settled in the industrial and industrializing cities in the North. By the 1940s about 1.6 million African Americans had made this journey, and by the 1970s another five million had joined them. They went in search of freedom, better working and living conditions, and a life for themselves and their families without the racism and violence they had experienced in the South. What they found in the North did not always meet their expectations as higher wages disappeared into higher rents; unemployment, hunger, and evictions remained a constant threat; and segregation persisted despite the absence of Jim Crow laws. In 1924 Charles H. Garvin, an African American physician practicing in Cleveland, Ohio, described how "just as soon as Negroes move into a neighborhood, even in our liberal northern cities, rents rise, promoting overcrowding, the sanitary standards are lowered, garbage collections and street cleanings become fewer." But Garvin also noted that among those individuals whose standard of living had improved, "diseases of civilization" were beginning to rise.[26]

By 1928, Dublin was also seeing what Garvin had noticed. Although the overall diabetes death rate in the United States still seemed to be lower in black populations than in white populations, the rate among Met Life's black policyholders had risen so rapidly over the course of five years that it had come to surpass that of the company's white policyholders.[27] Dublin considered two possible reasons for this shift: the greater concentration of black wage earners in cities, where diabetes rates tended to be high; and the relative lack of access to insulin treatment, which might have saved lives. Whatever the reasons, Dublin now realized that the data from Met Life indicated that African Americans were dying more often than whites from the disease.

In the South some new studies also appeared that revealed similar trends. In the same year that Dublin published his new findings, Harold J. Bowcock of Emory University's School of Medicine produced a study of one hundred cases of diabetes seen in the Colored Division of Grady Hospital and the Department of Medicine's J. J. Gray Clinic. Bowcock had decided to pursue this study after reading Lemann's publications and realizing that far too little was known about the burden of the disease on the country's black population. Hoping to "stimulate the further study of diabetes in large negro clinics," he reported his finding of a diabetes rate of 4.2 percent among black patients, a rate that was higher than the 3.4 percent Lemann had found. He also found no difference in the complications that black and white people developed as a result of having diabetes.[28]

In Baltimore, Eugene J. Leopold, a member of the Johns Hopkins Medical School faculty, was inspired by Lemann's and Bowcock's studies and began to collect data from Johns Hopkins Hospital's Out Patient Department Diabetic Clinic. Looking back over records kept between 1928 and 1930, he found that, of almost fifteen thousand blacks who sought care from the hospital's dispensary, 189 people were admitted to the diabetes clinic. This translated into an incidence of 1.27 percent, which he recognized was lower than Lemann's (3.4 percent) and Bowcock's (4.2 percent), but just a hair's breadth below the rate for whites who attended the Hopkins clinic (1.45 percent). Like Bowcock, he found no differences when it came to the complications associated with the disease; and like Dublin, he found that African Americans were dying at a higher rate from the disease than whites (20.8 versus 13.2 per 100,000). His conclusion could not have been clearer: diabetes was "not an uncommon disease among negroes," and it was "not different in any way from the disease as found among white people."[29]

Actually, there was one difference, which both Bowcock and Leopold acknowledged: over 70 percent of the black patients they treated were women, compared to the 55 percent that Joslin found among his white patients. To explain this they first turned to diet, blaming the high rates of diabetes on the consumption of such foods "as pork, cornbread, fat meats, and potatoes," which drove up rates of obesity. Women were more affected than men, they reasoned, in part because of their employment as maids and cooks. But Bowcock and Leopold, noting that "the elderly female is especially prone" to obesity, suggested that biology might matter as well.[30]

In subsequent years, other studies also mentioned increasing rates of diabetes among black women. One of the most impressive, which appeared in 1933, represented a joint effort by Joslin, Dublin, and another statistician, Herbert H. Marks, to learn what they could about global trends in diabetes morbidity and mortality over the previous several decades. Working closely with data from Met Life for the section of the study dealing with the United States, they noted that in contrast to the early twentieth century, when the mortality rate for men had exceeded that for women, the reverse was now the case. And nowhere was this transition more pronounced than among black women. Twenty years earlier their rate had been "barely half" that of white women, but it had "caught up." Even more troubling, this trend appeared to show no signs of stopping, and in recent years the mortality rate for black women had begun to surpass that of white women.[31]

The three diabetes specialists did not speculate on what might have been driving these changes in gender and race, but in the same study, they called the belief that African Americans were "relatively immune to diabetes" an "error." The data from Met Life, they argued, showed not only that the diabetes mortality rate of black wage earners between 1925 and 1930 had been just below that of whites, but that the closing of the gap reflected a "downward" trend among whites and an "upward" trend among blacks. Four years later, when Joslin brought out the sixth edition of *The Treatment of Diabetes Mellitus*, he made sure that anyone who turned to his textbook for advice— and thousands did—would know that "the mortality of colored persons [from diabetes] has been but little lower than that of the white race."[32]

The work of this small, yet influential, group of clinicians and researchers received some publicity. Dublin's 1928 study, for example, was the subject of an article that appeared a year later in the *New York Herald Tribune*.

Although the diabetes death rate among black people was not the focus of the article, the journalist nevertheless pointed out that it was clearly on the rise. The same was true of a *New York Times* article, which mentioned that the "upward trend" in the diabetes death rate among black wage earners insured by Met Life "refutes definitely the theory that the negro is much less susceptible to diabetes than the Caucasian." Four years later, Benjamin Jablons, head of the physicians' division of the American Jewish Congress, published an article in *Hygeia,* the American Medical Association's popular magazine, in which he announced that "diabetes is not a racial disease, as was one time thought." His evidence came from two recent findings: that it no longer "affect[ed] exclusively, or almost exclusively, the Jewish race," and that "the frequency with which diabetes is encountered in the Negro race has increased to a tremendous extent." To Jablons, diabetes was simply "a disease due to overindulgence in food." Thus higher rates of diabetes among African Americans had no other explanation than that the "improvement in the economic condition of the Negro race and other racial groups has increased the tendency to eat to excess."[33]

Although these early studies should have led to more awareness in the American medical community that African Americans were increasingly suffering from diabetes, they were largely overlooked. Almost as though they did not exist, other publications continued to report that black people had lower rates of the disease. A brief article in the *Journal of the American Medical Association* in 1931 even claimed that studies conducted by insurance companies demonstrated that black people are "less susceptible" to diabetes. (It is unclear whether the author had read studies other than Dublin's or was interpreting Dublin's publications differently.) Philadelphia's public health director announced in 1933 what he considered a "well known" fact: that "the Negroes are less prone to contract cancer and diabetes than the white race." Even Dublin himself claimed, in a 1936 article in *Scribner's,* that the disease "predominates among women in the most comfortable situated classes." Just one year later, two statisticians working for the U.S. Public Health Service went so far as to revive the claim that African Americans had a lower mortality rate from diabetes than whites. They published this in an edition of the *Journal of Negro Education* in which Dublin also published an article repeating his findings about the rapidly increasing rates of diabetes among black people.[34] That a single special issue on health included opposite claims—that African Americans had a lower rate of diabetes than whites, and that their rates surpassed those of whites—captures the confusion of the day.

Also working against the message of Dublin and others was the omission of data about diabetes rates among African Americans from government-sponsored studies of the disease. A particularly egregious example was the federal government's 1935–1936 National Health Survey, mentioned earlier, which had gathered detailed information about the disabilities preventing individuals from working, attending school, or engaging in other activities. Although the interviews included people of various races, the final report restricted its conclusions to one race alone. As the authors announced—without any explanation—they had "found [it] expedient to limit this report to data for white persons." Two years later, Mary Gover, associate statistician for the U.S. Public Health Service, in an article on mortality trends among African Americans in ten southern states, listed twenty-one "important causes" of death; diabetes was not among them.[35]

The excision and omission of data about African Americans from published studies provide the most blatant examples of how, in the decades prior to the publication of the 1985 Heckler Report, diabetes, and disabilities in general, in the black population were rendered invisible. But cultural assumptions added to the invisibility, making it difficult for clinicians and researchers to "see" what may have been in front of them. The persistent belief that blacks possessed a different, less developed, nervous system haunted writings on diabetes and race. Thus, in contrast to Jews, where assumptions about racial characteristics—in particular, the image of the nervous Jew—may have made diabetes more "visible" to observers, stereotypes about the slow-moving, slow-witted, "carefree" black person may have made it difficult to see diabetes until it had become fairly widespread.

Tellingly, even the writings of those who claimed diabetes rates were increasing among black people trafficked in negative stereotypes about the population they were studying. I have already pointed out contradictions in Lemann's writings as he put forth several inconsistent claims: that African Americans differed from whites in lacking "nervous strain"; that class, not race, best explained differential diabetes rates between blacks and whites;

and that race best explained the high frequency of diabetes among Jews. How Lemann might have made sense of these disparate claims remains unclear.

Dublin's writings also reveal his struggles to abandon negative stereotypes of black people, even though his views on race would have been considered progressive in his day. A student of Franz Boas, and a supporter of both the NAACP and the National Urban League, Dublin questioned the legitimacy of biological race, considered socioeconomic and environmental conditions better explanations of differential disease rates, and drew particular praise from black leaders for encouraging Met Life to sell insurance policies to black industrial workers. Like Lemann, Dublin also drew attention to the lack of evidence to support the claim that African Americans had immunity to diabetes. Indeed, he went so far as to question whether "*absolute* immunity to any disease" existed. To Dublin, the entire logic of racial immunity depended on the ability to accurately distinguish between the races. Yet so much "'crossing of the white and Negro bloods" had taken place, he contended, that it was no longer clear how to assign racial categories. "The mulatto, the octoroon, etc." were all classified as "'colored'" even though they possessed "both white and Negro blood," he wrote, making it "difficult if not impossible to determine" the true cause of differential rates.[36]

Yet Dublin still repeated older cultural scripts about diabetes and race. For example, despite rejecting the idea of "absolute immunity," he allowed that a "*relative* immunity (or resistance) or a *relative* susceptibility" to disease might still exist. The stumbling block, it seems, remained diseases of the nervous system, which continued to be ensconced in increasingly outdated racial hierarchies. Thus Dublin cited the work of World War I army investigators, who had interpreted lower rates among African Americans of such diseases as diabetes and neurasthenia as evidence "that the nervous system of Negroes shows fewer case [*sic*] of instability than that of the whites." This suggested to him a kind of relative immunity. Dublin also reproduced racial stereotypes when he compared African Americans living in urban areas, who were experiencing increased rates of diabetes, with "the more or less carefree rural Negro," who continued to be "more immune than the white man" to the disease.[37] In short, at the same time that he approached the idea of biological race skeptically, he reproduced without criticism the trope of the childlike, simple, and "carefree rural Negro" whose nervous system remained more impervious to stimulation than that of whites.

Similar stereotypes also appear in the writings of Leopold and Bowcock, despite both men showing considerable awareness of the ways that poverty contributed to the challenges their patients faced. They were particularly sensitive to the limited employment options for black women, which steered so many toward jobs as maids and cooks. They also noted the greater difficulties their patients encountered when trying to pay for prescribed foods and medicines. All in all, the two men offered a sympathetic picture of the hardships their patients endured as they struggled to get their diabetes under control. Yet despite mentioning their patients' intelligence and determination, what they highlighted was their obedience. In Leopold's words, they were "examples of the most complete co-operation, despite a meagerness of learning and lack of education." To Bowcock, the race's "ability for adaptation and imitation" and their "desire to cooperate" meant that they often served as models for "any patient who has become disgruntled or discouraged with a diabetic routine." Intended as flattery, such comments created one-dimensional figures, all of whom allegedly responded in the same way to a disease that must have produced feelings of dismay, anger, and fear at least some of the time. Denied a complex emotional life, the black patients who appeared in these medical writings bring to mind the "good slave." Particularly in the case of obese black women, they evoke an image of the kind, loyal, and grandmotherly "mammy," who never displayed anger at being enslaved. Absent from the medical writings is any image of emancipated individuals capable of thinking deeply, acting freely, and determining their own fate.[38]

Such images contributed to the invisibility of diabetes in black communities. Alongside the blatant omission of data about African Americans from official health reports, these images reinforced the idea that black people—relaxed, carefree, imitative, and compliant—were not advanced enough developmentally and emotionally to be at risk for the disease. Thus, to even begin to see diabetes in black communities, either African Americans' racial traits would need to be imagined differently, or the image of diabetes would have to change. When a small number of black physicians practicing in northern cities like Chicago, Cleveland, and New York began to notice declining infectious disease rates and increasing rates of "degenerative diseases" among their patients, they began the work of reimagining black traits.

In the first decades of the twentieth century, no more than a handful of black physicians drew attention to this change. Limited in number because of their exclusion from the vast majority of the country's medical and nursing schools, black health practitioners were usually stretched too thin to commit themselves to fighting both infectious and degenerative diseases. But several of those who turned their attention to diabetes in the interwar period wrote regular health columns, giving them a bully pulpit from which to redefine the relationship between disease and race. As they did, they painted a picture of African Americans that directly challenged the image of the "happy-go-lucky Negro." Instead, they showed that black people could be as nervous as anyone else. In so doing, they claimed one of the marks of civilization for themselves.

A Symbol of Progress and the Perils of Modern Life

In the 1920s, Dr. A. Wilberforce Williams was trying to figure out why diabetes was becoming so much more common in Chicago's black communities. He acknowledged that improved methods of diagnosis may have been allowing physicians to find the disease where it had previously been hidden, but he also noted that "the stress and strain" of modern life was driving up rates. In a health column he wrote regularly for the *Chicago Defender,* Williams told his readers that if they developed diabetes they had to find "freedom from worry, from physical and nervous strain." The only way to have any success at managing their disease was to calm down and cultivate "ease of mind."[39]

Dr. E. Elliott Rawlins, author of a health column for the *Amsterdam News,* had a similar message for his readers. The increasing rate of diabetes among blacks, he explained, stemmed from the same causes that were driving up the rate overall: "People in the United States live in more luxury, do less physical exercise, eat more food and have a greater nervous strain than in past years. This is especially so after 40 years of age." To

Dr. Mary F. Waring, modern efforts to get "contagious diseases under control" had proved so successful that it was now time "to turn to 'degenerative diseases.'" And for Dr. Charles H. Garvin, the increase in diabetes among black people was tied directly to their higher standard of living, which meant exposure to "civilization and its 'hustle and bustle' and 'burning the candle at both ends.'"[40]

These four physicians were all leaders in their respective communities and, with the exception of Garvin, all wrote regular health columns. Williams, who graduated from Northwestern University Medical School of Chicago in 1894, began practicing medicine at Provident Hospital immediately upon graduation and continued to do so until his death in 1940. He was appointed health editor of the *Chicago Defender* in 1911, and was the first African American physician to keep up a regular advice column on health and hygiene. Rawlins graduated from Long Island College Hospital in 1906 and began immediately to practice medicine in Harlem, where he remained until his untimely death in 1928. During the last five years of his life, he wrote the health column "Keeping Fit" for the *New York Amsterdam News*. Waring, who graduated from the Louisville National Medical College in 1894 and from Chicago's National Medical College in 1923, was chair of the Department of Health and Hygiene for the National Association of Colored Women (NACW). As part of her responsibilities she wrote a regular health column for the organization's publication, *National Notes*. Garvin, the only one not to write a regular health column, may well have been the most accomplished of the four. A graduate of Howard University's medical school in 1915, he achieved a number of firsts in his lifetime: the first black person to attend the Army Medical School; the first black physician the U.S. Army commissioned during World War I; and the first black physician to be on the staff of a white hospital in Cleveland, Ohio (where he settled after the war). Enjoying a national reputation, Garvin became a leading advocate for the advancement of rights and privileges for African Americans.[41]

The starting position for all four individuals was that diabetes was "no respecter of race or person." Evidence of this, they claimed, came from recent studies that challenged the idea that race explained the high rate of the disease among Jews, and that demonstrated rising rates among African Americans. In denying the role of race, they were echoing arguments that black health leaders had been making since at least 1906, when W. E. B. Du Bois's *The Health and Physique of the Negro American* appeared. In subsequent years, others followed Du Bois's lead and fought to discredit medical arguments that alleged to demonstrate racial inferiority. Williams, Rawlins, Waring, Garvin, and others contributed to this effort, yet they also had a different target and message. Previous writings had focused on infectious diseases, and on proving that high mortality rates from these diseases stemmed from horrific social conditions rather than racial traits. In Du Bois's words, the high death rate among blacks from infectious diseases was "without doubt a death rate due to *poverty* and *discrimination*."[42] In turning to diabetes, however, these figures were shifting from infectious to chronic, degenerative diseases; from diseases to which black people were believed to be susceptible to ones to which they were alleged to have immunities; and from diseases associated with poverty to ones associated with wealth.

High rates of infectious diseases symbolized filth, oppression, and racism; increasing rates of diabetes and other degenerative diseases signaled social advance. It meant that black people now lived in the urban fast lane rather than on a meandering country road or on the plantation, spent income rather than bartered for goods, and in general indulged in all that consumer culture had to offer, including the overconsumption of food. Similar to Jewish physicians' writings on diabetes, black physicians cast the higher rate of diabetes as the price of entry into the "hustle and bustle" of modern life. As Williams commented in 1935, after describing the increased tendency of African Americans to survive childhood and infectious diseases and to live "past middle life" and succumb to degenerative ones: "The Negro has learned how to live."[43]

Of course, not all "Negroes" had "learned how to live." Many continued to die disproportionately from infectious diseases. This concern led the organizers of National Negro Health Week, which had started in 1915, to sustain their efforts until 1952. It also motivated the Julius Rosenwald Foundation to fund a pilot treatment program in 1929 to try and reduce syphilis rates among poor blacks.[44] Such interventions took place primarily in the South, and often in rural areas. In contrast, the story of declining infectious disease rates and social advancement among African Americans took place in the urban North. The creators of this story, unlike Leopold and Bowcock, who were white university faculty members attending to poor black patients in their institutions' clinics, were black physicians catering primarily (although not exclusively) to a middle-class clientele. By the early 1930s there were almost four thousand black physicians in the United States, a miniscule number out of the roughly 150,000 physicians practicing in the country at the time, but a significant increase from the mere dozens who had practiced in the nineteenth century.[45] For them, increasing rates of the "diseases of civilization" heralded their entry into modern society, and proved that they could be as nervous as anyone.

Williams and Rawlins, the more prolific of the four, wrote numerous articles about nervous diseases for their health columns. The image they promoted countered the idea that black people were more resilient and carefree than whites. Instead, the stresses of modern life were leading them to suffer equally from nervous disorders. The "ideal environment at the present state of your civilization does not exist," Rawlins wrote, "and therefore the brain is continually injured, resulting in spiritual and physical abnormalities such as anger, fear, envy, selfishness, heart disease, diabetes, kidney trouble, neurasthenia, hysteria." To Rawlins, not even the "lowly hand workers" were immune from these pressures, and thus from diabetes, because they too "have a great deal of mental worry or responsibility" and thus "are now knowing the distress of the disease."[46]

Their patients bore no resemblance to the passive, slow-moving, compliant "Negroes" that Bowcock and Leopold had described. Instead, they proved difficult to control and were resistant to changing their ways. Williams, for example, admonished his readers that if they should develop diabetes they would have to learn "to be submissive and obey . . . [their] doctor in the minutest details of treatment." Stubborn and more inclined "to follow the advice of well-meaning but ignorant friends, neighbors or anybody who is impudent enough to suggest or give advice about things of which they know nothing," the patients Williams described could not have differed more from the "examples of the most complete co-operation" whom Leopold had praised.[47]

Undoubtedly, black physicians in the interwar years had their reasons for describing their patients as intractable and ornery. As members of a newly emerging professional middle class, they sought to establish their authority and to cultivate a paying clientele. Part of their strategy was to convince their readers that diabetes was, in Williams's words, "too serious a condition to be considered lightly." They also conveyed the message that only they possessed the knowledge that would lead to the successful management and treatment of disease, and that the best way to acquire this knowledge was through regular checkups with one's doctors.[48] But by and large the individuals they portrayed in their writings were independent and willful actors in their own lives, fully capable of exercising freedom of thought and action. It took little away from anyone's independence, they suggested, to accept the need for an expert hand to provide guidance, especially given modern society's constant bombarding of the senses, which itself could induce disease.

The black individuals portrayed in these articles were also fully capable of developing "civilized" diseases, like diabetes. The higher social status associated with increasing degenerative disease rates—and, by extension, the lower social status of infectious diseases—is particularly evident in the writings of Mary Fitzbutler Waring, who began her career as a leader in the battle against tuberculosis. As director of health for the National Association of Colored Women, a position she assumed in 1913, she was one of roughly 300,000 black women who joined clubs in the first decades of the twentieth century in order to effect change in their communities and encourage racial uplift. An accommodationist in the spirit of Booker T. Washington, Waring believed that full citizenship required achieving middle-class respectability, and she saw in public health and hygiene tools for accomplishing that goal. Ever since Washington had spearheaded National Negro Health Week, she and other black clubwomen had stepped up their involvement in public health work, convinced, in the words of one historian, that "the very survival of African Americans was at stake."[49] At a time when Jim Crow legislation denied African Americans health services that were available to their white neighbors, these women established hospitals and nursing schools in their communities and organized fundraising campaigns to supply these institutions with necessary materials and equipment. But more than anything else, they committed themselves to educating the poor about the value of hygiene and cleanliness. In 1917, when Waring was still fighting to gain control over infectious diseases, she encouraged her fellow clubwomen to "go into the backways and the tenement houses, into the alleys and basements, into the places unfrequented by garbage wagons and street cleaners and here help teach and preach 'cleanliness.'"[50]

Historians have documented the exacting nature of the work that black clubwomen performed in "the backways and tenements": they taught poor women how to keep their homes and themselves clean by removing piles of rubbish that attracted flies, sweeping and mopping floors, airing out the rooms where they slept, preserving and preparing food, washing hair, brushing teeth, and bathing. They also offered instruction in good manners, moral behavior, and the importance of a thrifty life. Confident that due to their middle-class upbringing they knew what was necessary to convince white people that African Americans deserved full citizenship, they preached a blend of public health and personal hygiene that promised to sanitize the backyards, homes, and minds of the poor. Gaining the upper hand over infectious disease rates and lifting up the race went hand in hand.[51]

This was a logic born in the impoverished environments of the poor, where infectious diseases claimed far too many lives. The enemies were flies and ignorance: the former because they carried disease, and the latter because with knowledge, disease-carrying insects could be killed or at least avoided. The battle against degenerative diseases, to which Waring turned in the late 1920s, had a similar logic—it, too, attacked impurities and ignorance. Yet instead of scouring the nooks and crannies of homes and backyards for germs, it demanded increased focus on the monitoring of bodily functions. As Waring explained, the degenerative diseases were "infections from within" rather than from the outside, and as such she considered it "imperative that more attention be given to the seemingly minor complaints and disorders as they develop." To accomplish this one had to begin by visiting a physician, who would conduct "a physical examination of eyes, throat, teeth, lungs, urine, functional tests, weight, blood, blood pressure and tension."[52] But that was not enough. One had to learn to monitor oneself, and the members of one's family, as well.

To Waring, this was women's work. In an article on "Degenerative Diseases," she announced that "the women of the country" were the ones responsible for "closer observance of small disorders and incipient encroachment of disease." Waring's ascription of a special role for wives and mothers fit with black clubwomen's embrace of the gendered division of labor. In the battle against infectious diseases, they, after all, had been the ones to enter the homes of the poor in an effort to teach new habits. Now she was challenging her middle-class readers not only to police the domestic spaces of the poor, but also to scrutinize the quotidian activities of their own families. Their social class meant that they were the ones who had advanced enough to be suffering from the degenerative diseases; thus they, and their families, were the ones in urgent need of change. Addressing them with language that acknowledged their new purchasing power and thus their participation in consumer culture, Waring encouraged her readers to tend to themselves with the same care that they gave to their possessions: "You look over your clothes and automobile and check up on their condition," she wrote; "do as much for your body."[53]

Waring's vision of degenerative diseases as both a sign of, and a vehicle for, racial uplift appeared in the writings of her fellow health columnists as well. In a piece on "What to Do for Diabetes," Williams insisted that treatment be not only medical, but also "hygienic and dietetic." For the medical side, he referred primarily to the use of insulin, but for hygiene and diet he included an expansive list of permitted and forbidden foods as well as the benefits of adequate rest, daily bathing, teeth cleaning after every meal, dressing properly, and avoiding alcohol, "sexual excesses," and any kind of "mental worry and overwork." For Rawlins the control of the emotions was paramount. In an article entitled "Keep a Cool Head and Save Your Ductless Glands," he described a link between an "ambitious person" who was thwarted in achieving what he or she "desires" and "organic and functional diseases, such as diabetes, arterio-sclerosis, heart disease and kidney disorders." In between were a host of emotions, including "continued worry, excessive anger, fear, envy and resentment," which made a lasting impression on "the sympathetic nervous system and cause[d] disfunction in the ductless glands." Later the same year, in his article "The Mind and Disease," Rawlins again held modern life and its stresses responsible for many of the new diseases, cautioning that emotions left unchecked caused havoc with one's mental and physical state. The solution he proposed might have come straight out of Haven Emerson, whom he referenced: "These mental reactions could be prevented by the self-education of the will-power, or by the persuasive influence of some other person."[54]

Rawlins's reference to Emerson draws our attention to similarities in the writings of black and white health professionals in the interwar years. Pitching their message primarily to middle-class readers, they shared a vision of diabetes (and other degenerative diseases) as a symbol of progress *and* a sign of the perils that a modern lifestyle posed to those who failed to practice self-restraint. Spelling out the strategies necessary to either prevent or manage diabetes amounted to producing a primer in self-restraint and bourgeois respectability. Only the constant and exacting examination of "habits of work, exercise, diet, play, recreation and sleep" promised to stave off the damage these diseases could cause, and help forge a path to middle-class respectability—for black and white people alike.

Yet there were also differences. Importantly, the residues of racial stereotypes that continued to appear in the writings of Dublin and others were absent in the writings of black practitioners. There was no back and forth between denying that race mattered and then reintroducing it to explain differences, as in Dublin's waffling between absolute and relative immunity. For black professionals, moreover, the consequences of succumbing to excess may have appeared more dire given that they were fighting to defend what many of them had only recently acquired: an education, a career, the possibility of purchasing a home, automobile, and other material goods, in short, the prospect of living a comfortable middle-class life. The danger now of overindulging lay not only in the possibility of developing diabetes, but also in the abandonment of hard-won claims to self-restraint and self-discipline that had supported African Americans' claims to full citizenship. Eight years before Hannah Lees suggested that "diabetics" made "better citizens" because those with "weak characters" died young, Waring concluded her article on degenerative diseases with a dire warning: "The world progresses, time sweeps on; only those who think and fight for right deserve to survive."[55]

Finding "Hidden Diabetics": The Oxford Study

During the late 1920s and 1930s, diabetes became more noticeable, and noticed, in black communities. Lemann, Bowcock, and Leopold observed the disease among poor African Americans in the South; Dublin documented it among industrial wage earners in the North; and Williams,

Rawlins, Waring, and Garvin saw it in the black middle class and to some extent among "lowly hand workers." In subsequent years, prestigious medical journals, such as the *New England Journal of Medicine* and the *Journal of the American Medical Association,* as well as the white and black press, occasionally advanced claims that the diabetes rate among black people was increasing faster than among whites.[56]

Nowhere was this more evident than among black women. What Leopold and Bowcock had noticed in the early 1930s had become a common refrain by the early 1940s: black women had a significantly higher rate of diabetes than either black men or white women. According to two physicians affiliated with the outpatient clinic of Harlem Hospital, the "sex distribution" among African Americans was four women to one man, compared to two to one for the white patients who attended their clinic. Also troubling was the pace of change in the diabetes mortality rate over the previous seven years: among black women it had jumped 76 percent compared to 26 percent for white women. In 1947, Hugh L. C. Wilkerson, the leading diabetes specialist in the U.S. Public Health Service, announced that the diabetes death rate among "non-white women" had increased 155.6 percent between 1920 and 1940, compared to 52.6 percent for white women.[57]

Wilkerson made this announcement just one year after the U.S. Public Health Service had initiated a study of diabetes in the small New England town of Oxford, Massachusetts, about fifty miles west of Boston. The Oxford Diabetes Study, begun in 1946, was an early step in an effort to uncover "hidden diabetes," which was itself part of a greatly expanded effort nationwide during the middle of the century to go beyond the 1935–1936 National Health Survey and gather more detailed information on the burden that chronic diseases posed to the nation. Convinced that many chronic diseases were preventable—Wilkerson believed that diabetes might even be reversible if caught early enough—health care providers and reformers from both the public and private spheres came together to brainstorm about how best to tackle increasing rates of chronic and degenerative diseases. But by choosing Oxford for its study of diabetes, the U.S. Public Health Service was declaring that a picturesque, racially homogenous, New England town could stand in for the rest of the nation: according to the 1950 Massachusetts Census, all of Oxford's roughly five thousand inhabitants were white. Indeed, the entire state of Massachusetts was over 98 percent white, with even Boston's nonwhite population comprising just under 5 percent of the total.[58]

There were, to be sure, good reasons to choose Oxford. Based on physical examinations of servicemen and inductees from the beginning of World War II, the designers of the study had become convinced that the National Health Survey had underestimated the prevalence of diabetes in the country by about half. The discrepancy, they suspected, had to do with the National Health Survey's reliance on self-reporting, which was particularly problematic for a disease like diabetes, of which so many people were unaware. They thus wanted a town that would allow them to examine everyone in the community, whether they had already received a diagnosis of diabetes or not.[59] To that end, they needed a high level of buy-in from whichever community they chose, and Oxford promised just that.

Elliott P. Joslin had grown up in Oxford and had strengthened his ties by purchasing a three-hundred-acre farm in his hometown. His relationships with local physicians and civic leaders would help the U.S. Public Health Service garner enough support to achieve a high level of compliance from the community. Indeed, the survey may have been Joslin's idea. Either way, the strategy worked: the U.S. Public Health Service was able to examine 70 percent of the town's inhabitants (3,516 of 4,983), and what it found was unexpected. Of the seventy people they identified as having the disease, only forty had previously been diagnosed. To the remaining thirty the result had come as a surprise. To Wilkerson and Leo P. Krall, who co-authored the first report on the study, this meant that 1.7 percent of the town had diabetes. It also meant that "for every 4 previously known cases there were 3 more hitherto undiscovered and unsuspected cases." Equally significant was their finding that diabetes was far more likely to appear in those who had a family history of the disease.[60] The question, though, was whether the results of the Oxford study said anything about the rest of the country.

Wilkerson and Krall thought so. In this same first report on the study's findings, they referred to Oxford not only as "a typical New England town," but also as "a typical American community." To support this, they pointed out that the "age composition [of] the population of the town closely parallels that of the country as a whole."[61] Since diabetes was largely a disease of the elderly, this was an important statistic to share. They also noted that the diabetes death rate in Oxford over the previous ten years had been "consistent" with that of the state of Massachusetts as a whole. (They did not say whether this was higher or lower than that for the country.) But when it came to other demographic categories, their message was unclear. As far as sex was concerned, they had found near parity in the morbidity rates for men and women, but said nothing about how this compared to data for any other region of the country. Given that one year later Wilkerson would draw attention to the much higher mortality rate of diabetes among "non-white women" than among white women, it is likely that Oxford's data were not representative of gender disparities in communities with demographics other than what one would find in "a typical New England town."

Wilkerson and Krall struggled most when they turned to race, but the absence of African Americans from their study is not what troubled them. Rather, reverting to early twentieth-century divisions of whites into distinct races, they worried that readers would consider Oxford atypical because "the predominant racial groups" in the town consisted of people of French and French Canadian descent. Of great concern, twenty-nine of the seventy people found to have diabetes hailed from this group. But rather than entertain the possibility that this had anything to do with this group's racial traits (as they might have had the group been black), they simply attributed the high rate to the fact that "this group is predominant in the tested area."[62] In other words, there may have been more of them in Oxford than elsewhere in the nation, but they were no different, biologically or otherwise, than anyone else.

But did this mean that individuals of French or French Canadian descent were no different than other whites or than all other "races"? A second U.S. Public Health Service study, begun in May 1947 in Jacksonville, Florida, seemed to provide an answer to that question. The goal of this project was to determine how a local public health department might, without a significant investment of resources, improve its ability to detect cases of diabetes early and so reduce the likelihood of complications. Since Jacksonville had 203,370 residents, public health officials could not reasonably examine every one, so they focused on relatives of people already known to have diabetes. They also paid attention to possible racial differences because roughly one-third of Jacksonville's population was black. What they found was that roughly the same number of undetected cases existed among black and white individuals. "It does not appear," they concluded, "that the racial composition of the group had an important effect on the rate of new cases observed."[63]

Thus, in their own ways, both the Oxford and the Jacksonville studies raised the possibility of racial differences only to declare them immaterial. True to that message, follow-up studies of these two sites did not even mention race. This does not mean that race was no longer a part of how diabetes was imagined and represented. On the contrary, the presumption was that since the different races had roughly the same prevalence of the disease, a town like Oxford, inhabited solely by whites and disproportionately by people of French or French Canadian descent, could legitimately stand in for the rest of the nation.

Wilkerson's decision to do a close-up study of a white New England town speaks volumes about both the visibility and invisibility of diabetes among African Americans in the years following World War II. It attests both to the growing sense that race no longer functioned effectively as a predictor of diabetes, and to how diabetes continued to be imagined as a white disease. In the postwar years, diabetes was not the only chronic disease to have a predominantly white "face": the first cohort study of coronary heart disease, begun in 1948, took place in the predominantly white New England town of Framingham, Massachusetts. And despite epidemiological studies that indicated increasing cancer rates among African Americans, cancer too continued to be associated with whites.[64]

The relative erasure of African Americans from discussions of diabetes is evident not only in written studies, but also in visual representations. Deeply concerned about the rapidly increasing rates of diabetes, Wilkerson set in motion a public health campaign, complete with educational films, to teach the nation about the seriousness of the disease. The first feature film, *The Story of Wendy Hill,* co-produced in 1949 with the American Diabetes Association, starred a young, middle-class white woman who had recently married. One of the film's primary goals was to assure young women like her that she could have children. As late as 1962, the film *Diabetics Unknown* described those who were most vulnerable as "fat, forty, familied, and fair."[65] Not until the 1980s did public health films make any mention of the disease in black communities.

* * *

On the surface it may seem that little had changed since the 1920s, when most writings on diabetes asserted that African Americans were immune and that whites suffered disproportionately from the disease. But a close look reveals that an important shift had taken place: few claimed any longer that African Americans were immune. Rather, the most common message, whether from epidemiologists, public health officials, medical research-ers, clinicians, or journalists, was that diabetes was increasing in black and white populations alike, and that the rapid pace of life and stress it pro-duced, the overconsumption of foods, and family history—not race—best explained the disease's distribution. In his historical study of cancer, Keith Wailoo, who identified a similar trend, wrote of "a generic, 'de racialized' whiteness" that populated epidemiological studies in the 1950s.[66] Read in this light, the decision to depict people with diabetes as white was not intended to describe the actual racial makeup of those who had diabetes; rather, a white individual was meant to represent everyone.

White individuals, in other words, had come to represent the "standard" human subject in medical research. Several developments contributed to the construction of this universal norm, not least being the rise of social science surveys that, in one historian's words, produced the idea of "the averaged American," as well as the growing push toward uniform standards within biomedicine itself.[67] But whatever benefits standardization may have provided came at the cost of rendering invisible anyone who did not look like the "norm."

For a period following World War II, then, diabetes appeared to be a uni-versal disease in which the perception of racial differences played a dimin-ished role. This would not last. By the 1950s—decades before the Heckler Report shocked the country by drawing attention to the great gap in dia-betes rates between whites and blacks—medical researchers with the U.S. Public Health Service "discovered" that several Native American tribes had extremely high rates of the disease, and talk of race began anew. These were the heady days following the discovery of DNA, when human genetics was becoming established as an academic discipline and research into the genetics of disease was receiving considerable attention and funding. When the geneticist James Neel hypothesized in 1962 that possession of a "thrifty gene" might explain high rates of diabetes, a link between race and diabetes was imagined once again, this time with Native Americans as the population believed to be most at risk. And as medical and public health personnel grappled with the meaning of this apparent shift, they began to think differently about the nature of diabetes itself. In the process, diabetes lost its status as a disease of civilization and slowly became a disease of "primitive" populations that were unable to adapt quickly enough to a Western lifestyle.

4

Native Peoples and the Thrifty
Gene Hypothesis

Nomadic tribes and peoples living in a primitive state rarely if ever
have diabetes. . . . It would seem therefore that diabetes is a product
of civilization.

John R. Williams, 1917

It has been speculated that natural selection might formerly have
favored diabetes-prone genotypes, and that these genotypes might
be most frequent in populations which recently lived under primitive
conditions.

T. D. Doeblin, 1969

LIKE AFRICAN AMERICANS, NATIVE AMERICANS did not suffer from diabetes. At least, that was the nearly universal belief in the first decades of the
twentieth century. Not that they were healthy. Tuberculosis was ravaging
their communities. Trachoma, enteritis, and other infectious diseases were
rampant as well. But diabetes, cancer, and cardiovascular ailments—the so-
called diseases of civilization—seemed to rarely claim a victim. Trying to
make sense of this disease pattern, professional and popular writers alike
drew on widespread tropes of "primitive" and "civilized." According to these
narratives, Native Americans, as a so-called primitive people, continued to
die of infectious diseases that flourished in unhygienic homes and communities, spread by individuals ignorant of modern hygienic codes of behavior.

These were the dirty diseases of "savages." As far as the "clean" diseases of the "civilized" were concerned, Native peoples appeared to be immune.[1]

These claims persisted until the middle of the century, when diabetes rates among Native Americans seemed to be rising, in some cases even surpassing those of whites. Yet few argued that Native peoples had finally become civilized. Instead, these increasing rates were attributed to their being biologically unequipped, as "primitive" peoples, to adapt to the challenges of civilization.[2]

How was it possible to read both low rates of diabetes in the early twentieth century and high rates of diabetes decades later as evidence of the primitiveness of Native Americans? What assumptions, arguments, and explanations worked to sustain an image of Native peoples as primitive, even as one of the markers of that alleged primitiveness shifted from *immunity* to diabetes to *an unusually high susceptibility* to the very same disease? The answer to these questions rests in the confluence of a number of developments, including the tendency to lump together tribes with different genetic ancestries into a single racial category, "Native Americans" or "American Indians"; the perception of Native peoples as an ideal laboratory for studying disease; the emergence of human genetics as a legitimate and highly revered scientific endeavor; and a reluctance by researchers and government officials to engage seriously with the direct health consequences of federal policies, which had been systematically decimating Native American lands, cultures, and communities for over a century.

None of this addresses the question of whether diabetes rates did, in fact, start out low among Native peoples, only to escalate rapidly as the century progressed. And while it is likely that diabetes rates did follow this pattern with some tribes, the paucity of reliable data, coupled with the ambiguity surrounding the category "Native American," provide ample reason to doubt diabetes's absence from Native populations in the early twentieth century. After all, for which of the thousands of Native American tribes might this have been true? As Kim Tallbear, an Indigenous Studies scholar, has pointed out, before contact with Europeans, "Native Americans" did not exist. Instead, there were thousands of small groups, each with its own language, history, and cultural traditions. European settlers erased these differences and placed all indigenous populations under one heading as part of their colonialist ventures, which then allowed them to rank different "races" in a hierarchy from least to most "civilized" and, thereby, to justify the forced removal of "primitive" peoples from their lands and homes.[3]

Such clear demarcations were never, however, stable. Intragroup differences—whether cultural, linguistic, geographic, historical, or genetic—consistently pushed against the totalizing nature of a single category. This was evident in political disputes between Native populations; the persistence of distinctive cultural traditions and rituals; and in noticeably different mortality and morbidity rates. In the diabetes literature, medical researchers certainly struggled throughout the century to make sense of differential rates between tribes, especially as unusually high rates of the disease were found among the Akimel O'odham (Pima), Cherokee, and several other Native populations in the decades following World War II. Nevertheless, despite comparatively low rates among a number of other tribes, including the Athapascan Indians, Eskimos, and Dineh (Navajo), professional and popular writers alike continued to claim that whites and Native Americans had different experiences of the disease. Ideas of racial difference in general, and the alleged primitivity of Native Americans in particular, proved difficult to let go.

This remained the case after World War II, despite attempts by physical anthropologists and population geneticists to change how race was understood. Wanting to distance themselves from their eugenic past, they declared their intent to replace fixed racial typologies with the idea of race as a population defined by "the frequencies of some gene or genes." In theory, this meant that an individual, or community of individuals, might belong to different "races" depending on the trait being studied. In practice, fixed typologies, and the racial hierarchies they represented, proved difficult to avoid. Ideas about "primitive" and "advanced" societies would continue to influence medical narratives about diabetes and indigenous societies for decades to come.[4]

No theory revealed this influence more clearly than the thrifty gene hypothesis. First proposed by the geneticist James Neel in 1962, it offered an evolutionary explanation for how a deleterious trait—a diabetic genotype—might have attained a high frequency in the human gene pool. Why, Neel wondered, did natural selection not result in a lower frequency of this trait?

Building on recent work that explained how the sickle cell trait conferred some protection against malaria, Neel suggested that a "thrifty genotype" might have helped early humans as they lived through repeated cycles of feast and famine by increasing the efficiency with which they stored fat when food was plentiful—and thus helping these "efficient" fat storers to survive and reproduce. According to this theory, when food became consistently available, this ability to store fat efficiently became a liability.[5]

What often goes unnoticed is that Neel did not offer his hypothesis as a way of explaining high rates of diabetes among Native Americans; in fact, he did not even mention them in his 1962 article. Instead, he was trying to understand the near universal distribution of diabetes. That is why he referred to "the first 99 per cent or more of man's life on earth, while he existed as a hunter and gatherer." For Neel, "man" referred to all the peoples of the world.[6] Yet Neel's hypothesis, which he first proposed in 1962 to explain the origin of diabetes in early humans, had by the late 1970s acquired the status of a highly plausible explanation, occasionally referred to as a theory, about why Native Americans had some of the highest rates of diabetes not only in the United States, but also in the world. Indeed, the idea of a close link between thrifty genes and indigenous peoples has persisted until today, despite Neel's abandonment of his own theory before his death in 1999, and despite the lack of any concrete evidence.[7] A belief in racial difference keeps it alive.

The history of Native Americans and diabetes provides additional evidence of the deep entrenchment of ideas of race in professional and popular writings on disease. It also opens a window onto one of the first sites where diabetes underwent a gradual transformation from a disease of "civilized humanity" to one that most afflicted those who lacked "culture."[8] Poverty, primitivity, and ignorance, not wealth, civilization, and education, became its defining traits.

A "Primitive People," a Convenient Storyline

In 1908 Aleš Hrdlička, the thirty-nine-year-old assistant curator in charge of the Division of Physical Anthropology at the U.S. National Museum, handed in his 460-page report. He had been on six expeditions between 1898 and 1905, visiting nearly every Indian tribe in the south-western United States and northwestern Mexico. Hrdlička was nothing if not thorough. A physician and a physical anthropologist, he had collected information about the Indians' physical environment, clothing, eating and reproductive habits, dwellings, occupations, physiology, and physiognomy. He measured heights, weights, and head sizes; took temperatures and pulse rates; and tested muscular strength. He also studied diseases, conducting examinations when possible and relying on the medical records of others when that could not be arranged. Pneumonia, tuberculosis, ophthalmias, rheumatism, arthritis, smallpox, measles, dysentery—these were the conditions he found most frequently among North American Indians. Cardiovascular problems, cancer, and nervous diseases, in contrast, were relatively rare. But the rarest was diabetes. During all of his expeditions, Hrdlička did not observe a single case of the disease, and he came across only one mention of it in the medical records of a physician practicing among the Akimel O'odham in Sacaton, Arizona. "Woman . . . Diabetes," appeared in the list of cases for January 1902.[9] That was all.

Little changed in the following decades. A survey conducted in 1933 on the health of the Seminole Indians in Oklahoma and Florida never mentioned diabetes. Four years later, C. G. Salsbury, medical director of the Sage Memorial Hospital in Ganado, Arizona, found that of the almost five thousand Dineh people treated there over a five-year period, only one had been diagnosed with the disease. The Alabama-Coushatta Indians of southeast Texas did not have a single case of diabetes until 1943. Such claims could also be read in the popular press. As one *New York Times* article relayed in 1951: "The Indians have been found to be fairly free from cancer, diabetes and the group of heart, brain and kidney disorders . . . which today comprise the major health problem of the white race."[10]

The evidence for these low rates was sporadic and occasionally anecdotal, but there is good reason to trust that diabetes was not yet the burden it would become for Native American communities. Since the life expectancy for Native peoples around the turn of the century was short, many did not live long enough to develop diabetes. Undernourished and hungry, they frequently lacked the physical strength to survive the harsh conditions of reservation life. During a particularly grueling winter in 1884, about one-quarter of the population on the Blackfoot reservation in Montana died of starvation. Infectious diseases flourished in this environment. At the beginning of the twentieth century, the tuberculosis death rate among Native Americans was roughly four times that of the white population. As late as 1949, Dineh children were still dying of diarrhea and enteritis at a rate twenty times greater than the rest of the nation. Lives were ending before the degenerative diseases could take hold.[11]

Such horrific conditions stemmed in large part from almost a century of federal policies that had destroyed the land, lifestyle, and livelihoods of the very people now dying at a far greater rate than the rest of the nation. The Akimel O'odham, for example, had successfully farmed along the Gila River for centuries, growing corn, cotton, wheat, squash, and beans, and trading surplus foods with white settlers and travelers alike. Two congressional acts—the Homestead Act (1862) and Desert Land Act (1877)—destroyed this bounty. Developed to encourage white settlers to move west and farm arid and semi-arid lands, these acts led to irrigation projects that dried up the Gila River, making it impossible, as one Akimel O'odham elder declared in 1914, "to irrigate all our fields."[12] By the last decades of the nineteenth century, they could no longer support themselves and became dependent on government subsidies.

Stories of other tribes followed a similar pattern. Thus, the Lakota (Sioux) Indians, who had hunted buffalo since the eighteenth century, were forced to rely primarily on farming after, as one government official admitted, being "herded into some of the most useless and barren lands of the nation," that is, after being resettled onto reservations. In this way, millions of people who had for millennia provided their own sustenance lost their ability to live independently and to nourish themselves adequately. Without the land, rivers, and forests that had once given them food and shelter, they struggled to ward off sickness. By the late nineteenth century, Native Americans were considered "a dying race."[13]

The dominant explanations for why Native people were dying off did not, however, hold the policies of the federal government responsible. Although the deplorable conditions of reservation life—including the extreme poverty, poorly built homes, and insufficient food and clean water—were all understood to stand in the way of efforts to improve the health of the reservations' inhabitants, officials with the Bureau of Indian Affairs (BIA) tended to hold American Indians responsible for their own plight. In 1929, M. C. Guthrie, chief medical director of the BIA, bemoaned the "ignorance, prejudice, and superstition" that led Indians to seek out the help of "so-called medicine men and other charlatans," rather than taking advantage of "trained personnel." To Guthrie, this was the mark of "a primitive people," a characterization with which few would have disagreed at the time.[14]

But what did "primitive" signify in this context? Guthrie's comment alluded to one meaning: the direct antithesis of Enlightenment ideals of rationality, science, and hygiene, each of which symbolized the ability to control nature. A photograph that Guthrie included in a 1929 *Public Health Report* captures this meaning in stark visual form (Figure 4.1). It juxtaposes a "trained" physician and an Apache medicine man, the physician leaning away from the medicine man, one arm behind his back as though he feared accidental contact, and the other arm caught in mid-action, moving forward toward the photographer. It is a pose that suggests action, in contrast to the medicine man, who stands with his arms hanging limply at his sides. Taller than the Indian Health Service physician, he is dwarfed by the huge headdress sitting atop his head, feathers shooting out in all directions. He wears a suit—might he be trying to "pass"?—but it is disheveled. Instead of a bowtie, he sports an Indian necklace and what appears to be a cross. The contrast is stark, and sends a clear message that the "Apache Indian medicine man," despite donning a suit, will forever remain wild, a stranger in the "civilized" world.

Contributing to this understanding of primitiveness was an idea about evolution that imagined different races as sequential stages in the development of humankind. According to this view, primitive peoples occupied the lower rungs of a ladder that led from non-human primates through the various human races on up to Caucasians, who occupied the uppermost rung.[15] As we have already noted, an important indicator of a race's position on the evolutionary ladder was the extent to which the nervous system had developed.

Primitive also often conjured up images of a people living close to nature. In its romanticized form, it brought to mind the noble savage, untainted by

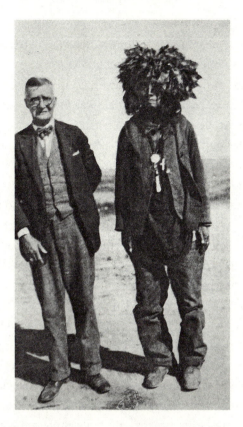

Fig. 4.1. An Indian Service physician and an Apache Indian medicine man. Reprinted from M. C. Guthrie, "The Health of the American Indian," *Public Health Reports (1896–1970)* 44, no. 16 (April 19, 1929): 945–957.

the evils and vices of modern life. In its brutal form, it transformed Indians into savages, justifying their expulsion from the land. Primitiveness was also aligned with the inability to protect oneself from nature's forces. Bertram Kraus, a physical anthropologist at the University of Arizona, produced a study of Indian health in 1954 in which he painted a picture of a people for whom "natural selection is still operative." Lacking knowledge of and access to modern medicine, they remained subject to "the weeding out of the biologically unfit . . . that has continued since the beginning of life on earth." Failing to recognize that the reservations where he conducted his studies were anything but "natural" environments, Kraus read the "high infant and child mortality rates" that emerged from his study as evidence that "the Indian populations are 'primitive'" and thus unable to protect their young ones from nature's harsh conditions.[16]

The various meanings of primitive appeared in one fashion or another in the disease literature. Indeed, so fungible was the concept of primitiveness that in the early decades of the twentieth century it was called on to explain not only low rates of diabetes among Native Americans but also high rates of tuberculosis. According to one popular explanation, Native Americans were dying in such great numbers from tuberculosis because they were forced to make the cultural transition from primitive to modern too rapidly. Whites, the story went, had had centuries to adapt to the changes marked by the agricultural and industrial revolutions, to learn how to use science and technology to gain control over the environment, and to absorb what it meant to leave superstition behind and embrace the rational mindset and disciplinary practices that were the hallmarks of modernity. Native Americans, in contrast, were experiencing a sudden encounter with "civilization," and thus lacked the luxury of time. As L. M. Hardin, an agency physician with the BIA, commented in 1898, "the transition from a stage of savagery to that of prospective citizenship within one generation furnishes a good field of operation for the tubercle bacillus."[17]

At the same time, primitiveness allegedly protected Native Americans from diabetes. We have already encountered this logic in explanations for why Jews suffered disproportionately from the disease. As noted earlier, Emil Kleen, author of one of the standard texts on diabetes at the turn of the century, had attributed the Jews' high rate to their "greater intellectual exertion, keener emotions, [and] higher nervous development." By the same token, he added, "among all people beyond the pale of culture, diabetes is very rare." Keen included in this group "Africans," "the Indians of America," and "the numerous and various aborigines of Australia, or in the English colonies of mixed but predominant colored population." For John R. Williams, a physician who presented his views to the Vermont State Medical Society in 1917, it was evident that "nomadic tribes and peoples living in a primitive state, rarely if ever have diabetes. . . . It would seem therefore that diabetes is a product of civilization."[18]

The conviction that Native Americans were being spared from diabetes and other diseases that afflicted whites led at least one BIA physician to claim that the Dineh had "with the exception of the diseases introduced by the white man, a good health record." Salsbury made this assertion in 1937, one year after the government published the results of a study conducted by the Public Health Service that claimed the Dineh suffered from higher rates of tuberculosis than any other Indian tribe. But Salsbury, as his own comment made clear, was not thinking about infectious diseases; instead, he was drawing attention to the relative absence of diseases that afflicted "the white man." In fact, Salsbury believed that by studying the Dineh he might be able to find "the solution of some of our most perplexing [health] problems."[19] "Our" clearly referred to the health problems of whites.

The widespread conviction in the first half of the twentieth century was that Native Americans differed racially from whites. This was not to deny some similarities. After all, if Indians and whites had nothing in common, a study of Indians would not reveal anything of use to "the white man." But difference—framed consistently as that between primitive and civilized peoples—informed the explanations offered to account for health disparities. As far as the diabetes literature was concerned, a robust conversation about the nature of these differences, including whether or not they even existed, did not occur until the 1960s. But decades earlier, a leading diabetes specialist had tried to question the allegedly lower rate of diabetes rates among Indians. No one, though, had listened.

From Immune to Especially Susceptible

Elliot Joslin was confused. From his own studies of diabetes he had become convinced that morbidity rates followed a clear pattern: the disease was prevalent where people were old and obese, women outnumbered men, and there was a high proportion of Jews. Yet recent studies had indicated that Arizona had a diabetes mortality rate one-fourth that of Rhode Island, despite any apparent differences in the demographics of the two states. Realizing that access to medical services and accurate death records could affect the reliability of the data collected, Joslin set out for Arizona in the late 1930s, convinced that "field work" could make sense of something that "armchair statistical studies" might overlook.[20]

Joslin had the support of the Arizona Board of Health, the Arizona State Medical Society, and the Veterans and Indian bureaus, all of which helped him to survey each doctor in the state either by mail or in person. He also visited prisons and mental institutions to ascertain the number of individuals diagnosed with the disease, and administered urine tests when he deemed it necessary to confirm a diagnosis. Joslin collected data on Indians, Jews, physicians, clergymen, prisoners, and the insane. In the end, he concluded that the diabetes rate in Arizona was every bit as high as that of Rhode Island. Previous surveys, he contended, had been wrong for three reasons: they had failed to adjust for age and sex; they had not canvassed the various populations in the state; and they did not recognize that Arizona death certificates rarely listed diabetes as a secondary cause of death.

To Joslin, the Native American population was just one of several groups whose rate of diabetes had been underestimated, but in no other case did his conclusion pose so direct a challenge to widely held beliefs. His confidence did not rest on solid data, which he confessed had been difficult to attain. Native Americans, he found, either avoided physicians and hospitals, or their homes were too dispersed for him to visit them all. Indeed, in a blunt statement that hinted at the prejudice with which he viewed those he was studying, he commented that "hunting diabetic Navajo Indians is a rather exhausting sport." In the end, Joslin found only seventy-three cases of diabetes in the nine tribes he surveyed. But reasoning that at best only one-half to two-thirds of the population had been included in the survey, he recalculated his data and concluded that "diabetes in Arizona is just as common among Indians as among the rest of the population."[21]

Joslin's entire perspective was shaped by his conviction that diabetes is a universal disease. This conviction had led him to reject claims that race had anything to do with the high rate of the disease among Jews, and it was now informing his interpretation of the data he gathered about Arizona Indians. To be sure, Joslin probably did uncover previously hidden cases of diabetes during his survey, which would have increased the rate he documented for Native Americans, but it is also evident that he had traveled to Arizona looking for support for his theory about the universality of the disease.

This became abundantly clear when he was trying to figure out why, of the seventy-three cases of diabetes he had found among the Native populations, only four had been Navajo, while ten were Papago, twelve were Apache, and twenty-one were Pima.[22] Even the way he posed the problem is telling, for raw numbers by themselves are meaningless. What if he had found only four individuals with diabetes among the Navajo because of the difficulty he had had collecting accurate information from the widely dispersed tribe? What if that number said nothing about the prevalence of the disease in the population? That Joslin, who possessed decent statistical skills, did not recognize this logical error suggests that he viewed this less as a puzzle and more as an opportunity to drive home what he already thought he knew about the disease—and the different tribes. He wrote: "the Navajos are no-mads and the Apaches herdsmen, and the Pimas depend on agriculture and I understand harvest their crops on shares, allowing the Papagos to do most of the work."[23] In other words, those who stay fit avoid diabetes, while those who do not engage in physical activity develop it.

One might imagine, given Joslin's prestige, that his message would have had an effect on the national conversation about Native Americans and dia-betes. But that did not happen, not even after he published his findings in the medical profession's flagship publication, *Journal of the American Medi-cal Association*. This is not to say that his article was ignored. In fact, his message about the universality of diabetes received considerable press. But near silence met his explicit assertion that Native Americans suffered from diabetes at rates comparable to those of whites. Later in the decade, Fred T. Foard, the newly appointed director of medical services at the BIA, was still naming high infant mortality, low life expectancy, and in particular deaths from tuberculosis and intestinal infections as the greatest challenges facing him at his new job.[24] He did not even mention diabetes.

Twenty years later, the situation was radically different. Study after study drew attention to the extraordinarily high rate of diabetes among Ameri-can Indians. The Akimel O'odham in particular had been shown to have high "postprandial blood sugars" at a rate "more than ten times the rate for the whole country," and they were not the only tribe for which this was true.[25] What had happened in those two decades to change the narrative so completely?

Had Joslin been alive—he died in 1962—he might have insisted that people were being diagnosed who had previously gone undetected, and in part he may have been correct. In the 1960s, when researchers began interviewing tribal members to gather data about family histories of the disease, they heard stories of older relatives who had diabetes. Interviews with the Akimel O'odham, for example, revealed that 44 percent of those who knew they had diabetes had a grandparent, parent, uncle, aunt, or child with the disease. Those conducting the study actually considered this a low estimate, reasoning that the "lack of medical enlightenment in earlier generations" may have meant that individuals who were asymptomatic were missed. And this led some to wonder whether the "'de novo' appearance of diabetes" in Native American communities might not be more apparent than real. At the very least, it suggested that the jump in rates should "be considered against a background of medical ignorance and limited medical care as well as a presumably shorter life span in times past."[26]

Yet it is unlikely that the discovery of hidden cases alone can explain the perceived rise in diabetes rates. As the previous comment suggests, more people were also surviving to an age when chronic diseases normally develop, in large part because the advent of effective antibiotics had reduced mortality rates from tuberculosis and other infectious diseases. We must also keep in mind that chronic diseases pose a disproportionate burden on populations living in grinding poverty. Thus, as conditions on reservations stagnated, as Native American populations became increasingly dependent on government subsidies, and as health care facilities on reservations continued to ignore the social determinants of health, diabetes rates inched up.[27]

By the 1960s, any talk of Native Americans' immunity to diabetes had disappeared. Native peoples were instead being reimagined as particularly susceptible to the disease, much as Jews had been decades before. Indeed, in the span of roughly a decade—between 1960 and 1973—over fifty Native populations became subjects of diabetes studies in the United States alone, much of the research funded by the U.S. Public Health Service. The motivation for these studies was in part to improve the health of Native Americans. But in the decades after World War II, as chronic diseases came to be defined as the greatest threat to the health of the entire nation, Native Americans emerged as ideal research subjects.[28] That this research occurred at roughly the same time that the discipline of human genetics was taking form meant that considerable attention would be focused on genes.

The Hunt for "Isolated Communities"

Thirty years earlier Native Americans had been identified as ideal research subjects for a different study—one on the efficacy of the bacillus Calmette-Guérin (BCG) vaccine in treating tuberculosis. The justifications for the vaccine trials, carried out in the 1930s, were largely repeated decades later when medical personnel shifted their focus from tuberculosis to diabetes. In both cases, researchers emphasized the unusually high disease rates in the Native populations. They also pointed to ease of access to the sick and their families, facilitated by the geographical containment of the populations on reservations, as well as the existence of a central medical infrastructure, in place because of the government's legal obligation to provide health care to its wards. Finally, low education levels among the reservations' inhabitants suggested that consent would not pose a problem. Put differently, researchers hoped that the individuals they were studying would ask fewer questions and be more trusting and compliant.[29]

Postwar diabetes studies also resembled those carried out earlier in the century by continuing to conceive of Native bodies as laboratories for the production of knowledge about disease. But instead of testing the efficacy of a specific treatment, scientists now probed Native bodies for insights into the genetics of a disease believed to have a significant heritable component. Such studies, they believed, would reveal much about the relationship among race, genetics, and disease.

Human genetics, at the time, was growing in stature as a field of study. It had been a long road. After the war, human geneticists had tried hard to make a sharp distinction between their goals and those of prewar eugenicists. In popular and professional journals, at conferences and public lectures, they joined anthropologists in denouncing the racism of their predecessors in general and the idea of fixed racial typologies in particular. Those preoccupied with race science, they contended, had assumed the existence of a specific number of human races and then searched for traits that could best explain the human divisions with which they had begun. The new understanding of race, in contrast, started with the data, and looked at the distribution of traits across the many different human populations for evidence of differences in "the frequencies of some gene or genes." As the British anthropologist Ashley Montagu announced: "This is a very different conception of race from that which until comparatively recently prevailed among most zoologists and anthropologists, who were accustomed to thinking of races in terms of absolute phenotypical differences rather than in terms of relative differences in the frequency distribution of traits or genes."[30] This meant, he pointed out, that an individual might very well belong to different races depending on the trait being studied.

Human geneticists also chided their predecessors for obsessing over such vague traits as feeblemindedness, and for advocating coercive measures aimed at limiting the reproduction of the eugenically "unfit." In contrast, they emphasized their commitment to the scientific study of the genetics of disease and their hope that the knowledge they produced would eventually translate into therapeutic interventions. In the best of all worlds, that intervention would involve the repair of damaged genes, but human geneticists recognized that the eradication of hereditary diseases would also have to involve decisions by disease carriers not to reproduce. They insisted, however, that the counseling they were promoting in the new genetics clinics cropping up around the country had nothing to do with the compulsory measures still on the books in many of the states. Instead, they emphasized voluntary decisions, made by an enlightened citizenry in consultation with their (informed) physicians, which would lead to a reduction in, if not elimination of, hereditary diseases.[31]

The lines that human geneticists were drawing were never as clear as they imagined. Fears about the deterioration of the human race and threats to the integrity of the human gene pool persisted throughout the 1950s and 1960s. Indeed, during a symposium on genetics at the 1958 annual meeting of the American College of Physicians, James Neel asked his colleagues whether "in our concern for the individual" we might have "forgotten to set up the team which has as its concern the species as a whole?"[32] Still, whatever blurring we may see today, Neel and his peers were evidently able to convince themselves—and others—that their goals were benevolent, not nefarious.

This ethical success was matched by innovations in research techniques, which solved several problems that had stymied genetics research in the first decades of the twentieth century. During those early years, those interested in genetics (following the heady rediscovery of Mendel's research on pea plants) had been limited to working with simpler study animals such as the fruit fly, or *Drosophila*, because no one had been able to figure out how to study human genetic material. According to Neel, the fruit fly "was small, easily manipulated, rapidly reproducing, and had only four pairs of chromosomes, which made assigning genes to chromosomal locations relatively easy." Developments in cytogenetics in the 1950s and 1960s, however, finally allowed those interested in studying humans to see inside the nucleus. Victor McKusick, a leading figure in medical genetics, rhapsodized that rendering the chromosomes visible meant that genetics now had its own "organ" and was, thus, akin to other medical specialties.[33]

But the path from rendering chromosomes visible to linking a particular genetic anomaly to a specific disease was long and arduous (and remains so even today). Diseases like sickle cell anemia, cystic fibrosis, and Tay-Sachs that are caused by a single-point mutation at a specific locus on a particular chromosome are extremely rare. Instead most diseases, diabetes among them, are far more complex, dependent not only on the interplay of many different genes but also on environmental factors. In such cases, searching for a genetic marker—a specific gene or DNA sequence that all individuals with diabetes would have—presented enormous challenges. Hence Neel's description in 1976 that diabetes is "a geneticist's nightmare."[34]

Human genetics research in the decades following the war thus encountered a host of obstacles. The difficulty of identifying genetic markers meant that much research continued to rely on the mapping of family pedigrees to determine whether specific diseases had been passed down according to standard Mendelian patterns of inheritance. As human geneticists well knew, the ideal populations for identifying this pattern were those who had "bred true," meaning that the genetic makeup of the trait under study was the same for every member of the population. Mendel had made sure that his tall pea plants and his short pea plants were true (homozygous) before conducting his famous experiments. The scientists who had studied *Drosophila* did the same. Since human geneticists could not control the breeding patterns of their study populations, they did the next best thing: they looked for population "isolates." These were groups of individuals living in geographic isolation who had a higher rate of intermarriage than usual, thus increasing the percentage of individuals who would be homozygous for a specific trait.[35]

Isolated communities throughout the world were sought for such studies. In the United States, human geneticists considered the Amish ideal for this purpose because they shared a common origin in Western Europe, were easily identified, and forbade marriage with members of other faiths, thus limiting genetic admixture. Still no group received as much attention as Native Americans, who excited researchers not only because their genetics, presumed to be simpler than that of other populations, promised to lead to greater knowledge of disease, but also because it was hoped that the study of their "primitive" bodies would shed light on the evolution of traits. At a meeting of human geneticists and physical anthropologists at Cold Spring Harbor in 1950, which drew scientists from all over the world, the level of anxiety was palpable as one researcher after the next voiced concern about developments that were leading "isolates to lose their identities," and in the worst cases to totally "break down and disappear." Almost twenty years later, Neel was still describing Native Americans as "one of the last great resources for the study of primitive man, one of the last opportunities to attempt to fathom the nature of the forces to which man was responding during the course of human evolution."[36]

Neel's comment makes clear that he and other scientists interested in studying Native Americans were imagining them as frozen in time at an earlier stage of human history. Anxiety about their disappearance stemmed from fear of losing a window onto the past that would allow them to study how natural selection worked to keep human populations in equilibrium with their environments. Of course, in theory, Neel and other human geneticists could have viewed "primitive" populations as simply having different gene frequencies than less "primitive" populations—perhaps as the result of becoming reproductively isolated at some point in time—but the claim that one population represented an early stage in another population's evolutionary development reintroduced not only the notion of stasis, but also of racial hierarchy. Native Americans, they were implying, did not have different gene frequencies because their paths diverged from that of whites; they had different gene frequencies because they had not changed, while whites had. Put differently, they were less evolved. This conviction, which remained unchallenged and indeed often unarticulated, led medical researchers in the postwar period to repeatedly explain away any evidence they encountered that these Native American "isolates" were neither as primitive nor as isolated as they needed them to be.[37]

The view of Native Americans as ideal research subjects, coupled with national concerns about rising rates of chronic disease, contributed greatly to the proliferation of diabetes studies conducted on reservations beginning in the 1960s. Added to the mix were specific worries about the state of Native health. Postwar surveys painted a harsh picture, with one study claiming that life expectancy for the average American Indian was a good twenty-five years behind that for non-Indians. Such alarming statistics revived a conversation, begun in the 1920s, about transferring the Indian Health Service from the Bureau of Indian Affairs to the U.S. Public Health Service. The U.S. Public Health Service had more resources, including a professional path that attracted a large cadre of nurses and physicians, university connections, and funding for research. In 1954 Congress approved the transfer, and almost immediately studies of Indian health increased.[38] Diabetes's secrets were about to be probed.

Unsettling Questions about Semantics and Categories

The U.S. Public Health Service did not waste time. That same year, in 1954, it sent John H. Parks, a physician with the Indian Health Service, to Arizona to evaluate health problems among the Akimel O'odham. Parks was particularly interested in diabetes, but in his attempt to gather information about the disease, he ran into immediate problems. "Differences in culture, language and diet, along with their acceptance of obesity and ignorance of modern medical concepts," lamented Parks, meant that the reservation's inhabitants lacked both knowledge of, and interest in, the disease.

To remedy this, he joined with another physician, Eleanor Waskow, and set up an educational program designed to spread the message that "diabetes mellitus is a potentially serious disease with serious complications." The two physicians also looked for volunteers who would submit to "a careful history, physical examination, and laboratory examination."[39] Their efforts paid off: of the 283 people known to have diabetes, ninety agreed to submit to further study.

Parks and Waskow scoured medical records and death certificates, gathered family histories and urine, and drew blood. What they found offered evidence of what they already suspected: at 4.1 percent, the incidence of diabetes among the Akimel O'odham was roughly three times greater than the 1.4 percent of whites documented during the Oxford study. To Parks and Waskow, this indicated a dire need for an effective public health program, but it also meant that the Akimel O'odham offered "a natural group for the critical study of diabetes." The combination of a high rate of the disease and being "inbred," they explained, meant that the Akimel O'odham made "it possible to trace a single gene back through all branches of the family— something that is impossible in a larger, more diffuse population."[40]

In thinking through how best to explain high rates of diabetes among Native peoples, Parks and Waskow had to contend with disagreements over whether heredity or the environment played a greater role. They knew that Joslin favored environmental factors, like diet and physical activity. But they were more enamored of the work of a physical anthropologist at the University of Arizona who had just completed a general health survey of American Indians living in the Southwest. Bertram S. Kraus, who had recorded significant differences in diabetes rates among the Tohono O'odham, Akimel O'odham, and Apache, admitted that neither the environment nor heredity had "much solid evidence to back it up."[41] But he reasoned that since other traits, like blood type and dentition, differed between tribes and appeared to be controlled by genes, it was likely that differences in diabetes would have a genetic foundation as well.

Kraus challenged Joslin directly in his study. He accused the senior physician of grouping together tribes in order to generate numbers that dampened differences in diabetes rates between Indians in Arizona and whites. He insisted, in fact, that the labels "Arizona Indians" and "United States

Indians" were misleading, since they obscured stark differences between tribes, which mattered when it came to public health.[42]

Kraus's critique of Joslin actually spoke to two issues. The first had to do with understandings of race. In emphasizing intragroup differences, Kraus was clearly working with the new definition of race. At least in theory, he was starting with the data (in this case, differential frequencies of diabetes) and working from there to construct populations, or "races," based on the relative frequencies of the disease. The starkly different rates among the Akimel O'odham, Tohono O'odham, and Apache thus led him to declare a category like "United States Indians" meaningless. Kraus was not, however, denying a link between race and diabetes. Thus, the second issue he addressed had to do with the role of genetics in explaining difference. For Kraus, diabetes even appeared to function as a kind of racial marker, helping him to figure out the relationship among tribes. It could serve this purpose because of his conviction that diabetes was fundamentally a genetic disease.

The differences between Joslin and Kraus were complex. Joslin, who emphasized the role of the environment and rejected the idea that diabetes had anything to do with race, did not hesitate to employ the categories of "white" and "Indian." Kraus, who insisted that heredity mattered more, raised serious questions about the meaning of the old racial categories. Just as they did for other studies of human genetics and chronic diseases in the postwar years, the categories of race, genetics, environment, and disease— their meanings, and their relationships to one another—came together in varied and unpredictable ways.

Drawing on Kraus's work, Parks and Waskow contended that diabetes was primarily a disease of heredity. But believing that genetics could explain the high rate of the disease among the Akimel O'odham did not mean that they knew how a "diabetes-producing gene" worked. They thus recommended "further research on the Pimans," insisting that this tribe and "other inbred Indian tribes with a high incidence of diabetes" formed "a fertile area for future diabetic research" and "a natural group for the critical study of diabetes." By "natural," Parks and Waskow may have meant little more than obvious. But as soon as we probe why they thought the Akimel O'odham made obvious research subjects, we are back at the image they painted of a population that was less evolved intellectually, culturally, and morally. Their repeated use of the word "inbred" reinforced this racial hierarchy and provided scientific justification for the research, since "inbred" populations possessed a degree of genetic homogeneity rarely found elsewhere. For Peter H. Bennett, who would spend forty years studying the Akimel O'odham, this Native group offered an opportunity to "study the nature of diabetes . . . under carefully controlled conditions." The knowledge thus produced, he hoped, would "be of benefit not only to the Pima and other Indians, but to diabetics throughout the world."[43]

Parks and Waskow published their study in 1961. In the following years, hardly a Native group escaped the gaze of medical researchers interested in diabetes. According to Kelly M. West, a leading figure in diabetes epidemiology, roughly eighty populations in North America and the Pacific Islands had been studied by the early 1970s. Explanations for their attractiveness repeated what had long been asserted: because they were confined to reservations, a "single source" provided most of their medical care; and since they tended to be "less mobile," it was easy to get a representative sample of the population. The opportunities for acquiring knowledge about diabetes were thus considerable. Improved care for "the native people," while important, took a back seat.[44]

Only a few of the initial studies of Native populations focused specifically on what might have been driving up diabetes rates. Instead, most investigators simply tried to figure out the disease's prevalence. Was it high, as among the Akimel O'odham? Low, as among the Apache? A table that West included in his 1974 review article brings home the great diversity uncovered (Box 4.1). Importantly, one of the questions that troubled many researchers at this stage of their work was whether the differences they were finding reflected variations in the methods they were employing, rather than actual differences in prevalence. Max Miller, whose team began studying the Akimel O'odham in the mid-1960s, went so far as to label as "arbitrary" the definition they were using of diabetes as "a venous plasma glucose level of 160mg/100ml or more two hours after a 75-gram glucose equivalent load." Indeed, he used "diabetes" with quotation marks to draw attention to the absence of a clear definition of the term. R. E. Henry and his colleagues, who studied the Cocopah Indians, also complained that researchers used different glucose loads in their tests, disagreed about the minimum concentration of blood glucose necessary to identify the presence of the disease, and even tested different bodily substances, some examining the plasma alone while others used whole blood. Thus, not only was there disagreement over the specific number that made someone a "diabetic"; there was also no consensus about what they were measuring. In what can only be considered a vast understatement, a team of researchers studying the Seneca Indians in 1969 remarked that "the nature of diabetes itself is obscure."[45]

Researchers also wondered whether they were dealing with one disease or several diseases. They were unsure because there appeared to be considerable diversity not just in rates but also in clinical symptoms. For example, as West pointed out, a good number of tribes seemed to have unusually low rates of ketosis, the juvenile form of diabetes, and coronary disease, and to tolerate high concentrations of blood glucose without becoming symptomatic. But to conclude that Indians and whites had different forms of diabetes left two problems unresolved: the stark intragroup differences that had mattered to Kraus would still need to be explained. And since the implication was that different diseases would differ genetically, there would need to be consensus that diabetes was, in fact, primarily a genetic disease.[46]

At the time that West wrote his review essay, few were fully convinced that genetics prevailed. To be sure, most researchers believed that diabetes was hereditary, but they were on the fence about whether heredity mattered as much as diet, nutrition, and physical exercise. The populations that gave them greatest pause were the Athabaskan Indians and Eskimos living in Alaska, both of whom appeared to have an unusually low rate of diabetes compared not only to other Native populations, but also to whites. By all accounts, the two Alaskan groups differed from one another ethnically and lived geographically apart, so there was little chance that intermarriage could explain the similarity in rates. What they shared, however, were active lifestyles and diets (heavy on protein with a moderate amount of fat and very little carbohydrates). In addition, Athabaskan Indians living in the southwest of the United States, and who followed a less active lifestyle and consumed a different diet, had higher rates of diabetes than their Alaskan

Box 4.1 Aboriginal populations with high and low rates of diabetes

High rates

Cherokees (North Carolina)
Alabama-Coushattas (Texas)
Choctaws (Mississippi)
Choctaws (Oklahoma)
Kiowas (Oklahoma)
Comanches (Oklahoma)
Pimas (Arizona)
Papagos (Arizona)
Yumas (Arizona)
Hualapis (Arizona)
Havasupis (Arizona)
Cocopahs (Arizona)
Chemehuevis (California)
Pawnees (Oklahoma)
Seminoles (Oklahoma)
Seminoles (Florida)
Washoes (Nevada and California)
Paiutes (Nevada and California)
Caddo (Oklahoma)
Senecas (New York)
Winnebagos (Nebraska)
Maricopas (Arizona)

Omahas (Nebraska)
Mojaves (California)
Sioux (Montana and Dakotas)
Assiniboines (Montana)
Passamaquoddy (Maine)
Cherokees (Oklahoma)
Creeks (Oklahoma)
Chickasaws (Oklahoma)
Cheyenne-Arapahos (Oklahoma)
Osages (Oklahoma)
Sauk-Foxes (Oklahoma)
Kickapoos (Oklahoma)
Shawnees (Oklahoma)
Polynesians
   Hawaiians
   Maoris (New Zealand)
   Rarotongans
Micronesians
   Chamorro females (Guam)
   Chamorro females (California)

Rates probably high

Poncas (Oklahoma)
Otoes (Oklahoma)
Potawatomies (Oklahoma)
Ft. Sill Apaches (Oklahoma)

Delawares (Oklahoma)
Wichitas (Oklahoma)
Kiowa-Apaches (Oklahoma)
Umatillos (Oregon)
Zunis (New Mexico)

Low rates

Eskimos
   Eastern and Western Greenland
   Eastern, Central, and Western
      Canada
   Alaska

Navajos (Arizona)
Hopis (Arizona)
Apaches (Arizona)
Western Shoshones of Nevada
   (1954 report only)

Chippewas (North Dakota)	Polynesians
Athapascan Indians	Ellice Islands
Canada	Pukapukans
Alaska	Western Samoans
Micronesians	Tongatapuns
Truk and Marshall Islands	Tahitians
Gilbert Islands	Melanesians
Paluans of Peleiu and	Fijis
Ngerchelong (Western	Natives of New Hebrides
Caroline Islands)	New Caledonia and the
Chamorro males of Rota	Solomon Islands
(Marianas)	Central American Indians
	Guatemala
	El Salvador

Source: Kelly M. West, "Diabetes in American Indians and Other Native Populations of the New World," *Diabetes* 10 (October 23, 1974): 841–855 (doi.org/10.2337/diab.23.10.841). Adapted with permission from the American Diabetes Association. Copyright 1974 by the American Diabetes Association.

kin. It seemed evident to those who studied these populations—and to those who read about them—that nutrition and physical fitness better explained this particular disease pattern. But was this true of other populations as well? Even the team of researchers who studied the Alaskan populations was reluctant to generalize, allowing for the possibility that "the explanation could be a genetic one."[47]

The flurry of studies conducted on Native Americans in the 1960s and early 1970s raised as many questions as they answered. Some of these were posed explicitly by researchers. West, for example, concluded his review with no fewer than a dozen questions, all of them touching on the reliability of the data. Were the differences even real? If so, how should they be explained? Other questions remained below the surface. For instance, researchers' confusion about new understandings of race became apparent when they tried to explain differences in disease rates. "Diabetes Mellitus in American (Pima) Indians" is the title of an article published in 1971.[48] But was this a study of the Pima, or of American Indians in general? The

implication of the title is that whatever researchers had learned by studying the Pima could be generalized to other (all?) American Indians. But
what happens then to the definition of "race" as a particular set of gene
frequencies?

As we have seen with Kraus, attempts to disaggregate the category
"American Indians" failed repeatedly, due to deep-seated beliefs that Native
populations were fundamentally different than "whites," and, therefore,
that it was permissible to group them together. The 102 citations covering eighty Native populations on which West based his review were filled
with references to difference, and specifically to the "primitive" nature of
the populations under study. This conviction allowed researchers to move
seamlessly from their worries about the methodological messiness of their
work, and their doubts about the reliability of their data, to serious conversations about how to explain the very differences they had just called into
question. Clearly the data alone were not driving their conclusions. If this
were so they would have recognized that only one of two conclusions was
possible at the time: either they knew far too little about the distribution
of diabetes across populations to make any claim about whether racial differences existed; or the stark differences among populations believed to
form a single "race" meant that race could not be a factor. Yet so strong was
the belief in racial differences that even West, who seemed agnostic about
whether race mattered when it came to diabetes, nevertheless believed that
the "evidence," shown in Box 4.1, demonstrated "that rates of diabetes were
higher or lower than in the general populations of North America and Western Europe."[49] In no case were they the same.

But were those differences genetic? In the early 1970s, the jury was still
out. But within a decade it would become common to trace high rates of
diabetes among Native Americans to their genes. To understand how that
happened we need to go back slightly in time to 1967–1968, when David
Rimoin, who would become a leading figure in human genetics, published
four papers offering evidence that Native Americans and whites had different forms of diabetes. Rimoin is still credited today with offering the first
evidence that diabetes was "a genetically heterogeneous group of disorders"
rather than the outcome of a "simple mode of inheritance." But his conclusions, as we will see, were only loosely based on scientific "facts."[50]

The Ascendency of Genetics

David Rimoin earned his M.D. in 1961 from McGill University and his Ph.D. from Johns Hopkins six years later. That was the year he published his first article on diabetes, with the simple title, "The Genetics of Diabetes Mellitus." Rimoin's goal was to figure out why the clinical signs of diabetes were so variable, for without an explanation clinicians would continue to disagree about who, in fact, "constitutes the diabetic patient." He was particularly interested in the marked variability between different ethnic groups when it came to the frequency with which ketosis and vascular complications occurred. Rimoin wanted to know whether these differences could be accounted for by genetics or the environment.[51]

For Rimoin—and for many other scientists of his era—environment meant little more than diet. So he compared the fat content and carbohydrate loads of the diets of eight different ethnic groups with the clinical symptoms most commonly found in their populations, and found no correlation. At this point, a cautious scientist who was not invested in a particular outcome might have considered other environmental factors. Why not explore stress, poverty, access to health care, and co-morbidities? Researchers knew that these factors affected disease rates, even if they did not study them as robustly. Instead Rimoin concluded that "ethnic variability in clinical disease, unrelated to significant environmental factors, suggests genetic heterogeneity."[52] The ease with which Rimoin reduced "significant environmental factors" to diet alone indicates the strength of his conviction that genetics provided the most promising explanation for the disease's clinical variability.

Rimoin did not, however, end his article with that statement. Rather, he went on to suggest several possible mechanisms of gene action that *could* be responsible for the development of diabetes. In other words, his paper offered a compelling case for the possibility—in his mind, the likelihood— that diabetes was "a genetically heterogeneous group of disorders." But it offered no proof, as Rimoin acknowledged. In the end, he admitted that all he had shown was that "genetic factors are important in the etiology of diabetes mellitus."[53]

Rimoin thus set out to find concrete evidence of genetic heterogeneity, and like other human geneticists at the time, he turned to a Native American population. Teaming up with John H. Saiki, who was not only a physician with the U.S. Public Health Service Indian Hospital in Fort Defiance, Arizona, but also his brother-in-law, he studied the Dineh, a population that Rimoin believed to be "genetically distinct."[54]

Rimoin and Saiki began by conducting a retrospective analysis of the 105 Dineh people who had received a diagnosis of diabetes at the Indian Hospital between 1958 and 1963; they also administered oral glucose-tolerance tests to twenty individuals with diabetes and thirteen who served as their control group. Their results confirmed the existence of clinical variability: the Dineh seldom had chronic vascular complications, and they also appeared to tolerate high blood-glucose concentrations without developing evident symptoms of the disease. Recognizing that they still lacked proof that this form of diabetes differed genetically from that of other populations, they designed another study: a comparison of the Dineh with a genetically distinct group. But despite their belief that the Dineh differed genetically from other Native American populations, they chose for their comparison "the European."[55]

One could only wonder about the appropriateness of comparing the Dineh to "the European" (which they also referred to as "white individuals"). Perhaps to resolve this inconsistency, but more than likely to make such a comparison methodologically feasible, they chose to have the Amish stand in for all Europeans, claiming that the Amish had "the typical European form of the disease with all of the acute and chronic complications."[56] Thus instead of limiting their conclusion to a comparison of these two populations—which might have been consistent with new understandings of race—their comparison of the Dineh and Amish became a proxy for comparing Native Americans and Europeans. In this way, old racial typologies slipped back in, operating alongside new understandings of race as a population.

In a final study, Rimoin returned to oral glucose-tolerance tests to determine the prevalence and characteristics of diabetes in the two populations. The results indicated stark differences in both the "clinical and metabolic features of diabetes," further supporting his belief that he was dealing with "distinct disorders." But did genetics explain these differences between the Amish and the Dineh? Rimoin realized that he still lacked such proof, but he believed that "evidence derived from other sources" suggested that genetics was more important than diet.[57] Yet a glance at his bibliography reveals that the source he cited in support of genetics' importance was none other than his own 1967 paper, which, as we have already seen, was about the *possibility* that genetic variability could explain clinical variability. By his own admission, he had not offered any proof.

The only way to make sense of the circularity of Rimoin's reasoning is to acknowledge the strength of his conviction that genetics could best explain clinical variability. Indeed, it was his conviction, rather than his evidence, that drove him to privilege genetics over environmental factors. This conviction also made it difficult for him to fully abandon older understandings of race, and to feel justified in having the Dineh stand in for all American Indians, and the Amish for all Europeans. Others engaged in diabetes research at the time revealed similar struggles. Max Miller, who was rapidly emerging as one of the leading figures in the study of diabetes among the Akimel O'odham, read Rimoin's publications and saw in them evidence that the frequency and types of complications associated with diabetes may "differ in the American Indian from those observed in the Caucasian and the Negro."[58] Rimoin had not, actually, asserted anything that clearly, but it was a short step from comparing the Dineh and Amish to erasing all intragroup differences and returning to the fixed racial typologies of the past.

Rimoin was not alone in drawing questionable links among genes, race, and diabetes. Nor was he alone in citing as proof a paper that had only presented a hypothesis. In 1988, a one-page article in the *Journal of the American Medical Association* summarized the results of a study conducted in San Antonio on diabetes in the Mexican American population. The study had revealed significant differences in diabetes prevalence in three different neighborhoods in the city: the highest, 15 percent, occurred in a predominantly Mexican American low-income neighborhood, followed by 12 percent in a middle-income mixed Chicano and Anglo neighborhood, and finally 7 percent in a largely white suburban neighborhood. But rather than explore whether income might be the determining factor, the researchers reasoned that since previous studies had shown that genetic factors contributed to the high rate of diabetes among the Akimel O'odham, it made sense to conduct genetic tests to determine the percentage of Native American ancestry in these neighborhoods. Sure enough, what they found

was that "in the low-income barrio, the percentage of Native American ancestry was 40% to 45%; in the middle-income area, 25% to 30%; and in the
suburban area, 15% to 20%."[59]

Yet the authors of this study also built their conclusion on questionable
evidence. The rational for conducting genetic tests had been their belief
that heredity best explained the high rate of diabetes among the Akimel
O'odham. In support, they cited a 1983 study by an accomplished human
geneticist, William Knowler. But Knowler and his co-authors had presented
nothing more than a hypothesis. In fact, they had labeled the last section
of their article "hypothesis," not "conclusion," in part because they had relied on family pedigrees for evidence and recognized that family members
who had the genotype but remained asymptomatic would not have been
counted. They did claim that evidence existed "for a genetic component
to diabetes in the Pima," and they cited research to back this up, but their
reference was to a two-year-old study that had "suggest[ed] that there may
be a gene . . . which plays a role in the expression of diabetes in the Pimas."
The authors of this early study had even cautioned that their data did "not
provide conclusive evidence" and had to be considered "an interesting, but
preliminary, report."[60]

In sum, as late as the 1980s little was known concretely about the genetics of diabetes mellitus. That diabetes was in part hereditary seemed probable, but attempts to establish the specific genetics of the disorder had been
unsuccessful. Claims to the contrary continued to populate the literature,
however, often in combination with assertions that the genetics differed
based on race and ethnicity. Joslin's attempt to erase biological differences
between Native Americans and whites had failed. Forty years after he reported on his Arizona findings, the popular explanation for Native Americans' high rate of diabetes centered on their possession of "thrifty genes."

Thrifty Genes—A Eugenicist's Musings

It may seem odd to discuss Native Americans, genetics, and diabetes
without delving into the thrifty gene hypothesis sooner. After all, Neel published his article in 1962 just as studies of diabetes and Native Americans
were gaining steam. But Neel's hypothesis received very little attention in

the decades following its publication.[61] This lack of interest stemmed in part from the absence of any mention of Native Americans in the original paper. Instead, the question driving Neel was how diabetes could have become so widely distributed around the world. He may not have mentioned Joslin's theory of the universality of diabetes in so many words, but he appeared to have a similar picture in mind: like Joslin, he thought of diabetes as a universal disease, not one that had anything to do with specific races. But where Joslin approached diabetes as a clinician, Neel approached it as a geneticist, interested in the evolution of the trait.

This suggests another reason the thrifty gene hypothesis did not have much of an influence on physicians and medical researchers in 1962: they were not Neel's intended audience. Publishing in the *American Journal of Human Genetics*, Neel was thinking about eugenics, not the health of Native Americans. Indeed, Neel concluded his article with a section entitled "Some Eugenic Considerations," where he imagined a future when a "thrifty" genotype might again be advantageous. Giving voice to widespread fears of a "population explosion" that would deplete the world's resources, he wrote of "the mounting pressure of population numbers" that might lead to "an eventual decline in the standard of living with, in many parts of the world, a persistence or return to seasonal fluctuations in the availability of food." If that were to transpire, he reasoned, "efforts to preserve the diabetic genotype through this transient period of plenty are in the interests of mankind. Here is a striking illustration of the need for caution in approaching what at first glance seem to be 'obvious' eugenic considerations."[62]

Neel's worries make more sense if we read them in conjunction with two articles he published in 1958, four years before he put forth his thrifty gene hypothesis. One was on "Medicine's Genetic Horizons," the other on "The Study of Natural Selection in Primitive and Civilized Human Populations." In both, Neel was working through the tensions he experienced as the result of wearing two hats, one as a physician and the other as a population geneticist. Perhaps nothing captures this tension better than the anxiety he expressed in 1958 when he worried that given medicine's "concern for the individual," physicians had "forgotten to set up the team which has as its concern the species as a whole."[63] Small wonder that Neel titled his biography *Physician to the Gene Pool*.

Neither article was about diabetes per se. Instead, Neel was interested more generally in constitutional diseases, which, he claimed, were taking up a lot of the physician's time and arose from people's inability to adapt to environmental changes. Such diseases, Neel noted, were increasing everywhere, but the populations manifesting some of the highest rates were those that were being forced "to make the cultural transition relatively rapidly." The narrative that Neel ended up constructing could have been lifted almost in its entirety from early twentieth-century explanations for why Native Americans had succumbed disproportionately to tuberculosis. Once again, underlying structural inequalities were ignored and the bodies of primitive peoples were imagined as being forced to deal quickly with changes to which more civilized populations had had ample time to adapt. In Neel's rendition of this story, the relevant changes resulted from "the Agricultural and Industrial Revolutions," which made control of the environment easier. But while the genetic systems of "civilized" populations had, through natural selection, slowly adapted to new environmental demands, "primitive peoples [were] being projected in a few generations from a Stone Age to an Atomic Age culture." Through this process, he added, they were being "called upon to telescope into a few generations biological and cultural adaptations which have extended over a period of thousands of years in Europe."[64] The impossibility of adapting that quickly, Neel was arguing, was evident in the increasing rates of hypertension, heart disease, and diabetes.

Neel, however, appeared to be less concerned about the health consequences of this rapid transition than excited about the "priceless opportunity" Native populations afforded to learn something about how genetic systems adapt to new circumstances. As we have seen, Neel's vision of such an experiment built on the assumption that "primitive" societies provided some approximation to early human societies, which were supposedly more subject to the forces of natural selection and lived in greater equilibrium with their environments. Thus, by studying those populations forced to adapt rapidly to changes associated with civilization, scientists "all over the world" had an opportunity to work together to study both the biological pressures on primitive populations and their biological responses. Distressed about what "civilization" was doing to the human race, Neel was convinced that a comparison of "primitive" and "advanced" societies would provide valuable information not only about how natural selection acted on human populations, but also about whether human actions might "unwittingly be thwarting the evolutionary mechanisms for ridding the human species of the undesirable genes which are constantly arising through mutation."[65]

This was the set of concerns that Neel brought to the table when he wrote about thrifty genes. He was trying to figure out how to make evolutionary sense of a widespread disease in order to determine the best way to improve the human race. Native American bodies, he believed, were useful in this endeavor, but it was because they possessed the same genetic system as all other humans. The thrifty gene hypothesis had nothing to do with genetic differences. At least not yet.

Linking Thrifty Genes to "Primitive" Populations

It was left to others to link thrifty genes to Native Americans, which a few researchers began to do shortly after Neel's article appeared. The first may well have been the geneticists John E. Johnson and C. Wallace McNutt, who in 1964 presented their study of roughly six hundred Alabama-Coushatta Indians living in southeast Texas. Johnson and McNutt revealed not only that about 10 percent of this population was "at risk" of developing diabetes (compared to 2 percent for the rest of the country), but also that this high rate had only recently occurred. It was in trying to explain this sudden increase that they turned to Neel's hypothesis, speculating that the "diabetic genotype" had until recently conferred "some survival value" to the Alabama-Coushattas, but that with improvements in diet and a reduction in physical activity, "subjects with the 'thrifty' genotype tended to become obese, to develop overactive anti-insulin homeostatic mechanisms, and eventually clinical diabetes."[66] But they did not think that this tendency was unique to the Alabama-Coushattas. On the contrary, like Neel, they viewed the thrifty gene hypothesis as a potential explanation for the widespread distribution of diabetes throughout humankind.

Gradually, though, other researchers began associating thrifty genes solely with Native Americans and other indigenous populations. In 1968, a geneticist with the National Institute of Dental Health drew on Neel's hypothesis when he speculated "a bit more than was perhaps warranted by

the data . . . that virtually all Indians may be of a genetic constitution especially susceptible to diabetes." Eight years later, an Australian endocrinologist also found the thrifty gene hypothesis helpful when trying to figure out
why four South Australian Aboriginal populations had unusually high rates
of diabetes. "It is conceivable," P. H. Wise wrote, "that the diabetic genotype
in the Aboriginal also conferred a survival benefit under native-dwelling
conditions, only to be rendered deleterious by urbanization." For the geneticist William Knowler, writing in 1981, thrifty genes helped to explain
high rates among the Akimel O'odham, as well as "other American Indian
tribes, Polynesians, and inhabitants of several other Pacific Islands, including Nauru." He also believed it might be responsible for high diabetes rates
among populations "following migration," such as Yemenites and Kurds in
Israel, and Japanese in Hawaii. But instead of considering that such a large
group might suggest a universal genotype, Knowler concluded that observations of all of them "are consistent with Neel's hypothesis that diabetes
results from the introduction of a steady food supply to people who have
evolved a 'thrifty genotype.'"[67]

Slowly, the number of studies mounted that linked thrifty genes specifically with "primitive populations." Newspapers picked this up as well,
informing readers that Native Americans were "at special risk because of
their history and genetics."[68] No one, however, advocated more fervently
on behalf of the thrifty gene hypothesis than the Australian Paul Zimmet.
Founder and director of the International Diabetes Institute, Zimmet published an article in 1979 in which he sounded an alarm about the "medical
effects of social progress" evident among Pacific Islanders. Worried about
rapidly rising rates of chronic degenerative diseases—and especially of diabetes—Zimmet noted that the rates were high only among those Pacific
Islanders who had "adopted a Western life-style" by shifting from a subsis-
tence to a cash economy. In contrast, the disease remained "rare in Mela-
nesians, and also in Polynesians, Micronesians, and Australian Aboriginals
who retain[ed] their traditional life-style." To Zimmet, who recognized the
important role played by rising obesity rates, reduced physical activity, consumption of processed foods, and stress, the greatest risk factor was by far
genetics. "It appears," he wrote, "that these people may have a 'diabetic
genotype' that is unmasked by the change in life-style."[69]

Much in Zimmet's article is reminiscent of Neel's 1958 article, in which the older scientist had grappled with the health consequences of rapid change. Thus, in trying to explain why rates of chronic non-communicable diseases among Pacific Islanders had recently surpassed that of whites, Zimmet referred to the "enormous social and technological revolutions" to which people in the West had had centuries to adapt, but which had left "Pacific Islanders and their social, cultural, and economic patterns . . . untouched." Then, however, "in the space of a few years, the Pacific Islanders were parachuted into the 20th century."[70]

Once again, the populations succumbing to disease in record numbers were being imagined as forced out of isolation after centuries of total stasis. Once again, they were cast as frozen in time, unchanging and backward, because they had neither initiated nor experienced the birth of Western science and technology. In this regard, Zimmet was simply recycling an image of native populations as primitive and thus unable to deal with the demands of modern society. Like Neel, despite being acutely aware of developments that had virtually destroyed local economies and infrastructures, he sought the reason for high rates of disease in the bodies of the sick. Yet in one significant way Zimmet broke sharply with Neel, for whereas Neel imagined a universal genotype, Zimmet insisted that "these people" alone possessed "a 'diabetic genotype,'" even while admitting he lacked concrete evidence. As he wrote: "While it has been difficult to prove to date, it seems apparent that Micronesians and Polynesians have a hereditary susceptibility to diabetes (i.e. diabetic genotype)."[71]

But to whom did this seem apparent, and based on what evidence? Since Zimmet recognized that he did not yet have proof, he had to assume that his readers would find his assertion reasonable, even probable. And well they may have. But doing so required his readers also to accept "Micronesian" and "Polynesian" as legitimate racial categories. Without that assumption, the entire edifice would have collapsed.

One might counter that Zimmet's claim was no different than asserting that Jews had a hereditary susceptibility to Tay-Sachs disease. But the genetics of Tay-Sachs, which is caused by a single autosomal recessive gene, was already known to be fairly simple in 1979, when Zimmet published his article. In contrast, the genetics of diabetes was still a "nightmare." Also, no one claimed that all Jews had a hereditary susceptibility to Tay-Sachs. Rather, the assertion was that this trait affected only Ashkenazi Jews; Sephardic Jews were no more likely to have the genetic disorder than any other population. In other words, the claims about Tay-Sachs and Ashkenazi Jews did not traffic in older racial typologies.[72]

Zimmet, however, in discussing the various factors that worked to "unmask" the diabetic genotype among Pacific Islanders, employed language that harkened back to early twentieth-century ideas about race and the nervous system. For example, when introducing the idea that "stress may be a diabetogenic factor," he asked his readers to imagine that "an easy-going Pacific Islander may find the change to a desk job or the responsibilities of a senior civil service post quite stressful in relation to his previous traditional lifestyle." Although Zimmet did not elaborate, his comment implied that Pacific Islanders had two choices: they could remain colonial subjects and escape diabetes, or they could expose themselves to the stresses that came with being a colonial power and experience a rise in their blood sugar. Diabetes became in this way not only a sign of a maladapted body, but also a cautionary tale about the costs of progress and a disciplinary tool.[73]

The Problem of Colonizers' "Strange Foods"

The link that Zimmet and others were making between "primitive" populations and rising diabetes rates did not go unchallenged. In the United States, as the Indian rights movement gained strength, Native American activists grew vocal in their demands for tribal sovereignty; for greater input into federal policies dealing with Indian affairs; for recognition of the harms they had suffered as wards of the federal government; and for an end to racist practices that had resulted in Native Americans having some of the lowest levels of education and some of the highest levels of poverty and disease in the nation. They also tackled head-on the meanings ascribed to "primitive" and "civilized," raising questions about how the actions of white people, which had led to the destruction of Native lands, lives, and livelihoods, could possibly be considered civilized.[74]

Activists who focused on Native American health did not shy away from tying rising rates of diabetes directly to colonialism and to the demise of traditional foodways. Thus Mike Myers of the Seneca Nation, who eventually became president and CEO at Network for Native Futures, issued a withering critique in the early 1980s of the actions of "so-called civilized" whites in general and of the Bureau of Indian Affairs in particular. To him the BIA had been little more than a colonial force, responsible for creating "disharmony" in the lives of Native peoples and bringing "strange diseases" to them. Diabetes, for example, had not been a problem until "invaders" stole Native lands, harmed the environment, destroyed traditional means of procuring foods, and forced Native peoples to rely on "strange foods from the colonizers," which made them sick.[75]

The plight of the Akimel O'odham drew particular attention. In a 1974 article in *Akwesasne Notes,* a publication of the Mohawk Nation dedicated to informing its 65,000 subscribers about general Indian affairs, readers learned that this tribe had "the highest recorded frequency of diabetes in the world." But they also learned that the Akimel O'odham had once prospered and been well nourished, using the Gila River to irrigate their lands and grow an abundance of food. The situation had changed in the late nineteenth century when "white settlers dammed and diverted the flow of the Gila River, making an agricultural existence impossible." These actions dried up the land, denuded the valley of trees, and led to mass starvation and, eventually, government rations. From this perspective, the problem was not thrifty genes or poor lifestyle choices, but rather "new diets, economic disaster, and social stress."[76]

The "new diets," which the government began providing in the nineteenth century, consisted primarily of flour, lard, coffee, sugar, salt, tobacco, beef, and salt pork. In the words of a Dakota woman, white people distributed these rations as "a way of assuaging the pangs of conscience" they felt for stealing Native lands. But she considered such food stuffs to be poor substitutes for the corn, squash, and beans that Native people had previously grown on their lands, and the wide variety of fruits, nuts, and edible roots they had once gathered. She also pointed out that enforced dependency on rations meant that Native people no longer engaged in the physical activity demanded by farming and hunting. To her, therefore, "the beginnings of diabetes" had to be located at the moment that "the Whiteman came and coveted the land." Later developments only made this unhealthy state of

affairs worse. As others pointed out, in the 1960s trading posts began adding to their shelves calorie-dense junk foods, such as chips, pre-packaged
sweets, and soda. Supermarkets with a more nutritious selection of foods
were often geographically inconvenient and financially out of reach.[77]

The Akimel O'odham had been farmers before being deprived of access
to the river that had made their lands arable. But they were not the only ones
who had suffered. Native Americans on the Great Plains, in the Northwest,
and in the East, who had hunted bison, fished and gathered berries, and
grown maize, squash, and beans on river banks, all had stories to tell of how
federal policies had either intentionally destroyed the natural resources
they had relied on for physical and spiritual nourishment, or had facilitated
and legitimized white takeover of Native habitats. The end result was forced
dependence on foods low in nutrients and high in sugar and fat.[78]

Thus for Native American activists, "strange diseases" like diabetes, kidney failure, and respiratory ailments were not evidence of their bodies'
primitive nature but rather were symbolic of white peoples' attempts to
eradicate them either through assimilation or by extermination. "It used to
be tuberculosis and other diseases that were brought to us," commented
one Dakota woman, "and now it is diabetes." Some even drew connections
between high mortality rates from diabetes and the near eradication that
Native peoples had suffered when white people had exposed them to smallpox. The method of delivery may have been less direct than transmitting a
smallpox virus, but the promulgation of policies that made Native peoples
"totally dependent on the colonizers" for food had been no less effective in
causing physical and spiritual harm.[79]

Native American activists highlighted as well the role of poverty in driving up diabetes rates. Peter MacDonald drew a link between the two in
1970 during a talk he gave at a nutrition conference in Fort Defiance, Arizona, just four months after he was elected chair of the Navajo Tribe. Viewing it as shameful that anyone in the United States—the richest nation in
the world—should go hungry, he pointed out that even those with enough
to eat can be malnourished. Diets rich in fats and carbohydrates and lacking in fresh fruits and vegetables can lead, he explained, to diabetes and
gallbladder problems. But rather than blame individuals for making bad
choices, MacDonald claimed that poverty mattered as much here as it did
in cases where people grew ill and died for want of any food. "Water short-

age, sub-standard housing, lack of refrigeration, dependence on high-priced trading posts [that] seldom have milk, eggs, and vegetables available" were all making it difficult if not impossible for Navajo people to grow their own produce or purchase healthy foods. No wonder "hunger and malnutrition" flourished. Dr. Taylor McKenzie agreed fully. The first Navajo to graduate from an accredited medical school, he pushed for passage of the Indian Health Care Improvement Act in 1976. Drawing attention to unconscionably high rates of tuberculosis, otitis media, and diabetes on Native reservations, he insisted that "the only reason" for so much sickness "is lack of money." A few years later, when giving the keynote address at a meeting on the health of the Navajo Nation, he grew even more pointed: how, he insisted, could anyone expect healthy choices from people whose per capita annual income was eight hundred dollars? The health of Native peoples, he insisted, depended on first raising their standard of living.[80]

In the case of diabetes, tackling poverty before anything else was all the more critical because inadequate resources raised levels of stress, which directly affected blood glucose levels. "I think I have gotten diabetes because I have been under so much stress with problems at home," commented one woman of the Devil's Lake Sioux Tribe.[81] She described a fractured family life, with children either dead or no longer in contact with her. A member of the Yurok tribe echoed her words, forging a similar link between stress and diabetes, although she tied it directly to racist policies advanced by the government. When she was interviewed in the early 1990s, she mentioned a flare-up of her disease, which she attributed to learning that her son had been killed, but for her this was also reminiscent of the violence that her mother—who also had diabetes—had experienced as a student.

Feeling thirsty, sleepy, and craving junk food, fat, sugar. . . . Sugar diabetes! Just like my mother, she couldn't take those memories either. Boarding Schools, you know what that's all about? Being kicked like a dog, slapped across the face for saying one little word in Yurok, feeling guilty about the very color of your skin. We, the redskins! You feel like giving up. No wonder your blood sugars go way up there![82]

This woman offered a radically different explanation of what was happening to her than the genetic model implied. She still spoke of inheritance, but rather than receiving "defective genes" from her mother, she inherited memories of being wrenched away from home and forced to attend board-ing school. Boarding schools, established on or near Indian reservations beginning in the 1860s, had been part of the government's plan to solve "the Indian problem" through education and assimilation. In theory, Native American children would improve their knowledge of English, embrace "American values," and acquire skills that would allow them to become eco-nomically self-sufficient. In practice, children encountered understaffed, underfunded, and unhygienic schools, where infectious diseases like tuber-culosis and trachoma flourished, and where they experienced harsh disci-pline and a frontal attack on all aspects of Native American life, including language, dress, diet, religious or spiritual beliefs, and history.[83] This Yurok woman may not have attended a boarding school, but she saw a direct link between her mother's devastating experiences at school and her son's vio-lent death. They were both part of the same story of dispossession, disloca-tion, and alienation. That was what was making them sick.

Native Americans who considered diabetes a product of their violent past were not so much denying a genetic component as suggesting its relative lack of importance. Whether they had heard of thrifty genes in the 1970s and 1980s is unclear, but if they had, they might have accepted its basic tenets: that some Native American tribes had a predisposition to the dis-ease that had been unmasked by historical events. But whereas Neel, Zim-met, and others described those historical events as parachuting "primitive" peoples into modern society—with the implication that to be modern was good—activists focused on the trauma that their ancestors had experienced as a result of their forced encounter with white settlers. This is the perspec-tive they wanted the next generation to learn, and once they began establish-ing their own schools in the 1970s, this is also what they taught.

Thus in 1981, one year after the Akwesasne Freedom School opened its doors on the Mohawk reservation in upstate New York, high-school students were introduced to a unit on health, colonialism, and native people. The school, along with freedom schools established on other reservations, was committed to teaching students the language, history, philosophy, and cul-ture of their tribe. Food—especially traditional foodways—was part of that education. To disseminate its curricular program widely, the Mohawk Na-tion provided a detailed description of the food unit in a section of their newsletter, *Akwesasne Notes,* dedicated to the "Native child." The title of the article, "Native People, Colonialism, and Food," said it all. It began with a description of the foods that Native peoples had once "hunted, trapped, fished, gathered . . . and raised," during which time they had been healthy, able to run great distances, give birth easily, heal quickly when wounded, and live to an advanced age. Only when colonizers destroyed the environment— including people, plant and animal life, air, water, wind, soil, grass, and weather—did Native people develop "cancer, diabetes, heart disease," and a host of other conditions. "Some people call colonialism 'progress' or 'civilization,'" the article continued, "but it is a process that causes destruction and damage to all living things. It is unhealthy. The colonizers justify the damage they bring, by saying that native people are 'primitive' and needed to be 'civilized.' These are very tricky words that they use to confuse us."[84]

Seeking to overturn standard definitions of primitive and civilized, Native American activists taught the next generation about the dark underbelly of "progress," where the remains of civilizations the "Whiteman" deemed unworthy of existence could be found. Fortunately, those civilizations could also be rediscovered, reclaimed, and revived. The central message was, therefore, that to improve their lives Native peoples had to focus not on their bodies, but on reclaiming material resources and recovering the rich and healthy past that colonizers had tried to destroy. This message remains at the heart of the current Native American food sovereignty movement, which sees Native control of indigenous foodways as critical to the promotion of health, nutrition, and economic stability, as well as to the restoration of Native cultures and identities.[85]

From this perspective, a focus on the genetic makeup of indigenous peoples appears narrow and misleading. In Kim Tallbear's words, it "deemphasize[s] the political histories upon which Native American sovereignty claims get articulated."[86] And that de-emphasizing or devaluing of the political past is exactly what proponents of the thrifty gene hypothesis continue to do, intentionally or not.

* * *

Lack of evidence has done little to quell interest in thrifty genes. Some of its staying power can be linked to the writings of the evolutionary biologist and popular science writer Jared Diamond. In a brief essay in *Natural History* in 1992 and in a more developed article in *Nature* eleven years later, Diamond drew heavily on the work of Zimmet as he drove a genetic wedge between those populations experiencing an explosive rise in diabetes rates and those "of European ancestry," whose rate appeared to be inching up much more slowly. Although he acknowledged that diabetes was a problem in populations around the world, and he offered an origin story in which he imagined a common genetic ancestry for all human populations, he nevertheless explained the inordinately high rate of diabetes among the Akimel O'odham, Nauru Islanders, and San Antonio residents who had a high "percent of Indian in their genes" to a combination of two factors: a greater frequency of "thrifty" genes as a result of their Indian ancestry, and the population's rapid introduction to a "supermarket-based" Western lifestyle. As a corollary to this story, Diamond hypothesized that the relatively low prevalence of diabetes among white Europeans might reflect an earlier and more slowly paced transition to this lifestyle, which allowed for the gradual "elimination" of "diabetes-related genes."[87]

Diamond and other proponents of the thrifty gene hypothesis always cite Neel's 1962 article, in which he first laid out his hypothesis, while rarely mentioning Neel's subsequent publications—in 1976, 1982, and 1999, one year before his death—when he shared his doubts about his own claims. Although he never fully abandoned the possibility that his general idea would prove valid, he admitted that he lacked a specific mechanism to explain how a "thrifty gene" might have functioned. He also worried that the division of diabetes into insulin-dependent diabetes mellitus (IDDM) and non-insulin-dependent diabetes mellitus (NIDDM), which officially took place in 1979, meant that distinct diabetes genotypes would have to have evolved independently, a possibility he considered unlikely. "If," he explained, "heterogeneity should multiply so that there are as many as, say, 100 entities, then their individual existence could be explained by simple mutation pressure, and the need for the thrifty genotype would disappear."[88]

Neel acknowledged in his later publications that "Amerindians" had an unusually high rate of diabetes. He also pointed out that rates were increasing among Polynesians, Micronesians, Yemenite Jews who had recently migrated to Israel, and the Japanese. Yet to Neel this was simply further evidence of a universal genotype being triggered by changes in the environment. Unlike Zimmet and Diamond, he saw no reason to invoke genetics to explain difference. In fact, by 1999, Neel had, for all intents and purposes, abandoned a genetic solution to the health problems plaguing modern society. Time was too short; the genetics of chronic degenerative diseases were too complex; morbidity rates showed no sign of slowing down; and nothing less than the future of the human race was at stake. Still clearly driven by eugenic concerns, Neel proposed "culture engineering," which, he explained, would involve "a conscious effort to develop in all dimensions the environment (in the broad sense) in which the human genome finds its optimal expression." But by "environment," Neel, like Rimoin before him, meant little more than a radical change in diet. And that change, he insisted, would "require personal discipline in societies that are increasingly hedonistic."[89] Thus, as different as Neel's "culture engineering" may have been from Zimmet's "genetic engineering," in one way they were exactly the same: both placed the source of the problem in the bodies, minds, and actions of those who were sick, failing to recognize the social and historical determinants of health.

Critics of the thrifty gene hypothesis have appropriately charged it with "geneticizing" a disease that is widely accepted to be heavily dependent on environmental triggers, and for "racializing" a disease by downplaying differences within study populations and accentuating differences between them.[90] In doing so, they have had to contend not only with researchers who continue to believe in the validity of the hypothesis, but also with Native Americans who have at times built the idea of thrifty genes into their own explanations of why their communities have such high rates of the disease. An ethnographic study conducted in 2012 with a Southwestern tribe, for example, revealed a diverse array of responses to the question of what caused diabetes. Diet, a sedentary lifestyle, and genetics were mentioned most frequently, and among those who brought up genetics, roughly one-quarter referred to thrifty genes. Yet study participants crafted their own narrative around what it meant to have a "very specific gene pool." Some even referred to their possession of a "survival gene," reading their successful adaptation to past environments as a strength they could use in battling diabetes. The meaning of thrifty genes had not, in other words, been fixed by Neel, Zimmet, Diamond, or any of the other advocates of the hypothesis. In the hands of some Native Americans it became instead a metaphor for "the inherent strength and resilience" of Native Americans "when facing historical challenges."[91]

Study participants also rarely mentioned genes alone. Instead, their responses pointed to an understanding of diabetes's etiology as multifactorial, and to an assessment of their current dilemma as grounded in the history of their tribe as much as in their genes and lifestyle choices. For them, genetics, behavior, and history could not be separated. It is in this vein that Tallbear and other scholar-activists who work at the nexus of race and disease write of "the co-constitution of natural and social orders." High diabetes rates among Native Americans may have a genetic component, but that component cannot be studied in isolation. For the authors of the twenty-chapter edited volume *Indigenous Peoples and Diabetes,* published in 2006, diabetes itself was approached "as a physiological response to adverse, traumatic or stressful life experiences, rather than as a disease in itself."[92] That is not the perspective that dominates today, however. Nor does it describe the approach of health researchers and public health officials who began, in the 1960s, to notice alarmingly high rates of diabetes not only among Native Americans, but among other "minority" populations as well.

5

A Nationwide Hunt for Hidden Disease

White, black, yellow, mulatto, chicano, Creole—respecter of no race or breed—rich, poor, bourgeois, laborer, banker, professor—no arbiter of caste or class—the genic substrate for the syndrome, diabetes mellitus, has become ubiquitous and in the best of us can be suspected as lying only dormant waiting for the right time.

C. P. Kimball, 1972

AS DIABETES DETECTION DRIVES GOT under way in the early 1950s, evidence of the disease in populations that had previously fallen under the radar continued to surface. There was a sense of urgency in finding these hidden cases: the 1947 Oxford study had sounded the alarm that the nation had to take rising diabetes rates seriously, and the postwar discovery of unusually high rates of the disease among Native Americans had only added to the public's concern.

The results of the detection drives were dramatic. By the 1960s, knowledge of diabetes in black communities had increased significantly; by the early 1980s, too, enough research on the disease among the country's growing Mexican American population had taken place that at least one physician assumed his Mexican American patients had "diabetes until proven otherwise." Within a decade, Asian Americans had also joined the list of those suffering disproportionately from the disease. By 1985, when the

U.S. Health and Human Services Secretary's Task Force on Black and Minority Health produced what most came to call the Heckler Report, decades
of research had suggested that whites no longer had a corner on diabetes.
In the words of members of the task force, diabetes had become a disease
that afflicted "minority groups."[1]

The Heckler Report marked the first time that the government pursued
a comprehensive and systematic examination of how racial and ethnic minorities' incidence of chronic disease, and the care they received for these
ailments, differed from the experiences of their white counterparts. Previous annual health reports, relying on variables such as infant and maternal
mortality and life expectancy, had told a story of consistently better health
outcomes for the nation's inhabitants. Margaret Mary Heckler, secretary of
Health and Human Services under Ronald Reagan, along with Thomas E.
Malone, deputy director of the National Institutes of Health, decided to ask
whether all Americans shared equally in this improvement. The results of
their study, released in October 1985, answered this question with a re-
sounding no.

The Heckler Report signified both an end and a beginning. By producing
what amounted to a ten-volume literature survey, it marked the culmination
of decades of research on health disparities. Yet it also sent "shockwaves"
through the nation and led immediately to the creation of the Office of
Minority Health. What surprised readers, and galvanized them into action,
was not the fact of health disparities but their severity so many years after
the civil rights movement had fought for the same rights and privileges
for all Americans that many white Americans could take for granted. For
the leaders of this movement, health care had been a civil rights issue. As
Martin Luther King Jr. had declared in 1966: "Of all the forms of inequality, injustice in health care is the most shocking and inhuman." Yet here,
twenty years later, what one historian has called a long "history of neglect"
had clearly not yet ended.[2]

By the time the Heckler Report appeared, diabetes no longer had a strong
association with middle-class whites; instead, it appeared to be burdening
minority groups disproportionately. This transformation occurred along
with the proliferation of diabetes detection drives, spearheaded by the
American Diabetes Association in 1948. According to an article in *Time*

magazine, these drives, launched to help "find the million unknown diabetics in the United States and Canada," amounted to "one of the biggest manhunts in U.S. History."[3]

That so many of those million were found among populations that were neither white nor middle class can best be explained by the civil rights movement's battle to get the nation to recognize—and then to eradicate—racial and economic injustices. In the words of the historian Michael B. Katz, "the movement transformed the historic links between race, poverty, and opportunity into a national disgrace." To address this disgrace, the Johnson administration had begun to implement policies and programs, most significantly the War on Poverty, which empowered the poor and wove them more firmly into the government's social welfare system. From Medicaid, which transformed "charity" patients into paying customers, to the Office of Economic Opportunity, which funded neighborhood health centers and thus brought physicians and other health care providers into the spaces where the poor resided, the War on Poverty shined a light on the health problems of poor minorities. The result was greater awareness of the burden of chronic diseases on populations whose acute health conditions had previously masked the slow physical deterioration that resulted from diseases like diabetes, cardiovascular ailments, and cancer.[4]

The transformation in the demographic image of diabetes also reflected the increased migration of people from rural to urban areas within the United States, and a second wave of major immigration, this time primarily from Mexico and Asia.[5] Urbanization made chronic diseases more visible among poor minorities as the makeup of America's poor became increasingly diverse. It bears repeating that Margaret Heckler had created a "Task Force on Black and Minority Health," an awkward title that nonetheless signaled the secretary's intent to explore health disparities among not only African Americans, but Native Americans, Hispanic Americans, and Asian Americans as well. Still, the task force addressed neither what these diverse populations had in common, nor what distinguished them from one another. In fact, the report rarely included comparisons among the populations; instead it almost always measured "disparities" in relationship to whites. But questions about the nature of the populations in the study, and their relationship to one another, clearly troubled members of the task force as they grappled with how best to understand the meaning of these health disparities for the nation.

Such confusion may have been inevitable, given the intense debates going on in the 1980s over how race and racial differences should be understood. Attacks on biological race that had begun in the 1930s and intensified in the 1950s had spawned vigorous discussions about the nature of race and its usefulness as an analytical category. The lack of clarity created particular problems for epidemiologists, who struggled with how to classify the populations they were studying, choosing at times to distinguish between whites and "the color groups," or, in an increasingly popular formulation, between whites and nonwhites. But none of these linguistic solutions proved satisfying, since they skirted the issue of why someone should be classified one way or the other. More often than not, "white" continued to be defined in accordance with the one-drop rule; accordingly, anyone believed to have some black ancestry was excluded. "Nonwhite" was even more problematic. As one epidemiologist complained, sometimes it meant "Negro" alone, and other times it included Japanese, Chinese, Indian, and more. Epidemiologists also worried, as two government researchers explained in 1947, that in using poorly understood racial categories they were reinforcing the idea that observed differences stemmed from "inherent racial differences," despite a lack of evidence that this was the case and even though racial classifications often hid "economic status."[6]

Epidemiologists struggled with these problems with each and every disease they studied. With diabetes, however, they had the added dimension that the disease itself was undergoing a significant reconceptualization in the late 1970s. After at least a century of noting that diabetes took different forms depending largely (although not solely) on the age of the person when it first appeared, medical experts sought to eliminate the vagueness and ambiguities in their description of the different types. Driven by a desire to bring increased standardization to the diagnosis and treatment of diabetes, and compelled by the increasing bureaucratization of health services, they officially divided diabetes into discrete types in 1979. Thereafter the medical community referred to the two most common forms as IDDM (insulin-dependent diabetes mellitus) and NIDDM (non-insulin-dependent diabetes mellitus). It also recognized gestational diabetes and MODY (maturity onset diabetes of the young) as discrete categories. Beginning in 1995, IDDM and NIDDM were renamed type 1 and type 2, respectively.[7]

The decision to divide diabetes into distinct categories right at the time that the disease was becoming associated primarily with poor minorities may have been serendipitous, but the consequences were serious nonetheless. This was especially so because the division between IDDM and NIDDM also became a division between races: as early as 1979, epidemiologists had contended that IDDM was more common among whites, while NIDDM was more common among minorities.[8] Eventually these two types would also generate quite different cultural images, with those with type 1 diabetes playing the part of the innocent victim, while those with type 2 were cast as irresponsible individuals making bad lifestyle choices. These different images were decades in the making, but by 1985, when the Heckler Report appeared, hints of this cultural divide were already evident.

The decades between 1950 and 1985 thus rendered diabetes visible among a wide array of peoples whose experiences with the disease had previously received little attention. Accompanying this increased visibility were a set of stories about why particular populations were at greater risk of developing the disease. Like the stories in the past, these were a mix of careful observations and unfounded assumptions and speculations. The most blatant assumption, enshrined by the Heckler Report, was that "minority groups" suffered more from diabetes than "whites"—a conclusion that required that one ignore the extremely high rate of diabetes found increasingly among poor whites. In the end, the omission of this population from the general narrative about health disparities, along with a lack of serious engagement with the role of poverty in driving up diabetes rates among "nonwhites," created a situation in which "hidden diabetics," when they came to light in the postwar decades, were identified through their racial and ethnic affiliations, while the roles of geography and class were left in the dark.

Flipping the Script: Race, Poverty, and Gender

In 1942 Julian Herman Lewis was still complaining that no one was paying attention to rising rates of diabetes among African Americans. A decade later, that was no longer the case. At the very least, diabetes had become a common topic in the black press. "Mrs. Clement Loses Limb" read the title of an article published December 9, 1950, in the Baltimore *Afro-American*. The person in question was seventy-year-old Emma Clarissa Clement, the first African American woman to win the Golden Rule Foundation's "American Mother of the Year" award, which she had received four years earlier. "Mrs. Clement," the reporter mentioned, "is said to be suffering from diabetes," although the reason for the amputation had "not been announced." Subsequent articles shared similar news of the devastation wrought by the disease. One piece, "Drive Opened to Aid Legless Artist," detailed the efforts of Nat Story, a former Saint Louis trombone player, to raise funds for a band member who had "lost both his legs as a result of diabetes" and needed a wheelchair.[9]

Other articles in the African American press focused less on tragedies and more on convincing readers of the importance of early detection for staving off complications and death. "Protect Your Health," an article in the *Black Worker,* shared a father's realization that he had diabetes after his daughter learned about the disease at school. "Medic Says Two Million, Now Well, Will Get Diabetes," announced the *Chicago Defender* as it reported on a talk that Howard University professor Riley F. Thomas had given at a health conference. An announcement about a planned exhibit at the Chicago Museum of Science and Industry, organized by the Chicago Diabetes Association, struck an unusually bright note, promising those who attended that they would receive "cheerful information" about "how to live" with the disease.[10]

It is possible that the increased attention diabetes received reflected an actual rise in rates among African Americans. As morbidity rates from infectious diseases continued to decline after the war, more individuals were living long enough to develop chronic diseases. The drop in infectious disease death rates was striking. Between 1940 and 1960, for example, the overall death rate for tuberculosis among "nonwhites" fell almost 90 percent. Even more impressive was the 95 percent drop among infants younger than one year. Not surprisingly over the same span of time, the life expectancy for African Americans increased by 20 percent from 53.1 to 63.6 years.[11]

Awareness of diabetes may also have been increasing because a far greater percentage of the black population was moving into urban centers as the labor they had once provided on farms became mechanized. In the short fifty-year period between 1910 and 1960, the ratio of African Americans living in rural as compared to urban areas shifted a full 180 degrees, changing from roughly 75 percent rural to around 75 percent urban.[12] With increasing urbanization came increased visibility.

Freedmen's Hospital in Washington, D.C., was one site where diabetes became visible among African Americans. Founded by the federal government in the year of the Emancipation Proclamation, the hospital was initially tasked with providing medical care to formerly enslaved people and training black physicians. By the middle of the twentieth century it boasted 351 beds, a separate tuberculosis wing with an additional 150 beds, and a six million dollar budget. In 1957, Thomas F. Riley, attending physician at the hospital and professor of medicine at Howard University, noted that the number of diabetes patients he was treating at the hospital had increased to three hundred from a mere twenty in 1937. Three years later Lewis K. Atkinson, a fellow in endocrinology at Freedmen's, drew attention to over five hundred black individuals who had been treated in the hospital's outpatient diabetes clinic. Atkinson was especially concerned about the individuals who had not attended the clinic because they were asymptomatic and thus unaware of the "chronic degenerative processes" that, although latent, were causing damage to their bodies. His solution was to recommend routine medical examinations as a way of diagnosing diabetes before it was too late.[13]

Thomas and Atkinson's concern signaled an increased commitment among black professionals to fight diabetes in their communities. This commitment was reflected as well in the National Medical Association's decision in 1950 to support the American Diabetes Association's Diabetes Week. The *Journal of the National Medical Association* also started to increase its coverage of the disease. In 1961, the association's president, James T. Aldrich, used the bully pulpit of his "President's Column" to emphasize that diabetes could be fatal, that anyone could get it, and that those most at risk were overweight, over forty years of age, and had a relative with the disease.[14] Aldrich mentioned nothing about race.

Thus, a full twenty years before the Heckler Report appeared, there was mounting concern that diabetes had become a serious burden on black communities. There was, however, no sense that the problem was more serious for black people than for other populations. If anything, the message was that African Americans could no longer be thought of as immune or protected; they suffered from diabetes just *the same* as anyone else. The claim that they were *more* prone to diabetes emerged gradually as knowledge of chronic health problems among the poor became more visible. But as the "face" of poverty became increasingly black, the role of poverty faded into the background and race became the primary focus.

The racialization and, as I will discuss later, feminization of poverty was, ironically, a partial consequence of New Deal legislation. Agricultural policies that paid land-owning farmers to let their fields remain fallow in order to raise the prices of the goods they produced deprived black tenant farmers of a major source of livelihood. One result was migration to northern cities, but unemployment ran high there as well. The exclusion of farm and domestic labor from the new Social Security benefits also affected the black population—and especially the black female population—disproportionately, denying them the safety net that many white laborers were beginning to enjoy. These policy decisions, along with other discriminatory practices, such as redlining, fueled increasing rates not merely of poverty, but of abject poverty, among black populations.[15]

The extent of the devastation became clear as the civil rights movement directed the nation's attention to the intimate link between political disenfranchisement and economic inequality, and the War on Poverty made government resources available to tackle the problems that were coming to light. When health activists and reformers traveled to the South, for example, they encountered towns where over 50 percent of the population was unemployed, 70 percent of the homes lacked running water, and only a few had toilets. Conditions in inner cities were also eye-opening. For all of these communities, the Office of Economic Opportunity's funding of neighborhood health clinics had a significant impact. From Mound Bayou, Mississippi, to Boston, Massachusetts, to Oakland, California, these clinics revealed the close connections among race, poverty, and disease, and made it clear that the so-called diseases of civilization no longer spared those living in extreme poverty. Writing specifically about diabetes, the director of a clinic in the Mississippi Delta claimed, first, that the disease had gone undetected in the area because there had been no health professionals who might have diagnosed it, and second, that high rates of obesity masked the fact that people were actually malnourished (Figure 5.1). Calories from "potatoes, beans and hominy grits"—a poor person's diet—do not, he pointed out, provide the nutrients people need to keep from getting sick.[16]

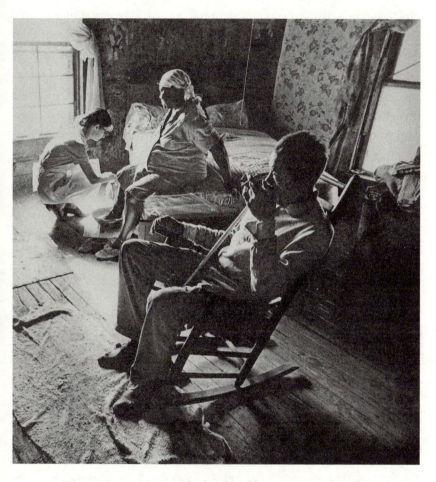

Fig. 5.1. Home visit, neighborhood health center, Mound Bayou, Mississippi. From H. Jack Geiger, "Health Center in Mississippi," *Hospital Practice* 4, no. 2 (1969): 68–81. Reprinted by permission of the publisher Taylor & Francis Ltd., http://www.tandfonline.com.

Neighborhood health centers in urban areas also documented and sought to address high rates of diabetes among poor African Americans. In 1963, for example, the City of Memphis Hospitals helped to create a decentralized network of seven neighborhood clinics and twenty satellite clinics to which the staff referred "patients with stabilized diabetes mellitus, cardiac or hypertensive disease." Five years later, a similar system was established in Atlanta. The clientele at both sites was more than 80 percent black. In time, other clinics opened their doors, and epidemiological studies, such as one begun in Alameda County, California, in 1965, kept repeating the same message: not only did people of color have higher rates of diabetes than whites, but also the gap between black and white people was increasing. By 1971, looking back over two decades of data, the head of the federal government's Division of Vital Statistics noted that between 1950 and 1967 the diabetes mortality rate had increased just 5 percent for whites but 44 percent for "the color groups." This message of disparity appeared as well in an official report delivered to Congress in December of 1975 that laid out a strategic plan for countering rising diabetes rates across the nation. The head of the task force, who had been appointed by the director of the National Institutes of Health the previous year, announced that someone who was "non-white" had a 20 percent greater chance of developing diabetes than a person who was white.[17]

Such statements may have been accurate, but they were also misleading, for they ignored data suggesting that poverty was linked to high diabetes rates as well. As far back as 1935–1936, the National Health Survey on Chronic Diseases and Disability had pointed out that individuals on relief were as much as 50 percent more likely to have diabetes as those "in comfortable circumstances." Roughly a decade later, even Elliott Joslin was noting that the "bulk of all diabetics" were coming from "the lower income group." In 1968, when the Department of Health, Education, and Welfare came out with a *Diabetes Source Book* to provide a concise summary of basic information about the disease to researchers and public health officials, it informed its readers that "diabetes prevalence rates are greatest in low income groups." One year later, public health departments in parts of Appalachia began reporting a diabetes mortality rate twice that of the nation as a whole.[18] Diabetes rates may have been higher among "nonwhites" because a larger percent of them lived in poverty, but the rates among poor whites appeared every bit as high.

The image of the person most at risk of becoming diabetic was not only shifting from middle-class to poor, and from white to black; it was also becoming increasingly feminized. What Leopold and Bowcock had noted in the 1930s, and Wilkerson had repeated in the 1940s, surfaced again in the 1960s as epidemiological studies revealed that the greatest disparity between blacks and whites occurred among women. This was evident in two back-to-back reports published in the early 1960s—one based in Florida and the other in Georgia—both of which noted not only that black women had the highest death rate of any group, but also that their death rate was peaking a full twenty years earlier than for white women. Researchers who mined national rather than state records uncovered similar patterns, noting in addition that the gap between white and black women had increased over time. A review of a quarter century of national data revealed, for example, that between 1949, when the diabetes mortality rate for black women had first surpassed that for white women, and 1957, the gap had nearly doubled from 5.4 percent to 10.4 percent. By 1969, the *Diabetes Source Book* was reporting that nonwhite females had roughly twice the rate of diabetes as white females and nonwhite males. Ten years later, a headline in *Ebony* magazine identified black women as the "No. 1 Victims" of diabetes. And by 1981, an article in the *New York Amsterdam News* warned that "except among certain Indian tribes, such as the Pima Indians, Black women suffer more diabetes than any other population groups." No one, however, pointed out that after Native Americans, black women had the highest poverty rate of any demographic group in the country. This was especially the case among the elderly, who were most prone to develop diabetes: statistics from 1981 revealed that while 20 percent of all elderly women lived below the poverty line, that number rose to 43.5 percent for black women.[19]

Why rates were increasing for African Americans, and especially for African American women, remained unclear. In fact, most studies at the time shied away from trying to explain the disparities they were identifying. Instead, they read like fact-finding missions, focused primarily on detecting and documenting the places and populations where diabetes seemed to be most prevalent. There were good reasons for waiting before drawing conclusions. William Peter Uprichard Jackson, a South African diabetes specialist, complained in 1970 that despite the increase in epidemiological studies, "there is apparently no good knowledge of any prevalence rate among American Negroes." Jackson, who was interested in the relationship between race and diabetes in different countries around the world, insisted that comparisons could not be made until standardized procedures were followed. Yet most studies relied on restricted and "biased samples," did not specify their methods, and did not explain their criteria for judging a particular result "abnormal." Studies that relied on death certificates were particularly problematic, he added, since "fashions change" when it comes to recording cause of death. None of this prevented him from providing an analysis of 125 articles on race and diabetes from a significant number of different countries, and concluding that "environmental factors, most clearly related to famine or feasting," were probably most responsible for whatever variations appeared. But he did not feel that he could rule out "intrinsic genetic 'racial' influences."[20]

Jackson's reluctance either to privilege biological race or to rule it out was common in writings on African Americans and disease in the 1970s and 1980s. The kind of genetically inflected theories that monopolized discussions of diabetes among Native Americans were simply absent. The epidemiologist Kelly West, who played a central role in drawing attention to high diabetes rates among Native Americans—and whose 1978 text, *Epidemiology of Diabetes and Its Vascular Lesions,* provided the most thorough and up-to-date compendium of knowledge on the disease—made clear his preference for "environmental rather than racial factors" in explaining diabetes rates among black people. The few researchers who did wonder about "innate" racial differences either expressed doubts or seemed hesitant, like Jackson, to make any definitive claims.[21]

Instead, discussions of risk factors tended to emphasize the same risks that appeared in writings on diabetes in other populations, namely heredity and obesity. Lewis Atkinson referred to them as "the two most important predisposing factors in the development of diabetes," clarifying that by heredity he meant "family history." Since he had analyzed patient records at Freedmen's Hospital, and not the individuals themselves, he lacked information on the family histories of those who had received care at the hospital, but he did have their weights, and he calculated that 72 percent had been obese before they had been diagnosed with the disease. Indeed, appearing to channel Joslin, he referred to diabetes as "largely a penalty of obesity," adding that "the greater the obesity the greater the likelihood of the penalty." His message was considered important enough that the *Atlanta Daily World*, the city's oldest black-owned newspaper, covered his research in an article titled "72% of 506 Diabetic Clinic Patients Previously Overweight." Clearly, the newspaper believed that this title would grab the attention of its readers.[22]

Atkinson said nothing about the distribution of obesity by sex, although his data showed that 72 percent of the 506 individuals who had diabetes were obese and that the same percentage was female. Other researchers were more forthright and attributed the gender disparity among black diabetes patients to women's greater adiposity. West believed the best explanation was that "black women are quite fat." To support the link he was establishing between fat and diabetes, he mentioned studies about the inhabitants of Malta and Hawaii, the New Zealand Maoris, several Native American tribes, Australian Aboriginals, Sumo wrestlers in Japan, and others. He also brought up earlier studies that had attributed high rates of diabetes among Jews to their propensity toward obesity. He did not, however, suggest that any of this had to do with inherent racial traits. On the contrary, although his position was unusual for the time, he seemed more inclined to attribute the high rate among black women to the fact that a high percentage of them lived below the poverty line. This is consistent, he added, "with the possibility that the US poor now have more diabetes because poor women have become very fat."[23]

West probably came closest among diabetes researchers to seeing poverty as a fundamental contributor to high diabetes rates, but even he was more focused on "fat" than on economics. His picture of fat was also decidedly racialized, as is evident in the populations he listed to support his claim that obesity and diabetes were intimately linked. He placed black women among Maltese, Hawaiians, Maoris, Aborigines, Native Americans, and Sumo wrestlers; obesity among poor whites is simply invisible. These populations, moreover, were exactly the same ones that appeared in articles promoting the thrifty gene hypothesis. West himself expressed considerable skepticism about the legitimacy of "'thrifty' genes," claiming that high diabetes rates among populations that "moved rapidly from primitive to modern conditions" might stem from environmental rather than genetic circumstances.[24] But the picture he painted still suggested that there was something about "nonwhites" that made them more susceptible to developing diabetes.

Claiming in the 1970s that the greatest risk factor for diabetes was "fat" also came with its own set of judgments. Of course, prejudice toward fat was not new. It was there in Joslin's recommendation that physicians use shame to get their diabetes patients to lose weight, and in Haven Emerson's tirade against those who were "dying of overeating." In the 1960s, the cardiologist Ancel Keys added his voice to this chorus, expressing his wish that "the idea . . . that obesity is immoral" be revived, believing that this is what might get those who were "fat" to change their ways.[25] But even if there was little that was new about attitudes toward fat in the 1970s, there was something different: these judgments were being ascribed more often to people of color living in poverty. The problem, as many physicians described it, was not only that their patients were obese, but also that they could not make the changes necessary to return to health. Fat, poor, and increasingly black, those with diabetes were also increasingly imagined as lacking the skills necessary to manage their own health.

From Intelligent to Incompetent

Already in 1958, Harold Dobson and several other members of the Department of Internal Medicine at Baylor University had drawn attention to the very different needs of patients who received care at Jefferson Davis Hospital, a charity institution, and those of "the average diabetic patient under private care." They based their claims on a study they had begun three years earlier, in which they had interviewed, and examined the charts of, roughly one-quarter of the 780 individuals with diabetes who appeared on the hospital's registry. Of the study participants, 63 percent were "Negro," 5 percent were "Latin American," and 32 percent were "white." Women made up 72 percent of the group; black women alone accounted for 48 percent of the total group. And because of strict eligibility requirements—a single person could not earn more than $100 a month and a couple no more than $125 a month to receive care at the clinic—they were all extremely poor.[26]

The writings of this small group of clinicians reveal tensions common to much charity work at the time: a combination of good intentions and considerable condescension toward those in need. Thus Dobson and his peers described with compassion how impossible it was for their patients to purchase the recommended protein-rich, low-carbohydrate diet, having to subsist instead on a diet of "margarine, gravy, fried foods, and cuts of meat that are almost pure fat." They lamented the inadequate staffing at the clinic, which meant that a single physician had to see fifteen to twenty-five patients in a three hour-period, and could often do little more than order blood and urine tests. Time for a thorough physical examination was simply lacking. As a result, complications arising from diabetes were often missed. What disturbed Dobson most was the way this system led physicians to treat "the blood sugar determinations and urine tests . . . , not the patient."[27]

Yet in addition to presenting this caring, compassionate perspective, Dobson also offered a vastly different picture of clinic patients than had predominated when the "typical diabetic" had been imagined as white, middle-class, and, quite often, a peer. The new patients—at least those who received care in the clinic—no longer possessed "greater intelligence than the average," as Hannah Lees had once claimed. Instead, Dobson described them as being "on the average in a lower intelligence group." He thus worried that they were not "mentally and physically capable" of controlling their diet, taking their insulin, and testing their urine on a regular basis. But his ultimate concern was that the lower intelligence, combined with extremely strained financial resources, would "decrease to a rather marked degree the ability of these patients to cooperate in the care of their diabetes."[28]

Dobson was giving voice to the great distance he felt between himself and clinic patients. And nowhere was this distance more evident than in the changes he and the other clinicians implemented to improve the quality of care in the clinic. To address the problem of understaffing, they decided to train medical students to "perform complete medical work-ups." It is not difficult to understand the appeal of such a solution: medical students would get a better education, medical school graduates who ended up as house physicians would arrive with experience, and presumably patients would get more care. Yet Dobson and his peers were also perpetuating a centuries-old system in which charity patients served as practice for physicians-in-training and thus risked getting inadequate care. Indeed, their claim that physicians who trained in charity hospitals were "the practitioners of tomorrow" suggests that they were aware of the two-tiered system they had just put in place.[29]

Other studies revealed a similar mix of good intentions, distancing, and condescension, once again revealing how the image of "the diabetic" was changing. In 1960 a team of researchers led by Robert S. Anderson, professor and chair of Internal Medicine at Meharry Medical College, conducted a study of seventy-one medically indigent diabetes patients (sixty of whom were female) who had received care at George W. Hubbard Hospital. The team was familiar with Dobson's work, although they were less worried about understaffing and more focused on gaining insight into the psychological, social, and clinical obstacles that prevented positive therapeutic outcomes. They were particularly concerned that medically indigent patients, who typically had less education than private patients, often felt hopeless and therefore were less likely to follow a physician's recommendations. Their goal, therefore, was to generate among their patients more interest and trust in a treatment regimen. They thought that paying close attention to "the individual's style of life," including "his emotional, intellectual, physical and financial resources," might produce beneficial results.[30]

The starting point for Anderson was the acknowledgment that the entire "traditional" approach to diabetes management had "been planned for the middle- and upper-class patient." As a first step toward devising an alternate management system for those living in poverty, he figured out which of the seventy-one patients in the study had good or excellent control of their diabetes, then set out to learn what he could about them: How much knowledge did they have of their disease? What specific regimen did they follow? What psychological traits or "inner resources" did they possess to help them through difficult times? Anderson relied on questionnaires, personal interviews, and a test called the Cornell Index, which measured an individual's "neuropsychiatric and psychosomatic disturbances" to gather answers to these questions. What he found was that about 10 percent of the patients had excellent control and another 28 percent had good control. He also found that almost three-quarters of the participants had poor knowledge of their disease and some kind of psychopathology. What he did not find was a significant correlation between successful control and either knowledge of diabetes or psychopathology.[31] The reasons some patients were better able to control their diabetes simply remained a puzzle.

Yet once again this research team revealed considerable ambivalence about the population under study, describing them as incapable of "abstract thinking," lacking "manual dexterity," and ignorant of "the concept of asepsis." Overlooking his own finding that knowledge of the disease was not a good predictor of successful control, Anderson recommended that future treatment programs keep all instruction simple: "Apparently," he wrote, "little more than administration of insulin or oral medication when required and the avoidance of concentrated starches can be expected from these patients." He made this assertion despite admitting that he did not know whether the medically indigent patients' "socioeconomic status limits their ability to apply the knowledge which they have." (One can only wonder at the thoroughness of any questionnaire that did not help the researchers to figure this out.) Yet despite these inconsistencies and uncertainties, Anderson concluded that with medically indigent patients, "the major responsibility for the control of the diabetes" could not rest with the individual, as was the case in the "traditional" approach, but had to reside "with the physician."[32]

Anderson's last statement captures the kind of reimagining of the diabetes patient that was taking place in the 1960s—at least of those diabetes patients who were becoming visible through institutions and programs dedicated to caring for the poor. Increasingly impoverished, uneducated, a person of color, and often female, the "new" diabetics had little in common with their providers, even when those providers were black, as was the case with the medical teams at Baylor and Meharry. Negative attitudes toward recipients of Medicaid (and other programs put into place through the War on Poverty) were not, it must be noted, unusual. And one could argue that describing medically indigent diabetics as requiring extra supervision was far superior to suggesting, as many did, that they were cunning and gaming the system.[33] But given the common perception that diabetes demanded more patient involvement than almost any other disease, the claim that medically indigent patients could not handle such responsibility placed them in a particularly subservient role.

The writings of Dobson, Anderson, and others point toward a bifurcation in diabetes "types" that would eventually resurface in how people thought about differences between those with type 1 and type 2 diabetes. The distinction, which resembled the one that Lees had made in the 1930s when she compared those who were "better citizens than the average" to those who "didn't live . . . to tell the tale," was now being employed to separate "private" from "medically indigent" patients. As is evident in Anderson's article, one of the core differences was the level of intelligence that diabetes patients were believed to possess, and the degree of independence they were, as a result, deemed capable of exercising.

The idea that those with diabetes varied in their ability to manage their disease had generated interest since at least the 1950s, when researchers had begun to explore the "emotional aspects" of treating patients and had distinguished between the "independent, intelligent and self-reliant" and the "excessively dependent" person. But this division had had nothing to do with race or poverty, and everything to do with personality types.[34] The goal of the research, moreover, had been to educate physicians about the great diversity among diabetes patients in order to aid these doctors in developing successful, individualized treatment plans. In Dobson's and Anderson's articles, the lesson about individual variation was lost. What emerged, instead, was a caricature of poor and medically indigent black diabetes patients as lacking intelligence, unable to understand anything but the simplest instructions, ignorant of such basic scientific concepts as germs, and most important, needing a professional to manage their disease. Lees's "diabetics" had been models of citizenship; the new patients, by contrast, required specific instructions and regular supervision to make sure that they came to no harm. In the eyes of the physicians providing care, they were no different than children.

"Corrosive Poverty" and a Push for Empowerment

An image of the sick poor as uninformed, dependent, and in some way responsible for their own illness and impoverishment was not the only one in circulation. The civil rights movement and the health activism it had spawned deliberately challenged this narrative by emphasizing not personal choice but instead institutional and political impediments to improving the health and well-being of black people. In 1965, the same year of the Watts riot and Malcolm X's assassination, the sociologist and anthropologist John Gibbs St. Clair Drake decried the "direct" and "indirect" victimization that African Americans experienced on a daily basis. This stretched from overt discriminatory practices, which created roadblocks that kept black people from gaining access to power, to the many indignities that flowed from these practices. For St. Clair Drake, high morbidity and mortality rates were prime examples of indirect victimization, for in his opinion they followed from discriminatory housing policies, job ceilings, an income gap, and blatant racism. Together they segregated black people into crowded, dilapidated, unsanitary ghettos; kept them out of white-collar jobs, leading them disproportionately into hazardous occupations; depressed wages and thus led to poor nutrition; and prevented them either from receiving emergency care close to their homes or, if they were admitted to a hospital, from receiving care comparable to that of whites. It followed for St. Clair Drake that the only solution was to abolish "corrosive poverty" by removing obstacles to "economic mobility." Improved health, he was convinced, would follow.[35]

Consistent with St. Clair Drake's pronouncements, activists committed themselves to serving the needs of the poor, convinced that race and class could not be disentangled. It was not only that breaking cycles of poverty would be impossible if basic health care needs were not first met; they argued that oppression and racism were themselves causing sickness. For these reasons, the Black Panther Party amended its platform in 1972 to include a demand for "completely free healthcare for all black and oppressed people," and put those words into practice by establishing free health clinics. As one physician described, most people arrived at the clinics with chronic diseases, such as "hypertension, ulcers, [and] diabetes," which had become progressively worse because of neglect. The staff thus began with "subtle everyday preventive medicine," which included basic tests for diabetes, high blood pressure, tuberculosis, and lead poisoning, as well as immunizations. Just as importantly, they educated people to be "more conscious about their health" and to learn how to advocate for change.[36]

Indeed, for many health activists a central role of neighborhood health centers was to empower poor people to take charge of their own health.

This was as true for centers established in poor white communities in Appalachia as it was for those launched in Watts, California, or Mound Bayou, Mississippi. Implementation may have proved more difficult than anticipated, but when Mud Creek Clinic opened its doors in 1972 in Harlan County, Kentucky, the intent of the organizers was to have the residents of the county participate in planning and running it. Like others inspired by community health centers, they envisioned "water systems, roads, schools, and other human services" as part of any effective health program. And they believed passionately that the road out of poverty and ill health had to come by empowering people to fight for themselves.[37]

This push for empowerment extended not only to those who were sick, but also to black health practitioners. That, at least, is what motivated the cardiologist Richard Allen Williams to edit a massive, nine-hundred-page text on health disparities in the black community ten years before the Heckler Report came out. Williams had been recruited to Watts in the late 1960s to assume a position as assistant medical director of the new 461-bed Martin Luther King Jr. General Hospital. Its founding had been an acknowledgment by the city of Los Angeles that the riot that had engulfed Watts in six days of violence in the summer of 1965 had stemmed, at least in part, from the absence of adequate health care services. In editing a *Textbook on Black-Related Diseases,* and in asking only black physicians and researchers to contribute, Williams was asserting black professionals' authority to lead the country in studying the "special medical problems of underprivileged minorities." He also considered them to be best positioned to eliminate "the rather paternalistic approach to the medical needs of Blacks . . . typical of many Whites." With his identity bound tightly to the established medical profession, Williams distanced himself from radical health activists by expressing his preference for "a new breed of doctor" who would be a "*medical evolutionary*" rather than a "social revolutionary," but he still saw his own intervention as part of a bigger effort to move "the Black community toward the goals of self-determination of its medical destiny."[38]

That journey, according to Williams, had to begin with knowledge of the degree to which high rates of disease were continuing to devastate black communities. For this reason, the first article of the volume, penned by the epidemiologist M. Alfred Haynes, was on the overall "Gap in Health Status between Black and White Americans." To drive home the magnitude of this gap, Haynes introduced the concept of "excess deaths," which was a way of measuring health disparities that would be picked up ten years later in the Heckler Report. As Haynes explained: "Assuming that the death rate of the Black is the same as that of the White at a specific age, one could expect a certain number of deaths. These are called *expected deaths*. The number of deaths which actually occur is far in excess of the deaths expected on the basis of the rate of the White population. . . . The difference between the expected deaths and the deaths that actually occur may be called *excess deaths*."[39]

Haynes calculated that 84,532 excess deaths took place in the United States in 1970 alone. And while cardiovascular diseases and malignant neoplasms accounted for most of them, diabetes was the only major killer where the mortality rate for women surpassed that for men. This was true, Haynes pointed out, for white as well as for black women, but whereas the gender gap among whites was insignificant, "the rate for the Black female far exceed[ed] that of the Black male."[40]

Haynes did not speculate about the reasons for this disparity. Indeed, in the few pages on diabetes mellitus that appeared in a separate chapter on endocrine diseases, the author Walter Lester Henry Jr. focused less on racial differences than on similarities between black and white people when it came to the expression of the disease. In the preface to the volume, however, Williams made clear his willingness to embrace biology, even genetics, as one among many possible reasons for health disparities, although he was just as clear in his rejection of all forms of biological reductionism. With a cautionary note to future physicians, he insisted that they learn to balance what the nineteenth-century French physiologist Claude Bernard had called *le milieu intérieur* with an equal focus on the "social, political, and economic ramifications" of the health problems of black people. In the end, Williams had his eyes on what he hoped would be the prize: that information about racial differences in health, "which was previously used against Blacks to institute, reinforce, and perpetuate patterns of institutional racism, will now be used on our behalf to eradicate these practices. Then we can say that the old stumbling blocks of oppression have metamorphosed into stepping stones of progress."[41]

As Williams was writing these words, the nation was gearing up for a battle "to address directly and fully the tragedy of diabetes mellitus." Just one year earlier, in 1974, Congress had passed the National Diabetes Mellitus Research and Education Act, which had allocated increased funding for diabetes and created a commission tasked with determining how best to proceed. Chaired by Oscar B. Crofford, director of the Diabetes-Endocrinology Center at Vanderbilt University's School of Medicine, the eighteen-member commission immediately set to work and published several volumes of findings within two years. Beginning with an overview of what was known about diabetes, it discussed the rapidly increasing number of Americans suffering from this disease, along with many of the complications that arose when it was left untreated, such as blindness, kidney disease, amputations, and heart disease. When it came to the demographic makeup of those most likely to develop diabetes, the authors also shared what anyone familiar with the literature would have known: "Women are 50% more likely than men to have diabetes, non-whites are one fifth more likely than whites to have diabetes, and poor people (incomes less than $5,000 per year) are three times as likely as middle-income and wealthy people to have diabetes."[42]

The question, though, was where to go from here. How should funds be allocated? What specific strategies should be employed? The commission's decision was to recommend that the National Institutes of Health take charge of coordinating and expanding the various efforts throughout the nation aimed at combating diabetes. And it charged the NIH to pursue three areas of focus: education of patients and providers, research, and translation of knowledge from science into practice. Nowhere in the recommendations were there any plans to eliminate poverty and racism, despite clear recognition that poor minorities suffered disproportionately from diabetes and other chronic diseases.

One Report, Two Diabetes Types

The lack of attention to poverty and race in the national commission's recommendation appears odd given that the members of the commission had gone out of their way to ensure that they gathered information from a diverse array of people. They had set up public hearings in Bethesda, Philadelphia, Los Angeles, Seattle, Atlanta, and Chicago, and invited interested parties around the country to share their stories and expertise. Concerned that "the poor and educationally deprived diabetic person" might not get wind of the hearings or, even if they were aware of them, might not be able to attend, they also sent interviewers out to clinics where the poor received care in order to take down their stories.[43] These interviews were taped and transcribed. Nine of them—presumably considered to be a representative sample—were included at the end of the commission's report. The picture they painted was dismal.

The individuals whose stories were reproduced were all middle-aged or elderly. We do not know anyone's sex or race, except for one person who identified herself as a "Negra." With the exception of one fifty-three-year-old who had had diabetes all his or her life, everyone had developed it as an adult. None was able to work; most had additional health problems, including kidney disease, arthritis, high blood pressure, and glaucoma. A few had suffered leg amputations, and several had difficulty with their vision. In response to questions about problems they had encountered because of economic hardships, the interviewees shared stories of missing doctors' appointments because they had no means of transportation, receiving the wrong kind of insulin at the pharmacy, or being refused insulin altogether. One woman explained that she failed to make an appointment because she had become ill and "wasn't able to go down to catch a bus." Another described having to travel 150 miles to the clinic because there was no medical facility closer to home. That person lived alone and had to take two buses and a streetcar to get to the clinic. Others talked about the expense of following the prescribed diet. Most received Medicaid or Medicare. Almost everyone had been waiting at the clinic for four hours or more without yet having seen a doctor. Several were illiterate.[44]

The inclusion of these nine stories in the commission's report was a way of making the plight of the poor visible to members of Congress. Yet by placing them at the end of the second volume of the commission's report, and separating them physically from the five hundred pages of testimony delivered during the hearings, the report drove a wedge between those who were poor and others with diabetes.

This gap was widened even more during the public hearings by the overwhelming focus in the testimonies on the juvenile form of diabetes. Many of the individuals who turned up to tell their stories or who sent in letters either had this form of diabetes or were parents of those who had it. A good number were also affiliated with the Juvenile Diabetes Foundation, which had been established in 1970 in order to find a cure for juvenile diabetes. Its founder, Leatrice (Lee) Ducat—who served on the eighteen-member National Commission on Diabetes and helped write the report—had become frustrated with what she perceived to be the American Diabetes Association's excessive concern with education, outreach, and training, and its concomitant lack of interest in research. To remedy this, she had started what turned out to be a rival organization, consisting primarily of parents of children with diabetes, who viewed the nation's conquest of polio as a model. Members of this organization turned out in droves to the public hearings and bombarded the commission with letters. One in particular, penned by the president of the Juvenile Diabetes Foundation's Washington, D.C., chapter, could not have been clearer about the organization's mission when he declared that "the single, overriding, most important problem in Diabetes today, is the long-standing neglect of research—not education, not training, not publications, not screening programs—but research."[45]

In 1976, three years before the official division of diabetes into IDDM and NIDDM, an emphasis on finding a cure for "diabetes" might have implied that everyone would benefit, regardless of the form they had. But that was not the way the testimonies played out. Instead, there was palpable tension in the words of parents of diabetic children who feared that funds would not be appropriated in ways that might most directly help their children and, perhaps, grandchildren. "I ask you to separate the problems of the juvenile diabetic from that of adult onset diabetes," wrote one father, as he described the devastation that had visited his family since his fifteen-year-old son had been diagnosed with the disease three years earlier. "The problems are vastly different," he explained. He understood that everyone who suffered from diabetes needed help, but he was also clear that his "main concern" rested with the "juvenile diabetic."[46]

Even those who seemed more sympathetic to people with the adult form ended up dividing those with diabetes into two types. This is evident in the testimony of Leo Krall, one of the head physicians at the Joslin Clinic, who emphasized that only a small number of the five to ten million people living with diabetes in the United States suffered from the juvenile form. The rest, he argued, could not wait "for the miracles and cures of the future"; what they needed today was to learn how "simply to survive and perform [their] normal daily functions." Krall was especially concerned about spreading this knowledge beyond the handful of institutions that served those with financial resources, pointing out that diabetes did not "confine itself to ethnic, education, economic or psychological boundaries." Yet despite stretching across these boundaries, Krall ended up erecting other walls in the way he characterized the challenge of educating the growing number of people with diabetes. The "old classical Chautauqua lecture method" no longer worked, he explained, because it was "geared to the motivated, Anglo-Saxon oriented, high school level educated person." In contrast, they were trying to educate "the masses who not only do not know what is available but also do not know what they do not know!"[47]

The commission's report thus effectively created two different groups. On the one hand were children (and their parents), whose stories filled the pages of the report. Their pleas were not only for a cure, but also for an end to stigma in school, at the workplace, and in social settings. They wanted the chance of having a "normal" life, one not dependent on needles and restrictive diets, one free of the complications that seemed inevitable and that might prevent them from getting married, having children, even grandchildren, and living long lives. On the other hand were, in Krall's words, the "masses," whose stories were largely absent from the testimonies, with some exceptions. One physician spoke up on behalf of Asian Americans; an American Indian wrote of the hardships and health problems that his people endured on reservations; and there were, of course, the nine testimonies included at the end of the volume, all of whose authors were poor and, in the case of at least one, black. But their voices were drowned out by the hundreds of testimonies, largely from middle-class whites, that dominated the report.

Reading through the commission's report, it becomes clear that poverty and race are both there and not there. They are present in the demographic data mentioned in the beginning of the report and in the testimonies included in the end. Throughout the rest of the report, however, they are invisible. There was certainly little in what the commission labeled its "Long Range Plan to Combat Diabetes" that suggested an interest in tackling the fundamental causes of poverty and racism. Instead it turned to medical research, education and outreach, and translation practices.

The clear articulation of a national program for addressing diabetes, which not only ignored both the demands of radical health activists and the measured approach of black physicians like Richard Williams, but also appeared indifferent to the concerns that had informed the civil rights movement and Johnson's War on Poverty, reveals much about the emerging political climate in the late 1970s. The War on Poverty may not have done much to redistribute wealth, but it had been an important step in funding government programs designed to help people suffering from poverty, disease, and malnutrition. Committed to finding a middle road between blaming individuals for their problems and condemning the nation's political and economic structures, reformers had focused on creating opportunities rather than attacking inequalities.[48] Still, by the late 1970s even this middle road had become the target of increased criticism.

Between the high costs of the Vietnam War, the 1970s oil crises, and the gradual deindustrialization of the nation's primary employment sectors, the U.S. economy had taken repeated hits and the financial optimism of previous decades had begun to fade. The economic downturn, alongside massive increases in health care expenditures, which were claiming an ever greater percentage of the nation's GDP, led to cost-saving measures that harmed poor minorities disproportionately. Outlays for health services also triggered a political backlash: Ronald Reagan would eventually be swept into power in 1980 by riding a wave of opposition to "big" government (as far as social services, not the military, was concerned) and by fueling racist sentiments.[49] For health care, this meant a switch from a vision of government as providing an essential safety net for those in need to a vision of informed individuals taking responsibility for their own health.[50]

By 1980, anyone who kept up with the news knew that diabetes had become a major health problem for the nation. Those who read past the headlines might also have learned that mortality and morbidity rates were highest among minorities, and that women were more affected than men. But after that, the message lost focus. Careful readers might have come across claims that the disease struck those living in poverty the hardest, although this did not receive much attention in either the popular press or in professional journals. The reasons for such disparities were also quite difficult to pinpoint, with the exception of the literature on Native Americans, which favored genetics. Otherwise, the tendency was to mention increasing rates of obesity and family history (or heredity), and to emphasize the importance of encouraging behavioral changes. Only the rare voice suggested that poverty and racism played a role.

The picture of diabetes became even more complicated in the 1980s. As a result of a second major wave of immigration, largely from Mexico and Asia, the image of the populations considered most susceptible to diabetes grew increasingly diverse. No longer did the claim that minority populations suffered disproportionately from diabetes refer primarily to Native Americans and African Americans; Hispanic and Asian Americans were joining the mix. And as the number of ethnic populations believed to be susceptible to diabetes increased, the number of different explanations for its exponential rise grew as well. Genetics, obesity, acculturation, nutrition, and even stress were frequent contenders. Poverty and racism, however, were seldom considered serious and legitimate contributors to the forces driving up diabetes rates.

Mexican Americans as a "Diabetic Race"

"The number of recent immigrants to the United States is greater than at any time in the past century," wrote the authors of a paper on cultural differences and nutrition.[51] The year was 1983 and the immigrants to whom they were referring were not European, as they had been at the beginning of the century, but Latin American and Asian. They were part of a second wave of immigration to the United States that had begun in 1965—when Congress passed the Immigration and Nationality Act, thereby repealing the national quotas it had put in place four decades earlier.[52] Doubling and tripling in number every generation, the new immigrants came to the attention of health providers, who struggled to care for individuals who hailed from cultures quite different than their own. For those interested in research, however, these often self-contained communities promised new opportunities to explore the fundamental causes of disease.

In 1979, Michael P. Stern, professor of medicine at the University of Texas Health Science Center in San Antonio, spearheaded two epidemiological studies of cardiovascular risk factors among Mexican Americans living in

Texas. The first, located in Laredo, a town on the border with Mexico, began in February. Six months later, he started a second study in San Antonio, which was considered at the time to have the highest concentration of persons of Mexican ancestry of any city in the country. Stern expressed concern that this rapidly growing population remained woefully understudied, despite accumulating evidence of serious health problems among them, which he deemed of considerable "public health relevance." He also argued for the scientific value of studying Mexican Americans, whom he described as being of "mixed European and native American ancestry." This "unique bicultural population," he argued, offers "an ideal 'laboratory'" for exploring the relative contributions of genes and sociocultural factors to disease patterns in different ethnic populations. His assumption was that since Native Americans appeared to have "a genetic predisposition to diabetes," and since "the Mexican American population was estimated to have a 30 to 40 percent native American contribution to its gene pool," a similarly high rate of diabetes among Mexican Americans would likely be attributable to their genes.[53]

Armed with these assumptions, Stern and his team traveled to Laredo. Focusing on two neighborhoods where low-income Mexican Americans resided, they used Spanish surnames and Spanish-language ability to identify the 389 individuals who ended up participating in the study. Participants filled out a questionnaire and agreed to have measurements taken of their weight, height, blood pressure, fasting blood glucose, serum cholesterol, and serum triglycerides. Stern then compared the results to data he had for both the Akimel O'odham and the nation at large. Although he exercised caution because the studies of these various populations had employed different sampling strategies and experimental designs, he still felt confident enough in the strength of the research to use it "to help place the Laredo Project results in perspective."[54]

Stern concluded that poor Mexican Americans in Laredo had levels of "overweight" and hyperglycemia that fell between those of the Akimel O'odham and the nation as a whole. What he could not determine was whether this pattern was "primarily due to sociocultural or to genetic factors."[55] The problem, as he saw it, was that diabetes and obesity were known to be linked, and sociocultural factors were known to affect levels of adiposity. But the Laredo study, he pointed out, had not been designed to distinguish between genetics and sociocultural factors. After all, the study participants were all poor Mexican Americans. Fortunately, that was not the case in San Antonio.

The San Antonio Heart Study, introduced earlier, was a much larger enterprise. The first phase alone involved interviews with roughly four thousand people and lasted from 1979 to 1982. Designed to tease out the relative contributions of "socioeconomic, cultural, life-style, and genetic factors" in explaining disease patterns among Mexican Americans, the study collected data from three different neighborhoods in the city: an affluent "suburb," whose population was roughly 90 percent Anglo American; a middle-class "transitional" neighborhood that was about 60 percent Mexican American and 40 percent Anglo American; and a low-income "barrio," which was primarily Mexican American. The interviewers went door to door gathering information about smoking, diet, exercise, and other personal habits, as well as family background, attitudes and beliefs about obesity and dieting, access to health care, and general knowledge of health and disease. Participants also received a free medical examination in a nearby mobile unit where the same measurements were taken as in Laredo. The results once again indicated that Mexican Americans had a higher prevalence of both obesity and diabetes than Anglo Americans, but not as high as the Akimel O'odham.[56]

Stern and his team believed they could do more with the data from San Antonio, since they now had information about Mexican Americans and Anglo Americans living in the same neighborhood, and information about each group from three different socioeconomic neighborhoods. In a series of papers they began publishing in 1982, the researchers showed that regardless of neighborhood, Mexican Americans had higher rates of obesity than Anglo Americans, although the gap decreased with increasing wealth. They also found that within each weight category (they had divided the subjects into "lean," "average," and "obese"), Mexican Americans had higher rates of diabetes. In other words, lean Mexican Americans had a higher prevalence of diabetes than lean Anglo Americans. They therefore concluded that something beyond socioeconomic status and obesity must be contributing to high rates among Mexican Americans. Their best guess was that the "residual" factor was the concentration of Native American genes.[57]

A paper published in 1984 engaged this question directly. The lead investigator, Lytt I. Gardner Jr., was an epidemiologist from the San Antonio research team. Lacking a genetic marker to determine Native American ancestry, which he would have preferred, Gardner followed standard practice among researchers at the time and turned to traits, like skin color, that were known to be "predominantly under genetic control." Based on the tests he ran, he concluded that the Mexican Americans he randomly selected from the barrio had a genetic admixture that was roughly 46 percent Native American; those from the transitional neighborhood had about 27 percent, and those from the suburbs had around 18 percent. Given that the diabetes rates declined from 14.5 percent to 10 percent to 5 percent in the same neighborhoods, respectively, and given that prior research had demonstrated that obesity alone could not explain this pattern, Gardner "speculated" that genetic factors played an important role. "The association of genetic admixture with NIDDM rates," he wrote, "suggests that much of the epidemic of NIDDM in Mexican Americans is confined to that part of the population with a substantial native American heritage."[58]

Note that Gardner no longer referred to "diabetes" in general, but rather to NIDDM. His use of this term reflected major changes, initiated by the National Diabetes Mellitus Research and Education Act, aimed at improving diabetes treatment and research. Along with the creation of the National Diabetes Advisory Board and diabetes research and training centers, stricter guidelines had been put in place to establish uniform diagnostic criteria. As mentioned earlier, one of the major goals was to eliminate the single umbrella term—diabetes mellitus—for the various forms of the disease, along with such vague descriptors as mild diabetes, severe or acute diabetes, or juvenile-onset and adult-onset diabetes, and to replace them with more clearly defined categories. Thus after 1979, clinicians and researchers referred either to NIDDM (type 2), which was the most common form, making up 90 to 95 percent of all cases; IDDM (type 1), which accounted for 5 to 10 percent of all cases; GDM (gestational diabetes mellitus); and several other minor types.[59]

This also meant that after 1979, studies of diabetes among "nonwhites" focused almost exclusively on NIDDM, since IDDM appeared to be far less of a problem in their communities. As a result, negative judgments about diabetes, which quickly became associated almost exclusively with NIDDM, also became associated more readily with minority populations.

Such judgments were evident in the papers produced by the scientists working in San Antonio. This happened despite the sophistication of their research, their acknowledgment that skin color was not a totally reliable indicator of genetic admixture, and their admission that absence of a genetic marker for NIDDM rendered their conclusions tentative. At times their judgments and condescension were obvious, as when Stern referred to Mexican Americans struggling with diabetes as an "ideal 'laboratory.'"[60] At other times, researchers' prejudices were less transparent, as in their obsession with finding out the percent Native American ancestry of the different socioeconomic groups they studied. Stern and his team may have presented Mexican Americans as a "bicultural population," but at no point in their many publications did they explore—or even mention—the impact of the population's European ancestry on disease patterns. They did not even bring this up for the suburban residents who, according to their own data, had an 82 percent European admixture. Why not write that European ancestry "protected" Mexican Americans from diabetes? Far from a trivial point, it reflects an overall tethering of Mexican Americans to Native Americans that made it difficult for Stern and his peers to imagine Mexican Americans as white. In fact, Mexican Americans' claim to "whiteness," like that of Jews in the early twentieth century, was far from settled.

Although officially classified as white in 1848 at the end of the Mexican-American War, Mexican immigrants encountered considerable discrimination when they attempted to purchase land, move into "white" neighborhoods, attend good schools, or seek remunerative employment—in short, when they tried to assimilate. Much of the prejudice they encountered derived from the color of their skin, which suggested ancestral ties to Native Americans. During a congressional hearing in 1926 on whether to extend the 1924 Restrictive Immigration Act to immigrants from countries in the Western Hemisphere, Congressman John Box of Texas, who favored stricter controls, argued that Mexicans were basically Indians "and very seldom become naturalized." To him, this meant that "they know little of sanitation, are very low mentally, and are generally unhealthy." Box's description, which both revived older images of Mexicans as disease vectors and expressed unabashedly the eugenic sentiments of his day, took on particular meaning during the Depression, when the economic downturn intensified animosity toward the influx of people from south of the border. Such racial animus resulted in the reclassification of Mexicans as a distinct race in the 1930 U.S. Census, although that was dropped by the next census. Still, in the very decades when national differences between Europeans gradually lost their association with race and all Americans of European ancestry simply became "white," Mexican Americans and others of Hispanic ancestry continued to be singled out. In the 1950 and 1960 U.S. Census, they were grouped under the heading "Persons of Spanish Mother Tongue"; in 1970 this was changed to "Persons of Both Spanish Surname and Spanish Mother Tongue"; and in 1980 to "Hispanic."[61]

Publications from the San Antonio study had none of the animus that radiated from Box's comment. What remained, however, was a sense of distance and confusion about how to think of the racial makeup of the study's subjects. This is evident in the way Stern and his team used quotation marks when comparing Mexican Americans to what they called "'other whites.'" The punctuation suggests that while they accepted Mexican Americans' whiteness, they still considered it somewhat different. They were not unusual in this regard. Some Mexican Americans even embraced an image of themselves as "another white race," finding the suggested hybridity useful for building group identity, fighting discrimination, and making sure that their health needs were met.[62] But there was a tradeoff, one that made it difficult for diabetes researchers to engage with Mexican Americans' complex ancestries. The only genetic link they seemed able to imagine was the one with Native Americans, and it was a link forged through perceptions of both groups as genetically predisposed to disease.

One must also wonder about the decision to compare Mexican Americans specifically to the Akimel O'odham, the Native American tribe with the highest rate of diabetes of all Native American populations in the United States. The data for the Akimel O'odham may have been the most robust, but that does not mean it was the most relevant, given the absence of any evidence that Mexican Americans—already a highly diverse population genetically—and the Akimel O'odham had common ancestors. Perhaps sensing that this was a potential weakness in their study, Gardner and his team claimed that they were extending the term "'native American' . . . to Amerindian tribes in general, and, . . . particularly to those indigenous to Mexico."[63] But this assertion was little more than rhetorical since their data about Native Americans came solely from studies of the Akimel O'odham.

In the end, attributing high diabetes rates among Mexican Americans in part to their Native American ancestry had little scientific evidence to support it; its "logic" drew instead on the assumption that if socioeconomic status and obesity could be held constant, then similarities in diabetes rates between Mexican Americans and Native Americans most likely stemmed from shared genetics. But this ignored the possibility that shared experiences of racism, dislocation, and poverty might also have driven up diabetes rates. Significantly, such a hypothesis did emerge in the narratives about Japanese Americans, as I will examine shortly. That Stern and his team did not entertain this possibility reveals as much about racial assumptions at the time as it does about disease trends. As in the case of Jews and diabetes, only some populations have been imagined to have nervous systems sensitive enough to be affected by discrimination and stress. In the 1980s, Mexican Americans were rarely among them.[64]

The ascription of high diabetes rates among Mexican Americans to their genetic kinship with Native Americans was, thus, tenuous at best. It was an appealing idea because it offered a genetics-based answer to what many had begun to consider a serious public health problem, but perhaps as well because it fit easily into an existing narrative. Gardner, for example, in the introduction to his article on Native American ancestry among Mexican Americans, mentioned thrifty genotypes and the work of Paul Zimmet and others who had studied the effect of diabetes on populations that had only recently become "Westernized" through contact or migration. By framing his article in this way, Gardner drew Mexican Americans into this tale of evolutionary biology, reinforcing an image of them as backward, uneducated, and not quite American. After all, the entire speculative apparatus constructed around "thrifty genes" assumed that the affected populations had only recently escaped a "primitive" culture to encounter a "modern" lifestyle. No matter how many generations people of Mexican descent had lived in the United States—and some could trace their ancestry back to 1845 when Texas became a state—this narrative and others would add to their struggles to be accepted as fully American.[65]

The studies in Laredo and San Antonio were not the only research projects designed to learn more about diabetes in Mexican Americans and other "Hispanic" populations, although they were among the first to draw attention to the paucity of knowledge about the "particular disease susceptibilities" of this rapidly growing group of individuals in the United States. Soon information emerged from California, New Mexico, Arizona, Colorado, Florida, and New York City that included other Spanish-speaking populations, such as those hailing from Puerto Rico and Cuba. Efforts arising from within Hispanic communities to improve health conditions in their neighborhoods drove these studies as well. Their concerns focused often on the need for greater access to health services as well as for bilingual materials and providers. They also showed greater awareness of the importance of material resources for securing good health than did the Laredo and San Antonio studies. Ramon Rivera, head of a survey about "the physical well-being of [the country's] growing Latino minority," was confident that "socio-economic factors" stood behind the high rates he expected to find not only of diabetes, but also of heart disease, drug addiction, and alcoholism. As he explained, the physical examination that accompanied the survey was, for many of the participants, the first they had had in their lives. "That's not to say," he added, that "they have never been ill, just that they could not afford medical care."[66] And people who lacked financial resources, he implied, could not be held responsible for their ill health.

But Rivera's perspective, which grew more popular as the Chicanx and Latinx civil rights movements gained ground, struggled against a narrative that, whether grounded directly in genetics or not, still placed the reason for high rates of diabetes in the bodies of Mexican Americans. In 1983, Francisco Bravo, a physician who practiced medicine for over forty-five years in the heavily Hispanic neighborhood of Boyle Heights in Los Angeles, referred to Mexican Americans as "a diabetic race." "I presume," he added, that "my patients have diabetes until proven otherwise." Roughly seventy years earlier, Joslin had suggested treating anyone with sugar in their urine as though they had diabetes, "until the contrary is proven." Bravo no longer needed a urine test; simply looking like a Mexican American had become enough.[67]

A Revealingly Different View of Asian Americans

The stories told about high rates of diabetes among Asian Americans, which also surfaced in the late 1970s, had much in common with the stories of other minority populations. Just as the Akimel O'odham represented Native Americans, and Mexican Americans dominated the scholarship on Hispanic Americans, Japanese Americans received the most attention of the different Asian American groups. Research revealed that this population, like other immigrant groups, experienced increasing diabetes rates in the years following migration, making them more prone to develop the disease than their peers in Japan. Researchers also attributed this increase to changes in diet and physical activity.

There, however, all parallels ended. Most striking is the absence of any speculation that increasing rates of diabetes might have stemmed from the "unmasking" of a genetic trait that predisposed Japanese individuals to diabetes. Instead, researchers assumed that differential rates had to stem from "environmental factors," such as diet and physical activity. A study conducted in the mid-1970s, comparing Japanese immigrants on the island of Hawaii with native Japanese in Hiroshima, was emblematic of this approach. The investigators consisted of scholars from the Hiroshima University School of Medicine, led by Ryoso Kawate, and several American researchers, including Peter H. Bennett and William C. Knowler, both of whom were experts on diabetes among the Akimel O'odham. Together, the two teams determined that Japanese migrants in Hawaii had a diabetes prevalence of 12.4 percent compared to 7.2 percent among those in Hiroshima. In trying to understand why this was the case, they decided to calculate the precise composition of the foods each population consumed, and to record their levels of physical activity. What they found was that despite consuming roughly the same amount of "total energy," the Hawaiian subjects ate far more animal fat and simple carbohydrates and far fewer complex carbohydrates than subjects in Hiroshima. They also moved less, since they tended to be less engaged in physically taxing work than the subjects in Hiroshima, whose jobs were primarily in agriculture and manual labor.[68]

Kawate's focus on diet and physical exercise is all the more striking because of his decision to link his findings to studies of other groups that had experienced "rapid progress from primitive to developed environments."

Thus, as in Gardner's case, he drew parallels to populations such as American Indians, Polynesians, Nauruans, and North African migrants to Israel. To fit Japanese migrants into this narrative, he chose 1950 as a point of radical disjuncture: before then, Japanese migrants lived mostly as "laborers and in poor economic condition"; afterward "their living standard improved rapidly," while their engagement in physical activity abated. The link that Kawate thus established to other dislocated groups was through a common experience of rapid environmental change. But he never once mentioned that American Indians and Nauruans, among others, were the very same groups featured in articles enamored of the idea that a "thrifty gene" might best explain rapid increases in diabetes rates in certain populations. In fact, the word "genetics" never appeared in the article.[69]

Kawate's attempt to cast the lives of Japanese migrants in prewar Hawaii as "primitive" in order to create some equivalence between the migrants and, for example, American Indians, was highly strained. The migrants' lives may have been difficult, but their history did not include being confined to reservations after their land had been stolen. Kawate was also ignoring the way his own narrative presented Japanese migrants as quite different than other migrant groups with high rates of diabetes: theirs was not a story of a (biologically) "primitive" population forced to Westernize more rapidly than their genes could tolerate; instead it was a story of a (socially) "primitive" population that had successfully assimilated into "Western" society, attaining levels of education, income, and social capital comparable and sometimes even surpassing that of white Americans. Similar to narratives that flourished at the beginning of the twentieth century, it was success that made Japanese immigrants vulnerable.

Not everyone agreed with this way of explaining high rates of diabetes among Asian Americans. A physician who tended to this population in Seattle argued that the assumption that Asians had "made it" had contributed to the neglect of this community, and had made it especially difficult to draw attention to the problems they continued to face with "adequate nutrition, discrimination in housing, job advancement, and medical attention." Others claimed that unusual "stress" played a significant role in explaining high rates of diabetes, especially among Japanese Americans. This hypothesis emerged from a study comparing "a native Japanese population" in

Tokyo and a "migrant pure Japanese population" in Seattle. The research-ers, who consisted of faculty from both the University of Washington in Seattle and the University of Tokyo, shared the assumption of their peers in Hawaii and Hiroshima that cross-cultural studies of migrant popula-tions permitted a more sophisticated analysis of the environmental factors influencing diabetes rates. This time, however, when listing environmen-tal influences on rising diabetes rates, the researchers added "psychosocial stress," explaining that they found it particularly pertinent for evaluating high rates among second-generation immigrants ("Nisei").[70] Although at the time of their study they had not yet had an opportunity to pursue this insight, the authors of the Heckler Report—as we will see shortly—picked up on this suggestion, drawing attention to the particular stress and strain the Nisei had experienced during their years of internment after the out-break of World War II.

When comparing research on the reasons for high diabetes rates among African Americans, Native Americans, Hispanic Americans, and Asian Americans, it is difficult to avoid the conclusion that genetics surfaced when researchers sought to explain high diabetes rates among populations imagined as not quite "modern" or "Western." The "failure" to assimilate, as in the case of Native Americans and Mexican Americans, became, as a result, a consequence of a group's biological makeup rather than the out-come of decades (or centuries) of racist and discriminatory practices.

The task force that Margaret Heckler and Thomas Malone created to ex-amine health disparities thus worked with a body of literature based on both observation and speculation. As a result, when they published the Heckler Report they not only exposed the horrific disparities that continued to burden minority populations in the United States; they also perpetuated several of the stereotypes and prejudices that burdened these populations.

The Heckler Report: Galvanizing and Imperfect

In April 1984 Margaret Mary Heckler, secretary of Health and Human Services, established a task force to study the nation's health disparities.[71] President Reagan had appointed her to the position just fifteen months earlier, and she had wasted little time in tackling what members of the task force called a "tragic dilemma in the United States." Heckler, who had a law degree from Boston College Law School and a reputation as a "Rockefeller Republican," had represented Massachusetts in Congress for sixteen years before she assumed this position. Although she lacked a background in public health, she had been a strong advocate for women's issues, including fighting for ratification of the Equal Rights Amendment, federal funding for childcare, and the financing of shelters for victims of domestic violence. To head up the task force, she turned to Thomas E. Malone, deputy director of the National Institutes of Health since 1977 and the first African American to hold this position. In turn, Malone pulled together a group of nineteen individuals (including himself), all of them in-house and thus all with the "programmatic authority" to make changes. Their charge was to determine the extent of health disparities in the nation, to identify the main reasons these disparities persisted, and to propose concrete actions to eliminate them. Secretary Heckler gave them one year to complete their task.[72]

The task force members had several decisions to make and very little time to make them. They had to figure out which measure to use for drawing comparisons between populations, which diseases and conditions to investigate, and how to contend with the relative paucity of information they had on the health status of Asian and Hispanic Americans. In the end, they chose as their measure "excess deaths." They defined the term, as Haynes had done before them, as the difference between the number of expected deaths, if the population were white, and the number of actual deaths. They then decided it made the most sense to concentrate on the six diseases and conditions that accounted for the vast majority of excess deaths, and chose, as a result, heart disease and stroke, homicide and accidents, cancer, infant mortality, cirrhosis, and diabetes. The members of the task force then worked with consultants and staff to gather as much information as they could. The final product was a ten-volume report that, much like a literature survey, provided, in their own words, "excellent reviews of research."[73] By putting together such a comprehensive report, and by coordinating literature on five different populations, the task force members believed they had produced something that would transform how the country thought about health disparities.

For anyone who had knowledge of the literature on health disparities, the Heckler Report may have held few surprises, but probably few readers had the big picture. Thus someone who knew that the life expectancy for African Americans was still only at the level that whites had reached thirty years earlier might still have been deeply troubled to read that "nonwhites" experienced roughly sixty thousand excess deaths per year. Pulling so much material together in one place thus proved galvanizing, and was remembered in subsequent years as the moment the government declared the elimination of health disparities a priority for the nation. Other evidence of this new priority included the establishment of an Office of Minority Health and a great influx of resources to support new research projects.[74] But those hoping to see funds allocated to improving the care of minority populations were sorely disappointed. Not only had Ronald Reagan recently slashed government spending for a host of social programs, including Medicaid and Medicare, but the administration had also made it clear that any new programs suggested by the task force would have to be "budgetarily neutral."[75]

The Heckler Report may, thus, have symbolized a beginning, but its ambitions were modest, focusing every one of its recommendations on research or education. The task force's goal was to generate more studies that would reveal the reasons for health disparities, and it wanted to get that information out to providers and patients more quickly and efficiently with the hope of effecting change. The recommendations, however, focused on lifestyle choices and behaviors, not on further desegregating medical institutions, improving access to quality health care, or increasing investments in preventive medicine. Heckler, when she traveled around the country to report on the task force's findings, was often rather blunt. Even before the full report appeared, she told attendees at the annual meeting of the National Association of Negro Business and Professional Women's Clubs that "changes in life style never come easy. But come they must if many black Americans are to live longer and healthier lives. . . . Some of these changes are personal and cannot be mandated by a government in a free society; they must be voluntary, but they must be made."[76]

Heckler's pronouncements encountered some resistance. African Americans in particular delivered sharp responses, taking Heckler to task for pointing a finger at the black community. Edith Irby Jones, president of the National Medical Association, chastised the secretary for implying that black people simply needed to "'behave'" in order to solve their health problems. Writing in 1986 in her "President's Column," which appeared in the *Journal of the National Medical Association,* she added: "Well, as black Americans, we know it is not as simple as all that. Blaming the patient will not cure the ills of America's underserved minorities. The diseases correctly identified by HHS [Health and Human Services] as affecting the health of the black community so devastatingly are in large measure the result of poverty, neglect, underlying prejudices, and the resulting stress. . . . We all know that while health education indeed may be helpful, as Mrs. Heckler suggests, what we really need is better nutrition in early life, better housing, and more and better jobs." One year later, when John E. Joyner succeeded Jones as president of the National Medical Association, he too criticized the task force for ignoring "the economic disparity that has a direct relationship between the status of one's health and the ability to pay for that health."[77]

To be fair to the task force, its report did mention the link between poverty and health disparities in the first volume, which provided an overall summary of the committee's findings. In a section dealing specifically with the "Social Characteristics of Minority Populations," the authors presented the four factors they believed to have the greatest influence on health: demographic profiles, nutrition and diet, exposure to environmental hazards at home and work, and patterns of coping with stress. There they drew attention to the much higher level of unemployment and poverty among minority families as compared to white families. They even mentioned "the shared characteristic of economic disadvantage among minorities." Yet few of these insights made their way into subsequent volumes where the task force explored the six health conditions in detail. Also, almost every time they brought up socioeconomic factors they quickly retreated, claiming, for example, that the link between unemployment and poverty remained unproven, and that despite shared "economic disadvantages," minority populations remained too diverse to permit a generic approach to improving health. Instead, they insisted that programs had to be designed to meet the unique needs of each group, and with this they returned to group behaviors and lifestyle choices.[78]

As a result, the Heckler Report continued the pattern of both mentioning and masking the role of poverty in producing and perpetuating health disparities. Such ambivalence toward poverty, it should be added, was not unusual for government health surveys, which had a long history of both collecting and downplaying demographic information related to class, such as occupation, education level, or income. What was favored instead were categories like age, sex, and race, each of which had purported biological legitimacy. This is exactly what Jones and Joyner were criticizing, as had many other health activists throughout the decades. But in the 1980s not only were critics up against tradition and inertia; they were also dealing with an unsympathetic political climate steeped in neoliberalism's emphasis on individual responsibility. Consequently, the government's first concerted effort to declare health disparities a national priority did little more than produce a flood of new research. Bench science, not neighborhood health centers, public health campaigns, or anti-poverty measures, came out ahead.[79]

The Heckler Report's specific volume on diabetes also contained few surprises. It repeated the troubling fact that diabetes mortality rates, when adjusted for age, were "50 percent higher in nonwhites than in whites." The report also specified that the Akimel O'odham had a tenfold greater risk of developing diabetes than whites; that among Hispanic Americans the chance of becoming diabetic was three times as great as among whites; that among African Americans the diabetes rate had tripled over the last two decades (compared to a doubling among whites); and that Asian Americans suffered disproportionately from the disease. To explain these disparities, the task force listed well-known risk factors, including age, sex, race, genetic factors, level of physical activity, pregnancy, and environmental issues. When it turned to the separate sections for each minority group, however, it did not draw evenly on the different risk factors. Genetics came up only in the sections on Native Americans and Hispanics; diet only in the sections on Native Americans and Asian Americans; and "psychosocial factors" only in the section on Asian Americans. (Oddly, there was no discussion of any risk factors in the section on African Americans.)[80] To be sure, since the task force was dependent on prior research, it could do little more than share what had previously been published. Its omissions and imbalances reflected the state of the scholarship. But by selecting the articles to feature (for example, by omitting available research on poverty and diabetes), and by offering their own commentary on the state of the scholarship, the members of the task force reinforced the legitimacy of thinking about the populations under study in markedly different ways.

The Heckler Report also reinforced and reified the populations themselves, although again, the members of the task force showed an awareness of the somewhat arbitrary nature of the groupings they employed. They drew attention, for example, to the "500 federally recognized American Indian tribes, 23 different countries of origin for Asian/Pacific Islanders, and three major places of origin for Hispanics." They realized as well that for three of the minority populations, they had been overly reliant on information about a single subpopulation, whether Pima Indians, Mexican Americans, or Japanese Americans. Yet, as I have already indicated, this awareness did not prevent them from making generalizations about the populations at large. What is also striking is the complete silence about diversity within the African American population, despite awareness of this diversity at the time. In his masterful work on the epidemiology of diabetes, for example, Kelly West had mentioned the "considerable differences among various populations with black skin in respect to physical attributes, genetic makeup, etc."[81] Yet no mention of this diversity appeared in the Heckler Report.

* * *

One year after the Heckler Report came out, sociologists Michael Omi and Howard Winant published a trenchant critique of contemporary scholarship on race, arguing that race needed to be understood as socially constructed, on the one hand, and as pervading all social relations and social structures, on the other. They coined the phrase "racial formation" to draw attention to the process through which particular understandings of race take root, and to emphasize that such understandings are always "being transformed by political struggle." They did not mention the Heckler Report in their book—they were not dealing with literature on health disparities—but they could easily have extended their critique to medical writings. For in the same way that social science literature had, in Omi and Winant's view, formed racial groups by creating "the 'native' where once there had been Pequot, Iroquois, or Tutelo," and "the 'black' where once there had been Asante or Ovimbundu, Yoruba or Bakongo," the Heckler Report helped to reinforce and reify populations such as "Black Americans," "Native Americans," and "Asian Americans" by collapsing a diverse array of peoples into discrete groups.[82]

The Heckler Report also participated in reifying the category of "whites." It appeared in all ten volumes as the population whose health statistics were consistently better than those of nonwhites. But had the task force disaggregated the data they had on whites—by paying attention, for example, to economic and regional differences—they would have produced a more complex picture. To be sure, the omission of poor whites from the Heckler Report made sense. The secretary's charge to the task force had been to assess the severity of health disparities experienced by racial and ethnic minorities—and in doing so, it helped make racial health disparities a national priority. But by omitting poor whites from the study, and by downplaying the impact of socioeconomic factors on health in other populations as well, the authors of the Heckler Report helped to create a picture of diabetes as "a disease of minority groups," while confining the reasons for disparities to the bodies of those who were sick and the behaviors they embraced. Whatever else may be said about the Heckler Report, it is clear that it played a significant role in the long history of the racial transformation of diabetes.

EPILOGUE

Diabetes and Race since 1985

SINCE THE MID-1980S, THE CENTRAL message in the United States has been that something about minorities makes them more prone to develop diabetes. This message has been communicated through posters, government websites, newspaper stories, and educational pamphlets. Consider a poster produced by the American Diabetes Association, most likely in the 1990s (Figure E.1). The populations that diabetes "favors" are portrayed as Native American, African American, and Hispanic. The poster lacks information about why these populations are more susceptible, but it implies that it has something to do with their respective racial identities. This message is reinforced by the omission of any sign that might indicate that these individuals represent populations with higher rates of poverty and more experiences of discrimination than whites. Indeed, the pride and determination in their faces create the impression that even if they have a genetic (racial) predisposition to diabetes, they are still empowered to make choices that will promote their health. Nothing in this poster suggests that there may be obstacles that would make "good" choices difficult. The power rests largely—even solely—in their hands.

Now imagine that the ADA had added a white person to the lineup. The message would immediately have changed by downplaying, if not eliminating, the possibility of a genetic (racial) predisposition to diabetes (although this very formulation reveals widespread assumptions that whites do not

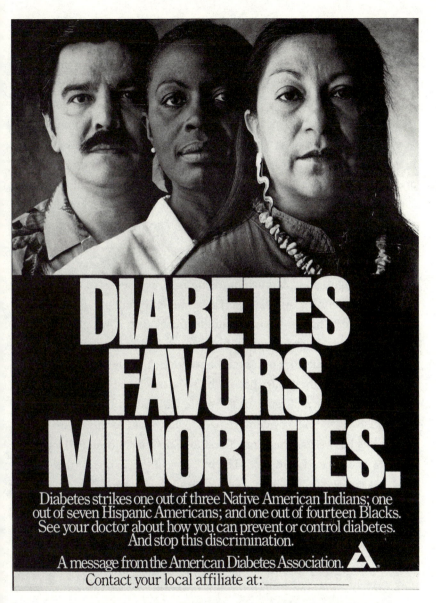

Fig. E.1: Poster from the American Diabetes Association, n.d.
From Digital Collections, U.S. National Library of Medicine,
A025996. Reprinted with permission by the American Diabetes
Association. Copyright by the American Diabetes Association.

have a race). And if geography had been included by portraying that person as living, for example, in Appalachia, then region and class would also have been introduced. By omitting poor whites—by rendering them invisible—this poster, like the Heckler Report before it, limited the way viewers imagined both the causes of, and the solutions to, the "diabetes epidemic." It should come as no surprise, then, that a newspaper article published in 2003 by the Gannett News Service had the headline: "Rising Diabetes Rates in Appalachia Shock Health Officials." The journalist shared statistics that put the rate of diabetes in West Virginia at 10.2 percent, a full 3.5 percent above the national average. A professor of endocrinology at Ohio University interviewed for this article claimed to have "been worried about this for 20 years."[1]

Since the beginning of the new millennium, more attention—although still not enough—has been paid to rising rates of diabetes in economically depressed regions like Appalachia. These studies invariably address the impact that poverty has on the health of the inhabitants, although that impact is often defined only in terms of the paucity of medical personnel and facilities, attitudes of fatalism, or lack of knowledge about the disease. The kind of radical critique that flourished in the 1960s, and that pointed to poverty itself as a fundamental cause of ill health, has had difficulty gaining traction. This was glaringly evident in a 2011 study that introduced the idea of a "diabetes belt" stretching from Texas to Ohio but concentrated largely in the U.S. Southeast (Figure E.2). Led by Lawrence E. Barker of the Centers for Disease Control (CDC), the research team that proposed this label dove beneath statewide data to examine what was going on at the local level in 640 counties throughout the country. The counties considered part of the diabetes belt, which included but were not confined to Appalachia, all had a prevalence of at least 11.2 percent (the national average was 8.5 percent) and were in close proximity to other counties with similarly high rates. The researchers also noted that the inhabitants of the counties in the belt had higher-than-average rates of obesity, sedentary lifestyles, low education levels, and "non-Hispanic African-American ancestry," all of which were considered risk factors for diabetes.[2]

Barker and his team published their results in the *American Journal of Preventive Medicine*. Nowhere in the paper did they mention poverty or

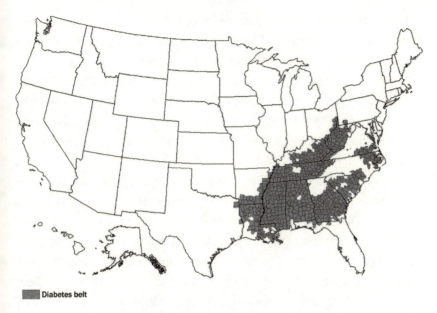

Fig. E.2: Diabetes Belt. Reprinted from Lawrence E. Barker et al.,
"Geographic Distribution of Diagnosed Diabetes in the U.S.: A
Diabetes Belt," *American Journal of Preventive Medicine* 40, no. 4
(2011): 437. Copyright (2011), with permission from Elsevier.

economic hardship. What excited them was their prediction that the diabetes rate could be lowered by 30 percent if people could be persuaded to
exercise more, eat better, and lose weight. They believed that by penetrat-
ing to the county level they had gained laser vision that would allow public
health officials to target their efforts more effectively. But those efforts had
everything to do with changing the behaviors of people who were sick, poor,
and uneducated, and little to do with altering the devastating conditions of
the counties located in the "diabetes belt."[3]

When various media sources picked up this story—and many did so immediately—the central message they communicated was that diabetes was a
disease of "lifestyle choices." Even acknowledging that "the area's economic
history" bore considerable responsibility for the high prevalence of diabetes
in the region—as Barker did during an interview—did little to encourage
an alternative explanation of the forces driving high diabetes rates. The economic history to which Barker referred was the decline in agricultural work

without a corresponding shift in dietary habits. He said nothing about the historic lack of investment in the regions of Appalachia or the long history of racist policies in the South, which had created obstacles to economic mobility and advancement. Similarly, when the director of the CDC's Division of Diabetes Translation put together a presentation on the diabetes belt, she included a map showing the tight link between "counties in persistent poverty" and high diabetes rates, but in her analysis of risk factors she prioritized obesity and race.[4]

Placing so much emphasis on obesity when trying to account for diabetes prevalence is not new. Joslin, we might remember, had called diabetes a "penalty of obesity." Still, as late as 1976, the National Commission on Diabetes felt the need to preface its statement that "obesity is strongly suspected to be one of the causes of diabetes" with a disclaimer that "the connection has never been conclusively established." By the mid-1980s, however, such caution had disappeared. The exact nature of the link remained unclear, but the association between the two had become a critical part of the public conversation about diabetes. By the mid-1990s, some even adopted the term "diabesity," which ostensibly erased any distinction between body size and disease. At the same time, obesity was being reimagined as a serious problem in its own right. From its designation as "a public health threat" in the mid-1980s, to perceptions that it was itself a disease, to fears that it was reaching "epidemic" proportions, obesity has been at the center of heated discussions over the relationship between body size and health. Members of the fat acceptance movement, in particular, have challenged the association of obesity with disease, and insisted instead that stigma and discrimination, not size, lead to many of the psychological and physiological problems common among people who are fat.[5]

Complicating this conversation further was the increasing association of obesity with poverty. According to a 2003 report from the Office of the Surgeon General, women of low socioeconomic status, regardless of race or ethnicity, were roughly "50% more likely to be obese than those of higher socioeconomic status." Yet despite the conflation of obesity, diabetes, and poverty, the deep connections among them were and are often dealt with superficially or simply overlooked. In the end, they are also often deemed consequences of "poor choices."[6]

The inclusion of "non-Hispanic African-American ancestry" as an important risk factor in articles about the "diabetes belt" brings home once more the powerful way that race continues to shape accounts of disease prevalence. Using the language of "ancestry," without also acknowledging that African Americans live disproportionately in poverty and continue to encounter racial discrimination in their everyday lives, has at least two serious consequences: it renders invisible the structural impediments that black people face, which give lie to claims that change depends on something as simple as "choice"; and it directs attention away from common obstacles that all poor people face—whether white, African American, Native American, Hispanic, or Pacific Islander—as they struggle to break cycles of poverty and advocate more effectively on their own behalf.[7]

Americans' obsession with race (but not racism) and ambivalence toward class have been reinforced historically by the government's tendency to collect information about race and ethnicity when conducting health studies, and to neglect other confounding factors such as class. This partial telling of the story is consistently reproduced on government websites designed to disseminate important information about diseases to the public. Thus, material about diabetes on the websites of the National Institutes of Health and the CDC informs readers that membership in certain racial and ethnic groups places them at high risk of developing diabetes while saying nothing about the risk of living in economically depressed inner-city neighborhoods and rural areas, or of encountering racism regularly. In this way, the picture that government organizations produce and reproduce of populations at risk for diabetes is at best misleading, and at worst evidence of how government messages can inadvertently reinforce structural racism by masking racial stereotypes within seemingly factual claims.[8]

The appeal of "race" as an explanation for health disparities has persisted throughout the history of diabetes, although the meaning of race has neither remained constant through time, nor has it been understood in the same way for all populations. Biological race was rarely contested as an explanation for high diabetes rates among Native Americans, while it was rarely mentioned as a reason for diabetes in the Asian American population. For Jews and African Americans, allusions to biological race have always engendered controversy.

The launching of the Human Genome Project in 1990 has only continued the pattern. Completed in 2000, the project to map the human genome has substantially transformed medical research by steering vast sums of money into the search for genetic variants that might explain health disparities between purported racial groups. In the process, it has also reinvigorated debates about the place of race in understanding the etiology of complex diseases. Advocates of this research insist that race is a strong predictor of health outcomes, and that a better understanding of race-specific genetic susceptibilities will increase the chances of reducing health disparities. Opponents counter that the focus on race ignores genetic diversity within groups, contributes to racial stereotyping, and diverts attention away from non-genetic explanations, like poverty, that might better explain differential rates.[9]

When diabetes first emerged as a public health concern in the late nineteenth century, it had a highly specific "racial profile" that linked the disease most frequently to whites in general and Jews in particular. Those populations no longer dominate the accounts we read of diabetes in professional journals and the popular press. African Americans, Hispanics, Native Americans, and Asian Americans have now replaced Jews and whites as the "races" most likely to develop diabetes, even as the meaning of "race" remains highly ambiguous and contested.

The racial profile of diabetes is not all that has changed. Diabetes is also no longer the same, and the various representations of the disease have undergone marked transformations. Most striking are the radically different portrayals of diabetes associated with type 1 and type 2. Characterizations of people with diabetes as "self-reliant," of "greater intelligence," and "better citizens than the average," which permeated the diabetes literature in the interwar years, have not so much disappeared as become channeled into representations of individuals with type 1. Some of the most compelling images for type 1 diabetes are of children who, before the advent of insulin pumps, had to learn how to give themselves injections, often multiple times a day. In contrast, the fears associated with overindulgence and conspicuous consumption, which also flourished in the interwar years, now burden individuals with type 2. "I really find it hard to take seriously the complaints of type 2 diabetics, who, in my view, brought this on themselves," commented a fifteen year old with type 1. He felt strongly that in contrast to the poor lifestyle choices of those with type 2 diabetes, he had a disease over which he "had absolutely no control." That type 1 diabetes is believed to be most prevalent among whites makes this contrast even more disturbing.[10]

A language of "choice" and "control" implies that all that someone needs to do to become healthy is decide to eat well, exercise frequently, visit a doctor regularly, and take prescribed medicines. Nowhere in this formulation is there any acknowledgment of the uneven distribution of resources that can make it difficult for even a well-intentioned individual to make what are considered healthy choices. Nor is there any recognition that racism and poverty are themselves fundamental causes of ill health, potentially exacerbating diabetes by raising stress and glucose levels, and certainly placing an additional burden on individuals who may already be struggling to make ends meet. Casting those with type 2 diabetes as responsible for their disease masks the structural inequalities that produce poor health and divides people with diabetes into those who are innocent and those who are guilty. It is not surprising that the mother of a young girl with type 1 diabetes expressed her "wish [that] it had a different name."[11]

* * *

The stories we tell matter. And the ones we tell about race matter in very particular ways, especially when they are undergirded by notions of innocence and guilt. The history of diabetes drives home the extent to which disease is a site for the absorption and reproduction of unsubstantiated claims about a population's alleged racial makeup. In the case of diabetes these claims were often shocking: Jews suffered disproportionately from diabetes because they were more modern; middle-class whites were more "civilized"; African Americans were less intelligent; Native Americans had primitive bodies unequipped to handle the demands of modern times; Japanese Americans experienced higher levels of stress. That the face of diabetes changed so frequently over the course of the twentieth century makes its history a rich resource for uncovering the deep entanglement of disease and race. Such entanglements are evident as well in the histories that scholars have produced of such diseases as schizophrenia, cancer, fetal alcohol syndrome, syphilis, tuberculosis, heart disease, and lung disease. And we are seeing them again in our recent discovery of an "opioid crisis." What is most striking about the history of opioid use and abuse in the United States is the stark contrast between the criminalization of drug abuse in the 1980s, when the affected population was imagined as being primarily black, and the emphasis on diversion programs and rehabilitation today, when the affected population is pictured as largely white and the victim of a pharmaceutical industry gone wild.[12] Placed in context with the other disease histories, the narrative of the opioid crisis becomes one more story of how deeply ideas of race penetrate conceptualizations of disease, from claims about causation, to strategies of intervention, to judgments about who does—and does not—deserve care.

Rivers Solomon, who penned the op-ed piece "I Have Diabetes. Am I to Blame?" discussed in the Introduction, described the confusion that people sometimes experience when trying to figure out which type of diabetes she has. Since she is young, some people think she has the type "that *just happens* for no reason." But because of her "fatness" and "blackness," others assume that she is "inherently lazy, deviant, sick, unclean," and, as a result, that she has brought this disease upon herself.[13] But why does it matter which type she has? My hope is that no matter the nature of her disease, we could agree that, like my father, she is not to blame for her diabetes.

NOTES

Introduction

1. Giving someone with LADA a diagnosis of type 2 diabetes is a common mistake. See Appel, "Misdiagnosed"; Unger, "Editorials."

2. This statement refers only to diabetes mellitus. Diabetes insipidus, a rare disease that results in the excessive production of non-sweet, dilute urine, was considered a different "species" of diabetes as early as the eighteenth century. See Swan, *Works of Thomas Sydenham*, 1:453. Throughout this book, when I refer to diabetes, I mean diabetes mellitus.

3. Feudtner, *Bittersweet;* Mauck, "Managing Care," 304–306.

4. National Institute of Diabetes and Digestive and Kidney Diseases, "Diabetes Overview."

5. Ahlqvist et al., "Novel Subgroups,"; Tuomi et al., "Many Faces of Diabetes"; Zaccardi et al., "Pathophysiology." Going in the direction of creating more rather than fewer categories, some have put forth a controversial suggestion that individuals with diabetes and Alzheimer's disease may have what they are calling type 3 diabetes. See Kandimalla, Thirumala, and Reddy, "Review"; Macmillan, "Researchers Identify."

6. Feudtner, *Bittersweet*. The standard account of insulin's discovery remains Bliss, *Discovery of Insulin*. See also Cooper and Ainsberg, *Breakthrough*. On diabetes before insulin, primarily in England, see Furdell, *Fatal Thirst*.

7. See, for example, Epstein, "Diabetes among Jews," 270.

8. For books that focus on scientific advancements in the history of diabetes, see Bliss, *Discovery of Insulin;* Tattersall, *Diabetes*.

9. The quotation from 1898 is cited in Pancoast, "Diabetes in the Negro," 41; Joslin, "Diabetic Problem," 727; Miller, Bennett, and Burch, "Hyperglycemia," 91; the California physician is cited in Sahagun, "Genetic Link," 1; National Institute of

Diabetes and Digestive and Kidney Diseases, "Risk Factors." See also Centers for Disease Control and Prevention, "Diabetes." In accordance with people-first language, I have avoided using the word "diabetic" as a noun unless it appeared in a direct quotation. I am grateful to Marion Nestle for her wisdom on this issue.

10. Stocking, "Turn-of-the-Century Concept of Race"; Jacobson, *Whiteness of a Different Color*; Stepan, *Idea of Race*; Barkan, *Retreat of Scientific Racism*; Reardon, *Race to the Finish*; Harmon, "Why White Supremacists Are Chugging Milk"; Hammonds and Herzig, *Nature of Difference*.

11. The literature on this debate is voluminous. For a particularly cogent description of the arguments for and against research on genetics and health disparities, see Fine, Ibrahim, and Thomas, "Editorial." See also Williams, "Race and Health"; Bloche, "Race-Based Therapeutics"; Epstein, *Inclusion*; "Is Race 'Real?'"

12. Phelan and Link, "Is Racism a Fundamental Cause?" See Pollock, *Medicating Race*, and Tallbear, *Native American DNA*, for exemplary studies demonstrating the impossibility of separating the biological and the social.

13. The following is just a sampling of works that deal with the history of race and disease in the United States: Jones, *Bad Blood*; McBride, *From TB to AIDS*; Kraut, *Silent Travelers*; Markel, *Quarantine!*; Humphreys, *Malaria*; Shah, *Contagious Divides*; Wailoo, *Dying in the City of Blues*; Jones, *Rationalizing Epidemics*; Roberts, *Infectious Fear*; Willrich, *Pox*; Pollock, *Medicating Race*; Reverby, *Examining Tuskegee*; McMillen, *Discovering Tuberculosis*.

14. Golden, *Message in a Bottle*; Metzl, *Protest Psychosis*; Wailoo, *How Cancer Crossed the Color Line*.

15. Joslin, "Prevention," 81–82; "Adiposity and Other Etiological Factors"; "Diabetes, Insulin, and Vitamin B." On the dating of the "obesity epidemic," see Saguy and Riley, "Weighing Both Sides"; Rasmussen, *Fat in the Fifties*.

16. Tallbear, *Native American DNA*, 11–13; Hatch, *Blood Sugar*; Krieger, "If 'Race' Is the Answer"; Williams, "Race and Health"; Smedley and Smedley, "Race as Biology"; Link and Phelan, "Social Conditions."

17. Solomon, "I Have Diabetes."

Chapter 1. *Judenkrankheit*

1. Seegen, *Diabetes Mellitus*, 125–126. On Seegen, see Efron, *Medicine and the German Jews*, 133. For statistics on Jews in Europe in 1900, see Crystall and Leitenberg, *Digital Maps*.

2. Efron, *Medicine and the German Jews*, 132–142. For a reference to *Judenkrankheit*, see Epstein, "Diabetes among Jews," 270.

3. Thomas, "Medical Treatment," 1451; Osler, *Principles*, 1st ed., 275; Wilson, "Increase in the Death Rate," 662–663; Morrison, "A Statistical Study," 57; Joslin, *Treatment*, 1st ed., 46.

4. Cited in Gabaccia, *We Are What We Eat*, 46–47, and in Diner, *Hungering for America*, 180, 185. For a more complete discussion of the immigrants' experience of food, see chapters 6 and 7 of Diner's book. See also Wood, *Foods of the Foreign-Born*, 89.

5. Fang et al., "Stressful Life Events"; Misra and Ganda, "Migration"; Acevedo-Garcia et al., "Integrating Social Epidemiology"; Ferreira and Lang, "Introduction," 10–11; Gebel, "Problem of Pounds."

6. Stern, "Mortality," 766; Epstein, "Diabetes among Jews," 271.

7. Quotations from Hopkins, "Letter to the Editor," 450–451, and Epstein, "Diabetes among Jews," 269. On the many possible causes of diabetes, see Joslin, *Treatment*, 1st ed., 49–53, and Osler, *Principles*, 1st ed., 295.

8. Comfort, *Science of Human Perfection;* Pernick, "Eugenics and Public Health"; Durrah, "Diabetes Mellitus," 242. For an early discussion of diabetes and Mendelian traits, see Cammidge, "Diabetes Mellitus and Heredity." A Mendelian trait refers to a trait that is influenced by a single locus on the gene; its expression follows the inheritance pattern established by the Austrian monk Gregor Mendel.

9. On the use of taste to diagnose diabetes, see Kirchhof, Popat, and Malowany, "Historical Perspective"; Joslin, *Treatment*, 1st ed., 17.

10. Tattersall, *Diabetes,* 180–184; Greene, *Prescribing by Numbers.*

11. "Adiposity"; Stern, " Mortality"; Efron, *Medicine,* 137. For a concise statement of the problems involved in defining "Jews," see Falk, "Eugenics."

12. I address these questions in a much abbreviated form in Tuchman, "Diabetes and Race."

13. Purdy, *Diabetes,* 18.

14. Wilson, "Study," 265; Wilson, "Increase in the Death Rate," 662–663. Wilson's views were criticized at the time. See Morrison, "Statistical Study," 55. See also Efron, *Medicine,* 134–135.

15. U.S. Congress, *Dictionary,* 1–5.

16. Singerman, "Jew as Racial Alien," 110, 117; Jacobson, *Whiteness,* 22; Ngai, "Architecture of Race," 81. On the long history of claiming Jews were oriental, see Kalmar and Penslar, *Orientalism.* On early twentieth-century racial hierarchies, see Stocking, "Turn-of-the-Century"; Brodkin, *How Jews Became White Folks;* Barkan, *Retreat,* 2, 19.

17. U.S. Congress, *Dictionary,* 5, 74; Abernethy, *Jew a Negro* (cited in Singerman, "Jew as Racial Alien," 117); Stoddard, "Pedigree of Judah" (cited in Singerman, "Jew as Racial Alien," 127); U.S. Congress, *Statements and Recommendations,* 48; Davenport is cited in Paul, *Controlling Human Heredity,* 105. See also Goldstein, *Price of Whiteness,* 108–115; Goldstein, "Contesting the Categories"; Goren, "Jews."

18. Wilson, "Crossing of the Races," 487–488, emphasis in the original.

19. Ibid., 488–495.

20. Fitz and Joslin, "Diabetes Mellitus"; Osler, *Principles,* 1st ed., 275; Lees, "Two Million Tightrope Walkers," 34; Emerson, "Sweetness Is Death," 24; Goldstein, "Unstable Other."

21. Emerson, "Sweetness Is Death," 24.

22. Ibid., 24–25.

23. Ibid.

24. Gilman, "Fat as Disability," 50. See also Hart, *Social Science,* chapters 3 and 4; Schwartz, *Never Satisfied;* Stearns, *Fat History.*

25. Emerson, "Sweetness Is Death," 25.

26. Barnett, *Elliott P. Joslin;* Epstein, "Diabetes among Jews," 273.

27. Joslin, "Diabetic Problem," 727.

28. Ibid., 728.

29. Joslin, "Prevention," 81–82.

30. Ibid., 81; Joslin, "Changing Diabetic Clientele," 305.

31. Gilman, "Fat as Disability," 51; Schwartz, *Never Satisfied,* 143.

32. "Diabetes as Jewish Peril."

33. Rosenberg, *Cholera Years;* Byers, "Diseases of the Southern Negro."

34. Kleen, *On Diabetes,* 15–19; Shattuck, "General Management," 367; Osler, *Principles,* 1st ed., 295. On "diseases of civilization" see Rosenberg, "Pathologies of Progress"; Martensen and Jones, "Diabetes"; Porter, "Diseases of Civilization." On similarly "positive" readings of angina pectoris, see Aronowitz, *Making Sense,* 97–101. On modernity and civilization, see Eisenstadt, "A Reappraisal of Theories of Social Change and Modernization."

35. Nott, "Physical History," 428–430; Beaulieu is cited in Gottheil, "Israel," 54; Baur, Fischer, and Lenz, *Human Heredity,* 667–674. See also Williamson, "Increased Death Rate," 458.

36. Jacobs and Fishberg, "Diabetes." On the Jewish medical community's general acceptance of Jewish diseases, see Hart, "Racial Science"; Hart, *Jews and Race;* Efron, *Medicine;* Efron, *Defenders.* On the *Jewish Encyclopedia,* see Schwartz, *Emergence of Jewish Scholarship.*

37. Fishberg, "Health and Sanitation," 177.

38. Jacobs and Fishberg, "Diabetes."

39. Graham, *Pathology and Treatment,* 82, 34–35; Jacobs and Fishberg, "Diabetes."

40. Goldstein, "Wandering Jews," 536; Jolly, *Handbuch,* 755; Jacobs and Fishberg, "Nervous Diseases."

41. Fishberg, "Health and Sanitation," 170.

42. Seegen, *Diabetes,* 126; Oppenheim is cited in Hart, *Jews and Race,* 107; Solis-Cohen is cited in "Adiposity," 1775–1776. See also Jacobs and Fishberg, "Nervous Diseases"; Epstein, "Diabetes among Jews," 274.

43. Epstein, "Diabetes among Jews," 270. In my analysis of Jews' reimagining of the meaning of diabetes, I have been influenced by Keith Wailoo's work on black activists and sickle cell anemia. See Wailoo, *Dying,* ch. 6.

44. On Lamarck's popularity in the United States during the early twentieth century, see Bowler, *Evolution;* Stocking, "Turn-of-the-Century."

45. Baur, Fischer, and Lenz, *Human Heredity,* 674–675; Fishberg, "Health and Sanitation," 170; Solis-Cohen is cited in "Adiposity," 1775–1776. See also Fishberg, *Jews,* 23; Lyon, *Diabetes;* Hart, *Social Science,* 11.

46. Epstein, "Diabetes among Jews," 269–274.

47. Beaulieu is cited in Fishberg, "Health and Sanitation," 177; Kleen, *On Diabetes,* 15; Williamson, "Increased Death Rate," 458; Roberts, "Nervous and Mental Influences," 23; Shattuck, "General Management," 367. See also Aronowitz, *Making Sense,* 88–89, 98; and Rosenberg, "Body and Mind."

48. Herskovits, *American Negro;* Krout, "Race and Culture," 183.

49. Barkan, *Retreat;* Taylor, "W. E. B. Du Bois's Challenge."

50. Stoddard is cited in Jacobson, *Whiteness,* 184; Fleure is cited in Stepan, *Idea of Race,* 162. See also Stepan, *Idea of Race;* Barkan, *Retreat;* King, *Race, Culture;* and Hart, *Social Science.*

51. Stepan, *Idea of Race,* 162; Ngai, *Impossible Subjects.*

52. U.S. President's Research Committee on Social Trends, *Recent Social Trends,* 1:xxiv; Brodkin, *How Jews Became White;* Jacobson, *Whiteness,* especially chapters 3 and 5; Goldstein, *Price of Whiteness,* 110–115.

53. Joslin, "Diabetes among Jews," 222; Ginzburg, "Frequency of Diabetes,"193. *The Jewish Post* covered this symposium in "Seventy-Five Per Cent of Diabetes Cases."

54. Joslin, *Treatment,* 8th ed., 106; Osler, *Principles,* 16th ed., 583; Grissom and Rosenlof, "Management," 461. See also "Diet or Die." I counted twenty-five articles, published between 1933 and 1954, that repeated this claim.

55. Schwartz, "Etiology"; Zisserman, "Diabetes," 314; Blotner, "Studies in Glycosuria."

56. Blotner, "Studies in Glysosuria," 1113. For a similar claim, see Dahlberg, "Swedish Jews," 109.

57. Reported in "Incidence of Diabetes," 886.

58. Steinitz, "Incidence of Diabetes"; Cohen, "Prevalence of Diabetes," 57.

59. Krikler, "Diseases of Jews," 688; Mendosa, "Jewish Diabetes."

60. Blotner, "Studies in Glycosuria," 1112.

61. Blotner, Hyde, and Kingsley, "Studies in Diabetes Mellitus," 891.

62. Wailoo and Pemberton, *Troubled Dream.*

Chapter 2. Whiteness

1. Dublin, "Recent Trends"; Hoffman, "Diabetes Record"; Wohl, "Diabetes"; "Diabetes Mortality Up," 24. The estimate from Met Life is mentioned in Joslin, *Treatment,* 6th ed., 26–27.

2. Emerson, "Sweetness Is Death," 24.

3. Tuchman, "Diabetes and 'Defective' Genes."

4. Wolfe, "Racial Integrity Laws"; Levine and Bashford, "Introduction," 6. On boundary work, see Gieryn, "Boundary-Work."

5. Williams, "Evaluation," 65; Emerson, "Sweetness Is Death," 25; Lees, "Two Million Tightrope Walkers," 38.

6. Wailoo, *How Cancer Crossed;* Aronowitz, *Risky Medicine;* Mooney, "Material Consumptive."

7. Elduff, "About Us."

8. Joslin, Dublin, and Marks, "Studies in Diabetes Mellitus II," 449; Dublin, "Modern Life," 40; Emerson, "Public Health," 1019; Joslin, *Diabetic Manual,* 1st ed., 17. See also Pollock, *Medicating Race,* 29–33, for an astute analysis of how race intersected with ideas of infectious and degenerative diseases.

9. Tuchman, "Biometrics and Citizenship."

10. Purdy, *Diabetes,* 18.

11. Wiebe, *Search for Order*.

12. Ibid., 42–43. On consumerism and culture, see Peiss, *Cheap Amusements*; Leach, *Land of Desire*; Nasaw, *Going Out*; and Dumenil, *Modern Temper*.

13. Gerstle, *American Crucible*, 93; Igo, *Known Citizen*; Rose, *Politics of Life*; Molina, *Fit to Be Citizens*; and Shah, *Contagious Divides*.

14. For excellent analyses of how early twentieth-century public health literature promoted the idea that health was a commodity that could be purchased, see Toon, "Managing," and Tomes, *Remaking the American Patient*.

15. Katz, *In the Shadow*; Linker, *War's Waste*; Kline, *Building a Better Race*.

16. Barnett, *Elliott P. Joslin*; Feudtner, *Bittersweet*.

17. Cited in Barnett, *Elliott P. Joslin*, 36. For biographical information on Joslin, see ibid. and Feudtner, *Bittersweet*. Joslin's textbook continued to be published after his death. The fourteenth edition came out in 2005.

18. Joslin, *Treatment of Diabetes Mellitus*, 1st ed., 364.

19. Albertson, "I Have Diabetes," 427; Feudtner, *Bittersweet*, 49, 124; Edison, Mina Miller, to Theodore Miller Edison, July 12, 1931.

20. Mentioned in Barnett, *Elliott P. Joslin*, 39. See also Feudtner, *Bittersweet*, 34.

21. Joslin, *Treatment*, 2nd ed., 54.

22. Joslin, "Shattuck Lecture," 836. Also, see Feudtner, *Bittersweet*, 131–132.

23. Joslin, "Prevention," 83.

24. Ibid., 84.

25. Williams, "Evaluation," 65. See also Wiley, "League," 190, who followed Joslin and blamed diabetes on "dietary indiscretions."

26. Osler, *Principles*, 1st ed., 298, emphasis in the original; Purdy, *Diabetes*, 47. On the widespread belief that diabetes was one disease, see Joslin, *Treatment*, 1st ed., 61–62.

27. Feudtner, *Bittersweet*.

28. Bliss, *Discovery*.

29. Cooper and Ainsberg, *Breakthrough*.

30. "Two Important Cures Announced."

31. Feudtner, *Bittersweet*.

32. Emerson, "Public Health Awaits," 1009; "McCann's Warning"; O-Day, "Blurring of Diabetes"; "Rip Van Winkles."

33. On "tight" control, see Mauck, "Managing Care."

34. My interpretation of these photographs draws on Feudtner, *Bittersweet*, 6–8.

35. Edison, Mina Miller, to Theodore Miller Edison, July 12, 1931. Mina Miller Edison penned several letters to her son Theodore Miller Edison in 1923 and 1931, describing Thomas Alva Edison's illness.

36. Edison, Mina Miller, to Theodore Miller Edison, April 9, 1923. I'm assuming that Edison was diagnosed in 1923 because in this letter, which is the first in which she mentions diabetes, Mina sounds like he had only recently received the diagnosis.

37. Albertson, "I Have Diabetes," 424; for Bunche, see personal note, November 1, 1958, and September 26, 1967, cited in Urquhart, *Ralph Bunche*, 298–299 and 394, respectively.

38. See, for example, Molina, *Fit to Be Citizens?*; Baynton, *Defectives in the Land*; Hirschmann and Linker, *Civil Disabilities.*

39. Baynton, "Disability" (Johnson is cited on 41); Hirschmann and Linker, "Disability, Citizenship, and Belonging."

40. Quotations by Albertson in this and the next three paragraphs are from Albertson, "I Have Diabetes."

41. Guttmacher, "Hereditary Counseling," 192; White, "Pregnancy Complicating Diabetes," 618.

42. Cited in Pernick, "Eugenics and Public Health," 1767.

43. White, "Pregnancy Complicating Diabetes," 637.

44. The literature on the history of eugenics is vast. See, for example, Kevles, *In the Name of Eugenics*; Paul, *Controlling Human Heredity*; Kline, *Building a Better Race*; Ladd-Taylor, *Fixing the Poor*; and Stern, *Eugenic Nation*. On the heyday of eugenic sterilization, see Reilly, *Surgical Solution*, 128; and Largent, *Breeding Contempt*, 77–80.

45. Laughlin, "Scope of the Committee's Work," 13; Jennings, "Health Progress," 271. On Jennings's opposition to eugenics, see Paul, *Controlling Human Heredity*, 70, 116; and Kevles, *In the Name of Eugenics*, 122–128.

46. Jennings, "Health Progress," 272.

47. Ibid., 275.

48. Ibid., 273. The paper that had the greatest influence on geneticists' assessment of the feasibility of eliminating a recessive trait was East, "Hidden Feeblemindedness." For a discussion of the impact of the Hardy-Weinberg principle on eugenics, see Paul, *Politics of Heredity*, 117–132.

49. Largent, *Breeding Contempt*, 72.

50. Skipper, "Diabetes Mellitus and Pregnancy," 370. I wish to thank Robert Tattersall for bringing this article to my attention. See also Kemp, "Danish Experiences"; "Heredity and Diabetes," 30; King, *In the Name of Illiberalism*, ch. 3. For a discussion of global eugenic legislation, see Bashford and Levine, *Oxford Handbook*. For a timeline of when European countries passed compulsory sterilization laws, see Klunker, "Genügen"; Proctor, *Racial Hygiene*, ch. 4; Weindling, "German Eugenics."

51. Klunker, "Genügen," 6. Some extremists recommended denying insulin to diabetes patients, thus removing, in their eyes, a medical treatment that was allowing the unfit to reproduce. This does not appear to have gained any ground. See Bertram, "Prophylaxe."

52. Bertram, "Prophylaxe," 1061-1062. See also Slater, "German Eugenics," 293. On the Marital Health Courts and the Genetic Health Courts, see Proctor, *Racial Hygiene*, 136–142; Weindling, "German Eugenics," 322; Slater, "German Eugenics."

53. Joslin, "Social and Medical Aspects," 1037–1038; "600,000 Diabetics," 297. In developing the ensuing argument, I have been most influenced by Pernick, "Eugenics and Public Health," and Paul, *Politics of Heredity*, 133–156. For an analysis of the development of the idea of "genetic risk" in the middle decades of the twentieth century, see Stern, *Telling Genes*.

54. Joslin, "Social and Medical Aspects," 1033. See also Joslin, *Treatment,* 6th ed., 88.

55. Joslin, "Social and Medical Aspects," 1033–1034.

56. Ibid.

57. Ibid., 1034–1035.

58. Ibid.

59. Bowcock, "Diabetic Negro," 109; White, "Diabetes in Childhood," 601–602; Klunker, "Genügen," 6; Lees, "Two Million Tightrope Walkers," 38; Leonard, "Diabetic's Disposition," 310; Frear, "Diabetes," 76.

60. Leonard, "Diabetic's Disposition," 310. See Wailoo, *How Cancer Crossed,* 85, for a similar conversation about cancer in the 1950s.

61. Joslin, *Diabetic Manual,* 1st ed., 17.

62. Joslin, "Prevention," 83; Joslin, *Treatment,* 8th ed., 16.

63. Rose and Novas, "Biological Citizenship," 1–3. For a brief overview of scholarship on this concept, see Mulligan, "Biological Citizenship."

64. Rose, *Politics of Life Itself,* 1–3, 22–27.

65. Molina, *Fit to Be Citizens?*; Shah, *Contagious Divides.* See also Roberts, *Infectious Fear.*

66. Lees, "Two Million Tightrope Walkers," 34–36. "Hotcha" refers to an expression of approval or delight.

67. Greene, *Prescribing by Numbers.* For several excellent studies of the challenges and rhetoric of diabetes's management, see Moore, *Managing Diabetes;* Bennett, *Managing Diabetes;* Hatch, *Blood Sugar;* and Mauck, "Managing Care."

68. Rose, *Politics of Life Itself.*

69. Grey, *New Deal Medicine,* 25.

70. Weisz, *Chronic Disease,* 92–94; Weisz, "Epidemiology." For the conversion from 1935 to 2017 dollars, I used the "Dollar Times," http://www.dollartimes.com/inflation/inflation.php?amount=3000&year=1935, accessed May 29, 2019.

71. U.S. Public Health Service, *Preliminary Reports, Bulletin 6,* 9–10; U.S. Interdepartmental Committee to Coordinate Health and Welfare Activities, *National Health Conference,* 46; Britten, Collins, and Fitzgerald, "The National Health Survey," 455; "Deaths among Poor," 26.

Chapter 3. Misunderstanding the African American Experience

1. Elliot, "Diabetes," 23; Birnie, "Influence of Environment," 249. On causes of mortality and morbidity among African Americans in the early twentieth century, see Savitt, *Race and Medicine;* Downs, *Sick from Freedom;* Byrd and Clayton, *American Health Dilemma,* 1:347.

2. Garvin, "Negro Health"; Du Bois, "Postscript"; Roberts, *Infectious Fear;* Smith, *Sick and Tired;* Beardsley, *History of Neglect.* The phrase "epidemiological transition" is from Omran, "Epidemiological Transition."

3. Humphreys et al., "Racial Disparities," 1770.

4. Smith, *Sick and Tired;* Byrd and Clayton, *American Health Dilemma,* vol. 2, chs. 1 and 2; Ward, *Black Physicians;* Hine, *Black Women.* On the history of tuberculosis

among African Americans, see McBride, *From TB to AIDS;* Roberts, *Infectious Fear.*

5. Williams, "Is the Negro Dying Out?," 662; Alexander, "Is the Negro Dying Out?," 673. See also Gover, *Mortality;* Wilkerson, *Warmth of Other Suns,* 10.

6. Gover, *Mortality,* 8; Hollinger, "Amalgation and Hypodescent"; Du Bois, "Post-Script." On the different criteria for determining the designation "Negro," see Davis, *Who Is Black?;* Wright, "One Drop"; and Fields, "Ideology and Race." For a discussion of different gradations of blackness, see Elliott, "Telling the Difference"; Zackondik, "Fixing the Color Line."

7. I discuss the Heckler Report in Chapter 5.

8. Smith, *Sick and Tired,* 58–59, 82. On the visibility and invisibility of disease, see Wailoo, *Dying.* On the invisibility of the black middle class, see Pattillo-McCoy, *Black Picket Fences;* Frazier, *Black Bourgeoisie;* Grahm, *Our Kind of People.*

9. Kleen, *On Diabetes,* 15–19; Futcher, "Frequency and Aetiology," 753, 755. The belief in racial immunities and susceptibilities was widespread. See Du Bois, *Health and Physique,* 98. For a similar logic in discussions of blacks and cancer, see Wailoo, *How Cancer Crossed.*

10. Hoffman, "Race Traits," 95. Emphasis in the original. For an analysis of race, malaria, and ideas of immunity, see Humphreys, *Malaria,* ch. 3.

11. Miller, *Review.* Other challenges to Hoffmann included Du Bois, *Health and Physique,* and a 1909 Symposium, "Is the Negro Dying Out?" For a discussion of Miller's critique, see Stepan and Gilman, "Appropriating the Idioms," 183.

12. *Proceedings of the St. Louis Medical Society,* June 7, 1884, 147–148. On race, evolution, and disease, see Savitt, *Medicine and Slavery;* Haller, *Outcasts from Evolution;* and Humphreys, *Intensely Human,* ch. 3.

13. Lemann, "Diabetes Mellitus in the Negro Race," 523–524. See also Morrison, "Statistical Study," 56.

14. Turner, *Ceramic Uncles;* Boskin, *Rise and Demise.*

15. Lemann, "Diabetes Mellitus in the Negro Race," 522, 525.

16. Lemann, "Diabetes Mellitus among the Negroes."

17. Lemann, "Diabetes Mellitus in the Negro Race," 523.

18. The three quotations were made during a discussion following Lehmann's paper. See Lemann, "Diabetes Mellitus in the Negro Race," 524–525.

19. Ibid.

20. Goldstein, "Diabetes in the Negro," 907.

21. "War on Diabetes," 20; Emerson, "Sweetness Is Death," 24; "Mortality from Diabetes," 42.

22. Lewis, *Biology of the Negro,* 282.

23. Mauck, "Managing Care," 149–155. On Dublin, see Bouk, *How Our Days Became Numbered,* esp. ch. 5; Dublin, *After Eighty Years.* See also Marquis, *Metropolitan Life.*

24. Dublin, "Mortality Statistics," 631. Dublin may not have "seen" the racial disparity because he was most interested in disrupting the dominant image of diabetes as a disease of the wealthy. See Marks, "Epidemiologists Explain Pellagra."

25. Dublin, "Health of the Negro," 77. On the willingness of Met Life to insure black wage earners, see Bouk, *How Our Days Became Numbered*, 184.

26. Garvin, "Negro Health," 341–342. For a similarly critical appraisal of how racial discrimination affected black health, see Williams, "Defender Health Editor Looks Back." On the migration of African Americans to the North, see Wilkerson, *Warmth of Other Suns;* Speak, *Black Chicago;* Robinson, *Disintegration.*

27. Dublin, "Health of the Negro," 77–85. According to one statistic, 87 percent of blacks in the North lived in cities with populations of ten thousand or more, compared to only 25 percent in the South. See Gover, *Mortality among Negroes*, 3.

28. Bowcock, "Diabetes Mellitus in the Negro Race." See also Bowcock, "Diabetic Negro."

29. Leopold, "Diabetes in the Negro Race," 292.

30. The quotation is from ibid., 289, but he is drawing on Bowcock, "Diabetes Mellitus in the Negro Race," 994.

31. Joslin, Dublin, and Marks, "Studies in Diabetes Mellitus I," 766.

32. Ibid., 764; Joslin, *Treatment*, 6th ed., 43.

33. "Rising Diabetes Death Rate"; "Industrial Health of Nation Surveyed"; Jablons, "Diabetes," 424. Jablons's affiliation with the American Jewish Congress is mentioned in "No Scientific Basis for 'Aryan' Race Theory." See also "Diabetes Gain Laid."

34. "Reaction of Negroes to Disease," 857; "Health Director Warns," 4; Dublin, "Modern Life," 40; Perrott and Holland, "Need for Adequate Data," 350. For similar resistance on the part of physicians to "recognize the African American cardiovascular disease in front of them," see Pollock, *Medicating Race,* 13.

35. U.S. Public Health Service, *Preliminary Reports, Bulletin 6*, 2; Gover, "Trend of Mortality."

36. Dublin, "Health of the Negro," 83. See, also, Wailoo, *How Cancer Crossed*, 61–62.

37. Dublin, "Health of the Negro," 85.

38. Leopold, "Diabetes in the Negro Race," 291–292; Bowcock, "Diabetic Negro," 109, 118. On caricatures of black women, see Turner, *Ceramic Uncles;* Walker-Barnes, *Too Heavy a Yoke*. I have been influenced by Keith Wailoo's discussion of the way medical writings on cancer denied black patients the "interior psychic space" ascribed to whites. See Wailoo, *How Cancer Crossed,* esp. the introduction and ch. 1.

39. Williams, "The Way to Health." See also Williams, "What to Do for Diabetes" and Williams, "Defender Health Editor Looks Back."

40. Rawlins, "Increasing Frequency of Diabetes"; Waring, "Degenerative Diseases," 6; Garvin, "Negro Health," 342.

41. On Williams, see Hamilton, "Williams." On Rawlins, see Whitney, "Harlem Mourns." On Waring, see Lawson, "Waring." On Garvin, see Gamble, *Making a Place*, 155–157, and "Garvin," *Encyclopedia of Cleveland History.*

42. Williams, "Diabetes," January 31, 1925; Rawlins, "Increasing Frequency of Diabetes"; Du Bois, "Postscript," 44. See also "Is the Negro Dying Out?"; and Gamble and Stone, "U.S. Policy on Health Inequities."

43. Williams, "Defender Health Editor Looks Back." See also Knadler, "Unsanitized Domestic Allegories"; Gamble, *Making a Place,* 9.

44. Quinn and Thomas, "The National Negro Health Week." The Rosenwald Foundation's funding ended in 1932 and one year later the USPHS redefined the program to gather information about the health consequences of untreated syphilis in the black community. The Tuskegee Syphilis Study continued until 1972. See Jones, *Bad Blood;* Reverby, *Examining Tuskegee.*

45. Williams, "Defender Health Editor Looks Back"; Starr, *The Social Transformation,* 167.

46. Rawlins, "The Mind and Disease" and "Diabetes."

47. Williams, "Diabetes," January 31, 1925.

48. Williams, "Diabetes," August 23, 1924. See also Williams, "Diabetes," June 18, 1927; Waring, "Degenerative Diseases." On the history of African American physicians in the United States, see Gamble, *Making a Place.*

49. Smith, *Sick and Tired,* 13. See also Gains, *Uplifting the Race;* Knadler, "Unsanitized Domestic Allegories"; and White, *Too Heavy a Load,* ch. 2. On Waring's accommodationism, see Lawson, "Waring"; Robinson, *Disintegration,* ch. 2.

50. Cited in Smith, *Sick and Tired,* 30–31.

51. Ibid.; Knadler, "Unsanitized Domestic Allegories."

52. Waring, "Degenerative Diseases." See also Williams, "Diabetes," August 23, 1924, in which he writes that regular medical exams are necessary for the "early diagnosis of many diseases that begin insidiously."

53. Waring, "Degenerative Diseases," 6. See also Smith, *Sick and Tired,* 18.

54. Williams, "What to Do for Diabetes"; Rawlins, "Keep a Cool Head;" Rawlins, "Mind and Disease."

55. Waring, "Degenerative Diseases."

56. See "Diabetes Gain"; Root and Marble, "Progress"; Dorn, "Changes"; Marks, "Recent Statistics."

57. Altschul and Nathan, "Diabetes," 251–252; Wilkerson, "Problems," 179. See also Cameron, "Observations." In 1951, researchers in Georgia also noted higher rates among black women. See McLoughlin, "Diabetes Detection." Keith Wailoo offers an excellent analysis of the category "nonwhite" in *How Cancer Crossed,* 102–104. I discuss this language in more detail in Chapter 5.

58. Wilkerson, "Problems of an Aging Population," 177; Wilkerson and Krall, "Diabetes," 210. On Oxford, see U.S. Bureau of the Census, "Report of the Seventeenth Decennial."

59. Wilkerson, "Problems of an Aging Population," 180. See also Mauck, "Managing Care," 182–188.

60. Wilkerson, "Problems of an Aging Population," 181; Wilkerson and Krall, "Diabetes," 213–216. Wilkerson and Krall found that while 38.6 percent of those who had diabetes had a close relative who had the disease, only 18.2 percent of those without diabetes had a diabetic relative. See also Mauck, "Managing Care," 15.

61. Wilkerson and Krall, "Diabetes," 211.

62. Ibid., 216.

63. Ford and Glenn, "Undetected Diabetes," 242.
64. Pollock, *Medicating Race*, 51–71; Oppenheimer, "Becoming the Framingham Study"; Wailoo, *How Cancer Crossed*; Hatch, *Blood Sugar*, ch. 3.
65. The films are available at the National Library of Medicine in Bethesda, Maryland. See, for example, *The Story of Wendy Hill* (1949) (NLM Unique ID: 8800594A); *Diabetics Unknown* (1962) (NLM Unique ID: 8800470A); *Diabetes and the Black Community* (1989) (NLM Unique ID: 9001323A).
66. Wailoo, *How Cancer Crossed*, 86–87. Further evidence of this shift was the decision in 1950 to cease production of the *National Negro Health News* because of a belief that Negroes' health concerns were no different than that of whites. See "Special Notice."
67. Igo, *The Averaged American*. See also Marks, *Progress of Experiment*; Epstein, *Inclusion*.

Chapter 4. Native Peoples and the Thrifty Gene Hypothesis

1. As late as 1951, a physician at the City Hospital in Cleveland referred to American Indians as "cesspools of infectious diseases." See "New Health Set-Up." On the link between American Indians and primitiveness, see Dippie, *Vanishing American*; Berkhofer, *White Man's Indian*; Deloria, *Playing Indian*; McMillen, "'The Red Man'"; McMillen, *Discovering Tuberculosis*; Jones, *Rationalizing Epidemic*. Joslin writes of diabetes that "unlike tuberculosis, it is clean and not contagious." See Joslin, *Diabetic Manual*, 1st ed., 17. Historical studies that address medicine's role in defining and sustaining distinctions between "primitive" and "civilized" populations are numerous. See, for example, Anderson, *Cultivation of Whiteness*; Jones, *Rationalizing Epidemics*; and Shah, *Contagious Divides*.
2. The idea that civilization was dangerous to American Indians goes back to the seventeenth century. See Mancall, *Deadly Medicine*.
3. Tallbear, *Native American DNA*, 5.
4. Dunn and Dobzhansky, *Heredity, Race and Society*, 101; Montagu, "Consideration," 317. McMillen tells a very similar story about race, tuberculosis, and Indians in *Discovering Tuberculosis*. On changing concepts of race in the twentieth century, see Stocking, *Race, Culture and Evolution*; Stepan, *Idea of Race*; Barkan, *Retreat*; Reardon, *Race to the Finish*.
5. Neel, "Diabetes." Jennifer Poudrier refers to the "thrifty gene theory" as "part of an ongoing and transforming story about race, genetics and disease" in Poudrier, "Geneticization," 239. For a brief biographical sketch of Neel, see Lindee, "James Van Gundia Neel." The best critique of the thrifty gene hypothesis is Paradies, Montoya, and Fullerton, "Racialized Genetics." See also McDermott, "Ethics, Epidemiology"; Fee, "Racializing Narratives"; and Krieger, *Epidemiology*, 249–261.
6. Neel, "Diabetes," 355.
7. Jared Diamond is one of the most popular proponents of this hypothesis. See Diamond, "Sweet Death" and "Double Puzzle." Like the thrifty gene hypothesis,

virgin soil theory and the slavery hypertension theory also attained the status of theory despite the absence of solid evidence. I am grateful to David Jones for pointing this out to me. See Jones, "Virgin Soils Revisited"; and Curtin, "Slavery Hypothesis."

8. Kleen, *On Diabetes*, 18–19.

9. Hrdlička, *Physiological and Medical Observations*, 182. For biographical information on Hrdlička, see Schultz, *Biographical Memoir*. "Pima" is the name Spanish settlers gave to this population; Akimel O'odham, meaning "River People," is the name that tribal members prefer.

10. Hamlin, "Health Survey"; Salsbury, "Disease Incidence"; Johnson and McNutt, "Diabetes," 123; "New Health Set-Up."

11. See Heat-Moon, "Stark Reminder"; Guthrie, "Health of the American Indian," 949–50; Foard, "Health of the American Indians," 1404; DeJong: "*If You Knew the Conditions,*" 15; Jones, *Rationalizing Epidemics*, 169–189.

12. Cited in DeJong, "Forced to Abandon," 29. See also DeJong, *Stealing the Gila*, 91.

13. Foard, "Health of the American Indians," 1403; Dippie, *Vanishing American*. On the plight of the Plains Indians, see Jones, *Rationalizing Epidemics*, 122–126.

14. Guthrie, "Health of the American Indian," 948–949. Dippie, *Vanishing American;* Berkhofer, *White Man's Indian*.

15. Berkhofer, *White Man's Indian;* Thomas, *Skull Wars*. On the way that ideas of "primitive" and "civilized" influenced theories about racial susceptibilities to tuberculosis, see McMillen, "'Red Man.'"

16. Kraus, *Indian Health*, 1, 137. See also Jacobson, *Whiteness of a Different Color*, ch. 6.

17. Hardin is cited in Jones, *Rationalizing Epidemics*, 141. A similar explanation would reemerge in the 1970s to explain why American Indians had such a high rate of diabetes.

18. Kleen, *On Diabetes*, 18–19; Williams, "Study," 396.

19. Salsbury, "Disease Incidence," 230; Jones, *Rationalizing Epidemics*, 176.

20. Joslin, "Universality," 2036.

21. Ibid., 2035–2037.

22. Ibid., 2036. Of the remaining twenty-six cases, eleven were unspecified, and the rest were distributed among the other five tribes. It is important to note that Joslin was not challenging the existence of racial categories. His claim was that disease—at least diabetes—was not a legitimate marker.

23. Ibid., 2036.

24. Foard, "Health of the American Indians," 1405. He refers to Indians as "a conquered race." See also Foard, "Federal Government."

25. Miller et al., "Prevalence." See also Stein et al., "High Prevalence," 844.

26. Parks and Waskow, "Diabetes," 102; Johnson and McNutt, "Diabetes," 122.

27. Joe and Young, *Diabetes*.

28. Ibid. Also West, "Diabetes." On the nation's increased worry about and investment in chronic diseases, see Weisz, *Chronic Disease*.

29. The view of American Indians as ideal research subjects dates back to the rise of anthropology in the nineteenth century and the concurrent development of the reservation system. I am grateful to Matthew Klingle for his insights on this topic. See Klingle, "Inescapable Paradoxes." See also Thomas, *Skull Wars*. On American Indians and the BCG vaccine, see McMillen, *Discovering Tuberculosis*, ch. 4; and Jones, *Rationalizing Epidemics*, ch. 7.

30. Montagu, "Consideration," 315. For an insightful and succinct discussion of this boundary work, see Reardon, *Race*.

31. Comfort, *Science*; Stern, *Telling Genes*; Paul, *Controlling Human Heredity*. Neel criticized the coercive nature of earlier measures in "Heredity."

32. Neel, "Editorial," 475. See also Stern, *Telling Genes*, and Wailoo and Pemberton, *Troubled Dream*.

33. Neel, *Physician*, 5. On McKusick's comments, see Comfort, *Science of Human Perfection*, 165.

34. Neel, "Diabetes."

35. See Meldrum, "David Rimoin." On *Drosophila*, see Kohler, *Lords of the Fly*. On the value of "isolates" for research, see the collection of papers in "Origin and Evolution of Man."

36. On isolated communities in other countries, see the discussion following Böök, "Clinical and Genetic Entities." On the importance of the Amish, see McKusick, Hostetler, and Egeland, "Genetic Studies," 211–214. On anxiety about disappearing "isolates," see Neel, "Opening Statement," 1; Oliver, "Concluding Remarks," 245; Böök, "Clinical and Genetical Entities," 124. This anxiety is a version of the trope of the "vanishing Indian." See Dippie, *Vanishing Indian*, and Brantlinger, *Dark Vanishings*.

37. Thomas, *Skull Wars*, 32; Iverson, "Blood Types."

38. DeJong, "*If You Knew the Conditions,*" ch. 7; Rhoades and Rhoades, "Public Health Foundation."

39. Parks and Waskow, "Diabetes," 100. According to Smith-Morris, the Akimel O'odham "are arguably the most studied ethnic group in the world." See her book *Diabetes*, 143.

40. Parks and Waskow, "Diabetes," 101, 105.

41. Kraus, *Indian Health*, 128.

42. Ibid., 94–95, 128.

43. Parks and Waskow, "Diabetes," 99; Bennett, "Diabetes," 5. For other comments about American Indians as ideal research subjects, see Miller et al., "Prevalence"; Miller, Bennett, and Burch, "Hyperglycemia," 103; Bennett, Burch, and Miller, "Diabetes," 128.

44. West, "Diabetes," 852.

45. Miller, Bennett, and Burch, "Hyperglycemia," 90–91; Henry et al., "Diabetes," 33; Doeblin et al., "Diabetes and Hyperglycemia," 625.

46. West, "Diabetes," 851.

47. Mouratoff, Carroll, and Scott, "Diabetes"; Scott and Mouratoff, "Diabetes."

48. Bennett, Burch, and Miller, "Diabetes."

49. West, "Diabetes," 843. It is worth noting that no one was trying to take apart the category of "white."

50. Rimoin, "Genetics," 346.

51. Ibid., 347, 349.

52. Ibid., 349.

53. Ibid., 350.

54. Rimoin, "Ethnic Variability," 695. The grant was a PHS graduate training grant, 5-TI-GM-624–04. Mentioned in Saiki and Rimoin, "Diabetes Mellitus. I."

55. Saiki and Rimoin, "Diabetes Mellitus. I," 2; Rimoin and Saiki, "Diabetes Mellitus. II," 9; Rimoin, "Ethnic Variability," 695.

56. Saiki and Rimoin, "Diabetes Mellitus. I," 5; Rimoin, "Ethnic Variability," 695.

57. Rimoin, "Ethnic Variability," 695, 699.

58. Miller, Bennett, and Burch, "Hyperglycemia," 89.

59. Raymond, "Diabetes."

60. Knowler et al., "Diabetes Mellitus in the Pima Indians: Genetic," 111–113; Williams et al., "HLA-A2," 462.

61. An Ngram search of Google Books does not show any activity until 1978, and even then interest remained moderate until the late 1980s. See also Poudrier, "Geneticization."

62. Neel, "Diabetes," 359–360. It is noteworthy that in his 1962 article, Neel does not cite a single article about American Indians or any other "primitive" populations. Most of his citations are, instead, to articles on diabetes and heredity, and a good number are focused specifically on diabetes and pregnancy. Importantly, one of the first mentions of his article was a brief paragraph summarizing his article in the *Eugenics Review* (a British journal) in July 1963. See "Periodicals." On geneticists' fears of "overpopulation," see Stern, *Eugenic Nation;* and Bashford, *Global Population.*

63. Neel, "Editorial," 475.

64. Ibid., 472–473; Neel, "Study," 59. On parallels to narratives about American Indians' susceptibility to tuberculosis, see McMillen, "Red Man," 621; Jones, *Rationalizing Epidemics.*

65. Neel, "Study," 59; Neel, "Editorial," 473–474.

66. Johnson and McNutt, "Diabetes," 120, 123. In "Racialized Genetics" (209), Paradies, Montoya, and Fullerton claim that this article was "one of the earliest" to mention the thrifty gene hypothesis.

67. Niswander, "Discussion," 134; Wise et al., "Diabetes," 196; Knowler et al., "Diabetes Incidence," 153. Knowler appears to have moved away from the thrifty gene hypothesis later in life. Instead, he argued that a combination of environmental factors and genes drove up diabetes rates among the Akimel O'odham, and that the risk factors were no different than those of other populations. See Knowler et al., "Diabetes Mellitus in the Pima Indians: Incidence."

68. Peterson, "Surge," A10. See also "Diabetes Theory," 118; Brody, "Tending to Obesity"; Shapiro, "Do Our Genes Determine," 1; Melillo, "Why Are the Pima Indians Sick?," 7; Gohdes, "Diabetes."

69. Zimmet, "Epidemiology," 144.

70. Ibid., 144–145.

71. Ibid., 147.

72. Wailoo and Pemberton, *Troubled Dream.*

73. Zimmet, "Epidemiology," 148; Anderson, *Colonial Pathologies.*

74. "Mike Myers."

75. Ibid. See also "Native People."

76. "New Hope." See also Smith-Morris, *Diabetes.*

77. The Dakota woman is cited in Lang, "In Their Tellings," 66. See also Justice, "History," 112–113; and Smith-Morris, *Diabetes,* 15–16 and ch. 9.

78. On the federal army's intentional destruction of the buffalo as a way of forcing dependence, see Smits, "Frontier Army." See also Vantrease, "Commod Bods."

79. The Dakota woman is cited in Lang, "Talking," 205. On a connection between diabetes and smallpox, see Brosseau, "Diabetes and Indians," 62; Tom-Orme, "Traditional Beliefs," 280. For a recent comparison between diabetes and small-pox, see Echo Hawk Consulting, *Feeding,* 31. On food as a colonial tool, see "Native People." As late as 1999, an article in the *Navajo Times* blamed federal dietary guidelines for the unhealthy eating habits found on reservations. See Barnard and Brown, "Traditional Diets."

80. MacDonald, "Hunger," 19. McKenzie's comments appear in "Indian Health Act," and in Adler, "Self-Determination." See also Donnan, "Employment," 5.

81. Cited in Lang, "Talking," 221. MacDonald directly linked stress and major ill-nesses in "MacDonald Challenges," 10.

82. Cited in Ferreira, "Slipping," 86. I wish to thank my graduate student Juliet Larkin-Gilmore, whose dissertation chapter on early twentieth-century Native American boarding schools deepened my understanding of the trauma described in this quotation. See Juliet C. Larkin-Gilmore, "Native Health on the Move: Pub-lic Health and Assimilation on the Lower Colorado River, 1890-1934." Ph.D. diss., Vanderbilt University, 2019.

83. Trennert, *Phoenix Indian School;* Trafzer and Keller, *Boarding School Blues;* Child, *Boarding School Seasons.*

84. "Native People," 24–25.

85. I am grateful to Dave Aftandilian for sharing his unpublished manuscript on this movement with me, "Merging Care," and for alerting me to the forthcom-ing book Mihesuah and Hoover, *Indigenous Food Sovereignty.* For an example of a recent intervention targeting social determinants of health among Native peo-ples in order to decrease health disparities, see Jernigan et al., "Multilevel and Community-Level Interventions." See also Centers for Disease Control, "Native Diabetes Wellness."

86. Tallbear, *Native American DNA,* 71.

87. Diamond, "Sweet Death," 2; Diamond, "Double Puzzle." For a trenchant critique of Diamond, see Rosenberg, "Pathologies of Progress."

88. Neel, "Towards a Better Understanding," 244; Neel, "Thrifty Genotype Revisited," 289–290. By 1982, NIDDM was itself no longer considered a single disease be-

cause of the discovery of what was referred to as maturity-onset diabetes of the young, or MODY. See Mauck, "Managing Care," 341, 344.

89. Neel, "'Thrifty Genotype' in 1998," S7.

90. For several excellent critiques of the thrifty gene hypothesis, see Paradies, Montoya, and Fullerton, "Racialized Genetics"; McDermott, "Ethics"; Fee, "Racializing Narratives"; Krieger, *Epidemiology*, 249–261; Poudrier, "Geneticization"; Hay, "Commentary."

91. Sahota, "Genetic Histories," 834.

92. Weiner, "Interpreting Ideas"; Olson, "Meeting the Challenges"; Tallbear, *Native American DNA*, 76, 84; Ferreira and Lang, *Indigenous Peoples*, 13. On ideas similar to "co-constitution," see Reardon, *Race to the Finish;* Braun, *Breathing Life;* and Pollock, *Medicating Race.* For a moving discussion of the impact of intergenerational and historic trauma on the health of Native people, see Emerson, "Diné Culture."

Chapter 5. A Nationwide Hunt for Hidden Disease

1. Sahagun, "Genetic Link"; U.S. Department of Health and Human Services, *Report of the Secretary's Task Force* (hereafter referred to as the Heckler Report). The report consisted of ten volumes. I draw on two of them—volume 1: Executive Summary, and volume 7: Chemical Dependency and Diabetes. This citation is from 7:193. For an excellent analysis of this report, see Gamble and Stone, "U.S. Policy." Some members of the black community refer to the report as the Heckler-Malone Report. See Joyner, "President's Inaugural Address," 1131.

2. The comment about "shockwaves" is from Gadson, "Health Equality"; for King's quotation, see Moore, "Tracking Down"; for the reference to a "history of neglect," see Beardsley, *History.*

3. American Diabetes Association, *Journey*, 40–43; "Missing Million." See also "Detecting Diabetes"; "Diabetes Data." On the founding of the ADA, see American Diabetes Association, *Journey*, 152–154; Striker, "American Diabetes Association."

4. Katz, *In the Shadow*, 252; Byrd and Clayton, *American Health Dilemma*, 2:291–392; Roemer, "Resistance," 1238.

5. Hirschman, "Immigration."

6. For the language of "the color groups," see U.S. Department of Health, Education, and Welfare, *Diabetes Mellitus Mortality*, 40; Goldstein, "Longevity and Health Status of the Negro American," 337; and Linder and Grove, *Vital Statistics*, 12. See also Sloan, "Ethnic Distribution."

7. Mauck, "Managing Care," 304–306.

8. Heckler Report, 7:214–216.

9. "Mrs. Clement"; "Drive Opened." The band member was George Morgan, who played the saxophone and clarinet.

10. "Protect Your Health"; "Medic Says"; "Diabetes Facts."

11. Grove and Hetzel, *Vital Statistics*, 309, 366, 381, 391. On page 43, they define white as "'persons stated to be 'white,' 'Cuban,' 'Mexican,' or 'Puerto Rican,'" and defined "nonwhite" as "all other persons."

12. Goldstein, "Longevity and Health Status of the Negro American," 340. This statistic was for "nonwhites." See also Smith, "Redistribution."

13. Stratford, "H.D. Doctor's Study"; Atkinson, "Early Diagnosis"; Cobb, "Short History." In 1868 Freedman's Hospital became the teaching hospital of Howard University Medical School. On the black hospital movement, see Gamble, *Making a Place*. For a discussion of Atkinson's research, see "72% of 506 Diabetic Clinic Patients."

14. Bethea, "Diabetes"; Aldrich, "President's Column," 78.

15. Katz, *In the Shadow*, 244–245.

16. Lyons, "Hunger and Sickness"; Daniel, "Blacks"; Dittmer, *Good Doctors*, 229–236.

17. Guthrie et al., "Clinical Nursing Conference"; Heckler Report, 1:153; Maty, James, and Kaplan, "Life-Course"; U.S. Department of Health, Education, and Welfare, *Diabetes Mellitus Mortality*, 1; National Commission on Diabetes (hereafter NCD), *Report*, vols. 1 and 2. In 1980 the staff of the Memphis clinic claimed to have logged over 500,000 visits, most of them by patients with diabetes. See Runyan, Zwaag, and Miller, "Memphis Diabetes," 385. On Alameda County, see also Wang, "Changing Face."

18. Comment from the National Health Survey is cited in Pate, "Public Health," 527, n.2; Joslin, "Unknown Diabetic," 303–304; U.S. Department of Health, Education, and Welfare, *Diabetes Source Book*, 49; Appalachian Regional Center for the Healing Arts, *Plan for Health Development*, part 1, 119. See also Acardi and Cross, "Mass Diabetes," 1.

19. Fulghum, "Diabetes"; Brown and Glover, "Diabetes Mellitus"; Tomasson, "Patterns," 382; U.S. Department of Health, Education, and Welfare, *Diabetes Source Book*, 10–11; Howell, "Diabetes"; Browne, "Diabetes Leading Cause"; Stallard, Ehrenreich, and Sklar, *Poverty*, 6–7; Katz, *In the Shadow*, 275.

20. Jackson, "Diabetes," 362, 397. He discusses methodological problems on 363–365.

21. West, *Epidemiology*, 203; Pettigrew and Pettigrew, "Race, Disease and Desegregation," 329. In *How Cancer Crossed the Color Line*, Keith Wailoo found a similar retreat from biological race in the literature on cancer.

22. Atkinson, "Early Diagnosis," 414–415; "72% of 506 Diabetic Clinic Patients." Atkinson did not cite Joslin, but rather Fineberg, "Obesity and Diabetes."

23. West, *Epidemiology*, 237, 277.

24. Ibid., 194–195.

25. Cited in "The Fat of the Land." On the history of attitudes toward obesity, see Schwartz, *Never Satisfied;* Stearns, *Fat History;* and Rasmussen, *Fat in the Fifties.*

26. Dobson et al., "Socioeconomic Status," 414–415.

27. Ibid., 414, 418, 421.

28. Lees, "Two Million Tightrope Walkers," 38; Dobson et al., "Socioeconomic Status," 414.

29. Dobson et al., "Socioeconomic Status," 420.

30. Anderson, Gunter, and Kennedy, "Evaluation," 74.

31. Ibid., 74–76, 80.

32. Ibid., 74, 81.

33. Douglas and Michaels, *Mommy Myth.*
34. Stearns, "Some Emotional Aspects," 472.
35. Drake, "Social and Economic Status," 773, 799. On Drake, see Bond and Drake, "Social Portrait." For an excellent analysis of the deep connections between Jim Crow legislation and health disparities, see Roberts, *Infectious Fear.*
36. Nelson, *Body and Soul,* 4, 106; Bassett, "Beyond Berets."
37. Couto, "Political Economy," 5–17. On the history of community health centers, see Sardell, *U.S. Experiment;* Lefkowitz, *Community Health.*
38. Williams, "Introduction to the New NMA President"; "Richard Allen Williams, M.D."; Williams, "Introduction," in Williams, *Textbook.*
39. Haynes, "Gap in Health Status," 4.
40. Ibid., 5.
41. Henry, "Endocrine Diseases," 319; Williams, "Introduction," in Williams, *Textbook,* xvii. Claude Bernard had coined the term *milieu intérieur* to refer to the capacity of the body's extra-cellular fluids to regulate the physiological processes vital to the body's proper functioning.
42. NCD, "Letter from Chairman Oscar B. Crofford to Carl Albert, Speaker of the House. Preliminary materials," *Report,* vol. 1, n.p; ibid., 2. See also Mauck, "Managing Care," 304, 323–329.
43. NCD, "Introduction," *Report,* vol. 2, n.p.
44. NCD, *Report,* vol. 2, part 2: Public Testimony and Biographical Sketches, 205–252.
45. NCD, *Report,* vol. 2, part 1: Public Testimony (Public Hearings 1–5), 19 (note that in the original document this entire quoted phrase was underlined); American Diabetes Association, *Journey,* 152–154. In 2000 the Juvenile Diabetes Foundation (JDF) became the JDRF (Juvenile Diabetes Research Foundation).
46. NCD, *Report,* vol. 2, part 1: Public Testimony (Public Hearings 1–5), 315–316.
47. Ibid., 43. The Chautauqua Movement was a successful adult education movement that flourished in the early twentieth century, spawned lectures and reading groups across the country, and because of its decidedly anti-immigration stance, appealed largely to Protestant audiences. See Canning, *Most American Thing;* Rieser, *Chautauqua Movement.* See also NCD, *Report,* vol. 2, part 1: Testimonies of Mr. Donald Moberg and Ms. Mary Abbott Hess, 55 and 151, respectively. Ms. Hess described the shift as one from a "'Melting Pot' to a 'salad bowl' of diverse ingredients."
48. Katz, *In the Shadow,* 254–256.
49. One example with particular consequences for the health of Americans was deployment of the myth of "welfare queens." See Roberts, *Killing;* Danziger and Haveman, "Reagan Administration's Budget Cuts."
50. Byrd and Clayton, *American Health Dilemma,* 2:291–392; Katz, *In the Shadow,* 254–261.
51. Freimer, Echenberg, and Kretchmer, "Cross-Cultural Medicine," 928.
52. Hirschman, "Immigration to the United States."
53. Stern et al., "Cardiovascular Risk Factors," 546–547, 553; Gunby, "San Antonio Heart Study," 225; "Ethnic Heart Problems."

54. For national data, Stern turned to the Health and Nutrition Examination Survey (HANES I and HANES II) because it "was designed to be representative of the entire US population." See Stern, "Cardiovascular Risk Factors," 549.

55. Ibid., 553.

56. Stern et al., "Knowledge, Attitudes, and Behavior." Stern's research was discussed in "Ethnic Heart Problems" and "Chicanos' Diabetes Risk."

57. Stern et al., "Knowledge, Attitudes, and Behavior"; Stern, Gaskill, and Haffner, "Does Obesity Explain Excess."

58. Gardner et al., "Prevalence," 86, 90.

59. Mauck, "Managing Care," 305–306; "Report of the Expert Committee"; Tattersall, "Maturity Onset Diabetes."

60. Gardner et al., "Prevalence," 86, 91. See also Hanis et al., "Diabetes."

61. Box's comment is cited in Molina, *Fit to Be Citizens?*, 118–119. I draw here on chapter 4 of Molina's book, as well as Ngai, "Architecture of Race"; Omi and Winant, *Racial Formation*, 1st ed., 82; Pachon and Moore, "Mexican Americans," 112; Gottlieb and Kimberling, "Admixture Estimates," 444. For census data, see U.S. Bureau of the Census, "History."

62. Stern et al., "Cardiovascular Risk Factors," 547, 552; Sheridan, "Another White Race," 125; Reed, "Ethnic Classification," 283.

63. Gardner et al., "Prevalence," 87.

64. For an analysis of how genetic epidemiologists continue to construct "ethnoracial taxonomic systems," see Montoya, *Making the Mexican Diabetic*. For a rare study that explores the role of stress in driving up diabetes rates among Mexican Americans, see Scheder, "Sickly-Sweet Harvest."

65. Gardner et al., "Prevalence," 86; Molina, *Fit to Be Citizens*, 180.

66. Cited in "U.S. Studies Latino Health." See also Reed, "Ethnic Classification," 283; Rodriguez, "Hispanic-Americans"; Sahagun, "Needed."

67. Bravo's comment is cited in Sahagun, "Genetic Link"; Joslin, *Treatment*, 1st ed., 17.

68. Kawate et al., "Diabetes," 161–162, 168.

69. Ibid., 169.

70. NCD, *Report*, vol. 2, part 1, 215–216; Fujimoto et al., "Type II," 137. Scholars had been studying the link between stress and diabetes for most of the century, although with the exception of early twentieth-century interest in Jews, diabetes, and nervousness, there was little interest in racial differences. Studies focused instead on why some individuals who were exposed to stressful situations experienced metabolic changes and others did not. See, for example, Treuting, "Role of Emotional Factors."

71. Gamble and Stone, "U.S. Policy."

72. Heckler Report, 1:1–2; O'Dea, *From Suffrage to Senate*, 338; "Thomas E. Malone, Ph.D." Malone received his Ph.D. in zoology from Harvard University in 1952.

73. Heckler Report, 1:3–7; Haynes, "Gap in Health Status," 4.

74. Gamble and Stone, "U.S. Policy," 105; American Heart Association News, "Much Done." Comments about excess deaths appeared repeatedly after the Heckler Re-

port came out. See Braithwaite and Lythcott, "Community Empowerment"; Dunea and Weiss, "Black-White Health Gap," Heckler Report, 1:2.

75. Cited in Dunea and Weiss, "Black-White Health Gap," 199. See also Jones, "President's Column," 486.

76. "Improved Health Habits."

77. Jones, "President's Column," 486; Joyner, "President's Inaugural Address." See also Gamble and Stone, "U.S. Policy," 105.

78. Heckler Report, 1:47–61; see also 1:7–8.

79. Goldstein, "Longevity and Health Status of Whites"; Kitagawa and Hauser, "Trends in Differential Fertility"; Dittmer, *Good Doctors;* Navarro, "Race or Class." Navarro argues that the U.S. government stands alone among Western developed nations in not gathering data on income, education, or occupation in any systematic way when it conducts health surveys.

80. Heckler Report, 7:193–194, 214–229.

81. Heckler Report, 1:18; West, *Epidemiology of Diabetes,* 203.

82. Omi and Winant, *Racial Formation,* 1st ed., 61, 68; 2nd ed., 66. On the ways that inclusion of minority populations in research studies in the 1980s encouraged an emphasis on differences between populations and a tendency to situate those differences in biology, see Epstein, *Inclusion.*

Epilogue

1. Wright, "Rising Diabetes Rates."

2. Tessaro, Smith, and Rye, "Knowledge and Perceptions of Diabetes"; Denham, Wood, and Remsberg, "Diabetes Care"; Barker et al., "Geographic Distribution," 438.

3. For an excellent recent study of how government policies aided the explosion of fast food restaurants in poor urban neighborhoods, see Jou, *Supersizing Urban America.*

4. Harmon, "County-Level 'Diabetes Belt'"; Albright, "Diabetes Characteristics."

5. NCD, *Report,* 1:15. Brody, "Panel"; Lawrence, "Framing Obesity"; Saguy and Riley, "Weighing Both Sides." A Google search reveals the use of the term "diabesity" as early as 1996 in connection with rodents, though it did not gain traction until decades later. See European Commission, "Diabesity."

6. Lawrence, "Framing Obesity," 73–74, n.6; Saguy and Riley, "Weighing Both Sides," 883–889; Aronowitz, "Framing Disease," 7.

7. For an example of the kind of study that creates bridges instead of walls, see Akins, "System Dynamics." The author found that rates of diabetes mellitus among white children on Medicaid in Kentucky were "approximately equal" to that of minority populations. For a study that found that racial differences in the prevalence of diabetes disappeared when populations of similar socioeconomic status were compared, see Signorello et al., "Comparing Diabetes Prevalence."

8. Navarro, "Race or Class"; Krieger, "Stormy Weather"; National Institute of Diabetes and Digestive and Kidney Diseases, "Diabetes Statistics"; Centers for Disease

Control and Prevention, "Diabetes?" For an excellent historical analysis of the way government data have created as much as recorded racial categorizations, see Nobles, "History Counts." See also Chaufan, "Poverty versus Genes."

9. On genetics and diabetes, see the sources cited in Maty, James, and Kaplan, "Life-Course." For the impact of genetics research on tuberculosis and cancer, see McMillen, *Discovering Tuberculosis;* and Wailoo, *How Cancer Crossed.* For a critique of the Human Genome Diversity Project, see Reardon, *Race to the Finish.* For arguments for and against research on genetics and health disparities, see Fine, Ibrahim, and Thomas, "Editorial"; Karter, "Race and Ethnicity"; Bloche, "Race-Based Therapeutics"; Epstein, *Inclusion;* Williams, "Race and Health"; Kahn, *Race in a Bottle;* Braun, *Breathing Life;* and Hatch, *Blood Sugar.*

10. Citations from Pérez-Peña, "Beyond 'I'm a Diabetic.'" On different meanings of type 1 and type 2, see Rock, "Classifying Diabetes." On racial disparities in type 1, see Centers for Disease Control and Prevention, *National Diabetes Statistics Report,* 7.

11. Pérez-Peña, "Beyond 'I'm a Diabetic.'" For recent efforts to address structural inequalities related to diabetes, see Hill, Nielsen, and Fox, "Understanding Social Factors."

12. Newkirk, "What the 'Crack Baby' Panic Reveals"; Shihipar, "Opioid Crisis."

13. Solomon, "I Have Diabetes."

BIBLIOGRAPHY

Abernathy, Arthur T. *The Jew a Negro: Being a Study of the Jewish Ancestry from an Impartial Standpoint.* Moravian Falls, NC: Dixie Publishing, 1910.

Acardi, Patrick, and Ruth B. Cross. "Mass Diabetes Detection Clinics in Henry County." *Communicator* 2, no. 18 (1971): 1.

Acevedo-Garcia, D., E. V. Sanchez-Vaznaugh, E. A. Viruell-Fuentes, and J. Almeida. "Integrating Social Epidemiology into Immigrant Health Research: A Cross-National Framework." *Social Science & Medicine* 75, no. 12 (2012): 2060–2068.

"Adiposity and Other Etiological Factors in Diabetes Mellitus." *Journal of the American Medical Association* 84, no. 23 (1925): 1775–1776.

Adler, Gail. "Self-Determination in Health Care." *Navajo Times*, August 25, 1977, A6.

Aftandilian, Dave. "Merging Care for People and Places through Contemporary Native American Food Sovereignty Movements and Traditional Worldviews." Unpublished manuscript in the author's possession.

Ahlqvist, Emma, Peter Storm, Annemari Käräjämäki, Mats Martinell, Mozhgan Dorkham, Annelie Carlsson, et al. "Novel Subgroups of Adult-Onset Diabetes and Their Association with Outcomes: A Data-Driven Cluster Analysis of Six Variables." *The Lancet: Diabetes & Endocrinology* 6, no. 5 (May 1, 2018): 361–369.

Akins, Victoria. "System Dynamics of Diabetes in the Presence of Social Determinants." Master's thesis, James Madison University, 2010, https://commons.lib.jmu.edu/master201019/413, accessed December 6, 2019.

Albertson, James. "I Have Diabetes." *American Mercury* 45 (1938): 424–428.

Albright, Ann. "Diabetes Characteristics and the Regional Epidemic." https://www.arc.gov/noindex/newsroom/events/Appalachian_Diabetes_Consultation_April_2014/Albright_Diabetes_Consultation_RegionalEpidemic%20_April2014.pdf, accessed May 28, 2019.

Aldrich, James T. "President's Column: Diabetes." *Journal of the National Medical Association*, 53, no. 1 (1961): 78.

Alexander, Walter G. "Is the Negro Dying Out?," *Colored American Magazine* 15, no. 1 (January 1909): 673–674.

Altschul, Alexander, and Arthur Nathan. "Diabetes Mellitus in Harlem Hospital Outpatient Department in New York." *Journal of the American Medical Association* 119, no. 3 (1942): 248–252.

American Diabetes Association. *The Journey and the Dream: A History of the American Diabetes Association.* Arlington, VA: American Diabetes Association, 1990.

American Heart Association News. "Much Done, Much Still to Do 30 Years after Heckler Report." *American Heart Association News Archive,* July 27, 2015. https://news.heart.org/much-done-much-still-to-do-30-years-after-heckler-report, accessed December 6, 2019.

Anderson, Robert, Lori M. Gunter, and Evelyn J. Kennedy. "Evaluation of Clinical, Cultural and Psychosomatic Influences in the Teaching and Management of Diabetic Patients: A Study of Medically Indigent Negro Patients." *American Journal of the Medical Sciences* 245, no. 6 (1963): 74–83.

Anderson, Warwick. *Colonial Pathologies: Tropical Medicine, Race, and Hygiene in the Philippines.* Durham, NC: Duke University Press, 2006.

———. *The Cultivation of Whiteness: Science, Health, and Racial Destiny in Australia.* Durham, NC: Duke University Press, 2006.

Appalachian Regional Center for the Healing Arts, Health Study Committee for the First Tennessee-Virginia Development District. *A Plan for Health Development.* Part 1: *Inventory of Health Resources* (Johnson City, TN, 1969).

Appel, Susan J. "Misdiagnosed with Type 2 Diabetes." *Clinical Advisor,* March 14, 2007, http://www.clinicaladvisor.com/clinical-challenge/misdiagnosed-with-type-2-diabetes/article/337390, accessed October 5, 2019.

Aronowitz, Robert. "Framing Disease: An Underappreciated Mechanism for the Social Patterning of Health," *Social Science & Medicine* 67, no. 1 (August 2008): 1–9.

———. *Making Sense of Illness: Science, Society, and Disease.* Cambridge, UK: Cambridge University Press, 1998.

———. *Risky Medicine: Our Quest to Cure Fear and Uncertainty.* Chicago: University of Chicago Press, 2015.

Atkinson, Lewis K. "The Early Diagnosis of Diabetes Mellitus." *Journal of the National Medical Association* 52, no. 6 (1960): 414–419.

Barkan, Elazar. *The Retreat of Scientific Racism: Changing Concepts of Race in Britain and the United States between the World Wars.* New York: Cambridge University Press, 1992.

Barker, Lawrence E., K. A. Kirtland, E. W. Gregg, L. S. Geiss, and T. J. Thompson. "Geographic Distribution of Diagnosed Diabetes in the U.S.: A Diabetes Belt." *American Journal of Preventive Medicine* 40, no. 4 (2011): 434–439.

Barnard, Neal D., and Derek M. Brown. "Traditional Diets Prove More Healthy for Native Americans." *Navajo Times,* April 8, 1999, A5.

Barnett, Donald M. *Elliott P. Joslin, MD: A Centennial Portrait.* Boston: Joslin Diabetes Center, 1998.

Bashford, Alison. *Global Population: History, Geopolitics, and Life on Earth*. New York: Columbia University Press, 2016.

Bashford, Alison, and Philippa Levine, eds. *The Oxford Handbook of the History of Eugenics*. Oxford, UK: Oxford University Press, 2010.

Bassett, Mary T. "Beyond Berets: The Black Panthers as Health Activists." *American Journal of Public Health* 106, no. 10 (2016): 1741–1743.

Baur, Erwin, Eugen Fischer, and Fritz Lenz. *Human Heredity*. Trans. Eden Paul and Cedar Paul. New York: Macmillan, 1931.

Baynton, Douglas. *Defectives in the Land*. Chicago: University of Chicago Press, 2016.

———. "Disability and the Justification of Inequality in American History." Pp. 33–57 in *The New Disability History*, ed. Paul Longmore and Lauri Umansky. New York: New York University Press, 2001.

Beardsley, Edward H. *A History of Neglect: Health Care for Blacks and Mill Workers in the Twentieth-Century South*. Knoxville: University of Tennessee Press, 1987.

Bennett, Jeffrey A. *Managing Diabetes. The Cultural Politics of Disease*. New York: New York University Press, 2019.

Bennett, Peter H. "Diabetes in the Desert: The Pima Indians of Arizona." *ADA Forecast* 25, no. 3 (1972): 1–5.

Bennett, Peter H., Thomas A. Burch, and Max Miller. "Diabetes Mellitus in American (Pima) Indians." *Lancet* 2, no. 7716 (1971): 125–128.

Berkhofer, Robert F., Jr. *The White Man's Indian*. New York: Vintage, 1978.

Bertram, Ferdinand. "Die Prophylaxe der Zuckerkrankheit." *Medizinische Welt* 10, no. 30 (1936): 1061–1065.

Bethea, Dennis A. "Diabetes, Killer No. 8, a Major Health Problem." *Afro-American*, January 7, 1950, A5.

Birnie, C. W. "The Influence of Environment and Race on Disease." *Journal of the National Medical Association* 2, no. 4 (1910): 243–251.

Bliss, Michael. *The Discovery of Insulin* (1982; Chicago: University of Chicago Press, 2007).

Bloche, M. Gregg. "Race-Based Therapeutics." *New England Journal of Medicine* 351, no. 20 (2004): 2035–2037.

Blotner, Harry. "Studies in Glysosuria and Diabetes Mellitus in Selectees." *Journal of the American Medical Association* 131, no. 14 (1946): 1109–1114.

Blotner, Harry, R. W. Hyde, and L. V. Kingsley. "Studies in Diabetes Mellitus and Transient Glycosuria in Selectees and Volunteers." *New England Journal of Medicine* 229, no. 24 (1943): 885–892.

Bond, George Clement, and John Gibbs St. Claire Drake. "A Social Portrait of John Gibbs St. Claire Drake: An American Anthropologist." *American Ethnologist* 15, no. 4 (1988): 762–81.

Böök, J. A. "Clinical and Genetical Entities in Human Populations, with Some Remarks on Schizophrenia, Manic-Depressive Psychosis and Mental Deficiency in a North Swedish Population," *Cold Spring Harbor Symposium on Quantitative Biology* 15 (1950): 123–128.

Boskin, Joseph. *The Rise and Demise of an American Jester.* New York: Oxford University Press, 1986.

Bouk, Dan. *How Our Days Became Numbered: The Risk and the Rise of the Statistical Individual.* Chicago: University of Chicago Press, 2015.

Bowcock, H. M. "Diabetes Mellitus in the Negro Race: A Study of One Hundred Consecutive Cases." *Southern Medical Journal* 21 (1928): 994–998.

———. "The Diabetic Negro." *Diabetes* 1 (1933): 109–118.

Bowler, Peter J. *Evolution: The History of an Idea.* Berkeley: University of California Press, 1984.

Braithwaite, Ronald L., and Ngina Lythcott. "Community Empowerment as a Strategy for Health Promotion for Black and Other Minority Populations." *Journal of the American Medical Association* 261, no. 2 (January 13, 1989): 282–283.

Brantlinger, Patrick. *Dark Vanishings: Discourse on the Extinction of Primitive Races, 1800–1930.* Ithaca, NY: Cornell University Press, 2003.

Braun, Lundy. *Breathing Life into the Machine: The Surprising Career of the Spirometer from Plantation to Genetics.* Minneapolis: University of Minnesota Press, 2014.

Britten, Rollo H., Selwyn D. Collins, and James S. Fitzgerald. "The National Health Survey: Some General Findings as to Disease, Accidents, and Impairments in Urban Areas." *Public Health Reports* 55 (March 15, 1940): 444–470.

Brodkin, Karen. *How Jews Became White Folks & What That Says about Race in America.* New Brunswick, NJ: Rutgers University Press, 1998.

Brody, Jane E. "Panel Terms Obesity a Major U.S. Killer Needing Top Priority." *New York Times,* February 14, 1990, A1.

———. "Tending to Obesity Inbred Tribe Aids Diabetes." *New York Times,* February 5, 1980, C1, C5.

Brosseau, James D. "Diabetes and Indians: A Clinician's Perspective." Pp. 41–66 in *Diabetes as a Disease of Civilisation: The Impact of Culture Change on Indigenous Peoples,* ed. Jennie R. Joe and Robert S. Young. Berlin: Mouton de Gruyter, 1994.

Brown, Charles H., and Dan H. G. Glover. "Diabetes Mellitus—A Public Health Problem in Georgia." *Journal of the Medical Association of Georgia* 53 (1964): 243–244.

Brown, W. L. "Diabetes in Relation to Ductless Glands." *Journal of Nervous and Mental Diseases* 53, no. 6 (1921): 473.

Browne, Zamgba. "Diabetes Leading Cause of Death among Blacks." *New York Amsterdam News,* December 19, 1981, 20.

Byers, J. Wellington. "Diseases of the Southern Negro." *Medical and Surgical Reporter* 43 (1888): 734–737.

Byrd, W. Michael, and Linda Clayton. *An American Health Dilemma: Race, Medicine, and Health Care in the United States, 1900–2000,* 2 vols. New York: Routledge, 2000–2002.

Cameron, Paul. "Observations on the Negro Diabetic." *Journal of the Oklahoma State Medical Association* 36 (1943): 517–520.

Cammidge, P. J. "Diabetes Mellitus and Heredity." *British Medical Journal* 2, no. 3538 (1928): 738–741.

Canning, C. *The Most American Thing in America: Circuit Chautauqua as Performance.* Iowa City: University of Iowa Press, 2005.

Centers for Disease Control and Prevention. "Diabetes. Who's at Risk?," https://www.cdc.gov/diabetes/basics/risk-factors.html, accessed December 6, 2019.

———. *National Diabetes Statistics Report, 2017: Estimates of Diabetes and Its Burden in the United* States, https://www.cdc.gov/diabetes/data/statistics-report/index.html, accessed December 6, 2019.

———. "Native Diabetes Wellness Program. Traditional Foods Project, 2008–2014." https://www.cdc.gov/diabetes/ndwp/traditional-foods/index.html, accessed December 6, 2019.

Chaufan, Claudia. "Poverty versus Genes: The Social Context of Type 2 Diabetes." *Diabetes Voice* 49 (2004): 35–37.

"Chicanos' Diabetes Risk Higher Than Anglos,' Study Says." *Los Angeles Times,* March 6, 1982, A6.

Child, Brenda J. *Boarding School Seasons: American Indian Families, 1900–1940.* Lincoln: University of Nebraska Press, 1998.

Cobb, W. Montague. "A Short History of Freedmen's Hospital." *Journal of the National Medical Association* 54, no. 3 (1962): 271–287.

Cohen, A. M. "Prevalence of Diabetes among Different Ethnic Jewish Groups in Israel." *Metabolism* 10, no. 1 (1961): 50–58.

Comfort, Nathaniel. *The Science of Human Perfection: How Genes Became the Heart of American Medicine.* New Haven: Yale University Press, 2014.

Cooper, Thea, and Arthur Ainsberg. *Breakthrough: Elizabeth Hughes, the Discovery of Insulin, and the Making of a Medical Miracle.* New York: St. Martin's, 2010.

Couto, Richard A. "The Political Economy of Appalachian Health." Pp. 5–17 in *Health in Appalachia: Proceedings of the UK Conference on Appalachia.* Lexington: University of Kentucky Press, 1988.

Crystall, Sandy, and Laurence Leitenberg. *Digital Maps of Jewish Populations in Europe (1750–1950) for Online Viewing by the Public: Final Report,* International Institute for Jewish Genealogy and Paul Jacobi Center, February 2014, https://www.iijg.org/wp-content/uploads/2014/06/LeitenbergCrystall-JewishPopulationsMaps-Report-3-2-f.pdf, accessed December 6, 2019.

Curtin, P. D. "The Slavery Hypothesis for Hypertension among African Americans: The Historical Evidence." *American Journal of Public Health* 82, no. 12 (December 1992): 1681–1686.

Dahlberg, Gunnar. "The Swedish Jews: A Discussion of the Basic Concept." *Acta genetica et statistica medica* 3 (1952): 106–117.

Daniel, Leon. "Blacks in Mississippi Still Poorest of the Poor." *Afro-American,* July 28, 1984, 6.

Danziger, Sheldon, and Robert Haveman. "The Reagan Administration's Budget Cuts: Their Impact on the Poor." *Challenge* 24, no. 2 (1981): 5–13.

Davis, F. James. *Who Is Black? One Nation's Definition.* University Park: Pennsylvania State University Press, 1991.

"Deaths among Poor Exceed Others 100%." *New York Times*, October 6, 1937, 26.

"Deaths Due to Diabetes." *Journal of the American Medical Association* 223, no. 5 (1973): 566.

DeJong, David H. "Forced to Abandon Their Farms: Water Deprivation and Starvation among the Gila River Pima, 1892–1904." *American Indian Culture and Research Journal* 28, no. 3 (2004): 29–56.

———. "*If You Knew the Conditions*": *A Chronicle of the Indian Medical Service and American Indian Health Care, 1908–1955*. Lanham MD: Lexington Books, 2008.

———. *Stealing the Gila: The Pima Agricultural Economy and Water Deprivation, 1848–1921*. Tucson: University of Arizona Press, 2009.

Deloria, Philip J. *Playing Indian*. New Haven: Yale University Press, 1998.

Denham, S. A., L. E. Wood, and K. Remsberg. "Diabetes Care: Provider Disparities in the U.S. Appalachian Region." *Rural and Remote Health* 10, no. 2 (April–June 2010): 1320.

"Detecting Diabetes." *Newsweek*, November 1, 1948, 49.

"Diabetes as Jewish Peril." *New York Times*, April 14, 1926.

"Diabetes Data." *Newsweek*, February 7, 1949, 48–49.

"Diabetes Facts Presented in Special Exhibit." *Daily Defender*, November 10, 1959, 19.

"Diabetes Gain Laid to Rise in Mode of Living." *New York Herald Tribune*, November 16, 1935.

"Diabetes, Insulin, and Vitamin B." *British Medical Journal* 2, no. 3334 (1924): 961.

"Diabetes Mortality Up 58% in 30 Years." *New York Times*, April 30, 1933, 24.

"Diabetes Theory: Frugal Genes." *Science News* 115, no. 8 (1979).

Diamond, Jared. "The Double Puzzle of Diabetes." *Nature* 423 (June 5, 2003): 599–602.

———. "Sweet Death." *Natural History* 101, no. 1 (1992): 2–5.

"Diet or Die." *Time Magazine*, August 31, 1942.

Diner, Hasia R. *Hungering for America. Italian, Irish, & Jewish Foodways in the Age of Immigration*. Cambridge, MA: Harvard University Press, 2001.

Dippie, Brian W. *The Vanishing American: White Attitudes and U.S. Indian Policy*. Kansas City: University Press of Kansas, 1982.

Dittmer, John. *The Good Doctors: The Medical Committee for Human Rights and the Struggle for Social Justice in Health Care*. New York: Bloomsbury Press, 2009.

Dobson, Harold L., Harry S. Lipscomb, James A. Greene, and Hugo T. Engelhardt. "Socioeconomic Status and Diabetes Mellitus." *Journal of Chronic Disease* 7 (1958): 413–421.

Doeblin, T. D., Kathleen Evans, Gilliam B. Ingall, Kathleen Dowling, M. E. Chilcote, W. Elsea, and R. M. Bannerman. "Diabetes and Hyperglycemia in Seneca Indians." *Human Heredity* 19 (1969): 613–627.

Donnan, Marcia. "Employment Means Better Future for Pine Ridge Mothers, Children." *The Indian* 1, no. 11 (1970): 5.

Dorn, Harold F. "Changes in Mortality Rates, 1930 to 1940." *National Negro Health News* 11, no. 2 (1943): 1–3.

Douglas, Susan, and Meredith W. Michaels. *The Mommy Myth: The Idealization of Motherhood and How It Has Undermined All Women*. New York: Free Press, 2005.

Downs, Jim. *Sick from Freedom: African-American Illness and Suffering during the Civil War and Reconstruction*. New York: Oxford University Press, 2012.

Drake, John Gibbs St. Claire. "The Social and Economic Status of the Negro in the United States." *Daedalus* 94, no. 4 (1964): 771–814.

"Drive Opened to Aid Legless Artist." *Afro-American*, March 29, 1958, 19.

Dublin, Louis I. *After Eighty Years: The Impact of Life Insurance on the Public Health*. Gainesville: University of Florida Press, 1966.

———. "The Health of the Negro." *Annals of the American Academy of Political and Social Science* 140 (1928): 77–85.

———. "Modern Life Takes Its Toll: The Story of Diabetes," *Scribner's* 100 (1936): 40–43.

———. "Mortality Statistics of Diabetes among Wage Earners, with Observations on the Comparative Incidence of the Disease in the General Population." *Medical Record* 94 (1918): 631–632.

———. "Recent Trends in Diabetes Mortality." *Bulletin of the New York Academy of Medicine* 9, no. 9 (1933): 540–546.

Du Bois, W. E. B. *The Health and Physique of the Negro American*. Atlanta: Atlanta University Press, 1906.

———. "Postscript: Our Health." *Crisis* 40, no. 2 (1933): 44.

Dumenil, Lynn. *The Modern Temper: American Culture and Society in the 1920's*. New York: Hill and Wang, 1995.

Dunea, George, and Kevin B. Weiss. "Black-White Health Gap in the USA." *British Medical Journal* 294 (January 24, 1987): 199–200.

Dunn, Lawrence Clarence, and Theodosius Dobzhansky. *Heredity, Race and Society*. Baltimore: Penguin, 1946.

Durrah, Fred F. "Diabetes Mellitus." *Journal of the National Medical Association* 13, no. 4 (1921): 242–248.

East, Edward M. "Hidden Feeblemindedness." *Journal of Heredity* 8 (1917): 215–217.

Echo Hawk Consulting. *Feeding Ourselves: Food Access, Health Disparities, and the Pathways to Healthy Native American Communities*. Longmont, CO: Echo Hawk Consulting, 2015.

Edison, Mina Miller, to Theodore Miller Edison, April 9, 1923–July 12, 1931. In *The Miller Family Papers: Theodore Miller Edison Correspondence, 1923, 1931*. Chautauqua, NY: Chautauqua Institution Archives, Oliver Archive Center, boxes 7G2 977–979.

Efron, John M. *Defenders of the Race: Jewish Doctors and Race Science in Fin-de-Siècle Europe*. New Haven: Yale University Press, 1994.

———. *Medicine and the German Jews: A History*. New Haven: Yale University Press, 2001.

Eisenstadt, S. N. "A Reappraisal of Theories of Social Change and Modernization." Pp. 412-429 in *Social Change and Modernity*, ed. Neil J. Smelser and Hans Haferkamp. Berkeley: University of California Press, 1992.

Elduff, John. "About Us." *Collier's*, https://colliersmagazine.com/about-us, accessed May 29, 2019.

Elliott, Arthur R. "Diabetes Mellitus: The Limitations of Its Dietetics Treatment." *Journal of the American Medical Association* 42, no. 1 (1904): 19–23.

Elliott, Michael A. "Telling the Difference: Nineteenth-Century Legal Narratives of Racial Taxonomy." *Law and Social Inquiry* 24 (1999): 611–636.

Emerson, Haven. "Public Health Awaits Social Change." *American Journal of Public Health* 24, no. 10 (1934): 1005–1022.

———. "Sweetness Is Death." *Survey* 53 (1924): 23–25.

Emerson, Larry W. "Diné Culture, Decolonization, and the Politics of Hózhó." Pp. 49–67 in *Diné Perspectives: Revitalizing and Reclaiming Navajo Thought*, ed. Lloyd L. Lee. Tucson: University of Arizona Press, 2014.

Epstein, Albert A. "Diabetes among Jews—Its Cause and Prevention." *Modern Medicine* 1 (1919): 269–275.

Epstein, Steven. *Inclusion: The Politics of Difference in Medical Research*. Chicago: University of Chicago Press, 2007.

"Ethnic Heart Problems." *Atlanta Daily World*, March 19, 1982, 6.

European Commission. "Diabesity: A World-Wide Challenge. Towards a Global Initiative on Gene-Environment Interactions in Diabetes/Obesity in Specific Populations." Luxembourg: Publications Office of the European Union, 2012, https://ec.europa.eu/research/health/pdf/diabesity-conference-report-022012_en.pdf, accessed May 28, 2019.

Falk, Raphael. "Eugenics and the Jews." Chap. 27 in *The Oxford Handbook of the History of Eugenics*, ed. Alison Bashford and Philippa Levine. Oxford, UK: Oxford University Press, 2010.

Fang, Carolyn Y., Guenther Boden, Philip T. Siu, and Marilyn Tseng. "Stressful Life Events Are Associated with Insulin Resistance among Chinese Immigrant Women in the United States." *Preventive Medicine Reports* 2 (2015): 563–567.

"The Fat of the Land." *Time*, January 13, 1961.

Fee, Margery. "Racializing Narratives: Obesity, Diabetes and the 'Aboriginal' Thrifty Genotype." *Social Science & Medicine* 62 (2006): 2988–2997.

Ferreira, Mariana Leal. "Slipping through Sky Holes: Yurok Body Imagery in Northern California." Pp. 73–103 in *Indigenous Peoples and Diabetes. Community Empowerment and Wellness*, ed. Mariana Leal Ferreira and Gretchen Chesley Lang. Durham, NC: Carolina Academic Press, 2006.

Ferreira, Mariana Leal, and Gretchen Chesley Lang. "Introduction: Deconstructing Diabetes." Pp. 10–13 in *Indigenous Peoples and Diabetes: Community Empowerment and Wellness*, ed. Mariana Leal Ferreira and Gretchen Chesley Lang. Durham, NC: Carolina Academic Press, 2006.

———, eds. *Indigenous Peoples and Diabetes: Community Empowerment and Wellness*. Durham, NC: Carolina Academic Press, 2006.

Feudtner, Chris. *Bittersweet: Diabetes, Insulin, and the Transformation of Illness*. Chapel Hill: University of North Carolina Press, 2003.

Fields, Barbara. "Ideology and Race in American History." In *Region, Race, and Reconstruction*, ed. J. Morgan Kousser and James M. McPherson. New York: Oxford University Press, 1982.

Fine, Michael J., Said A. Ibrahim, and Stephen B. Thomas. "Editorial: The Role of Race and Genetics in Health Disparities Research." *American Journal of Public Health* 95, no. 12 (2005): 2125–2128.

Fineberg, S. K. "Obesity and Diabetes: A Reevaluation." *Annals of Internal Medicine* 52 (April 1960): 750–760.

Fishberg, Maurice. "Health and Sanitation of the Immigrant Jewish Population of New York." *The Menorah: A Monthly Magazine for the Jewish Home* 33, nos. 1–3 (1902): 37–46, 72–82, 168–180.

———. *The Jews: A Study of Race and Environment*. London: Walter Scott, 1911.

Fitz, Reginald H., and Elliott P. Joslin. "Diabetes Mellitus at the Massachusetts General Hospital from 1824 to 1898: A Study of the Medical Records." *Journal of the American Medical Association* 31 (1898): 165–171.

Foard, Fred T. "The Federal Government and American Indians' Health." *Journal of the American Medical Association* 142, no. 5 (1950): 328–331.

———. "The Health of the American Indians." *American Journal of Public Health* 39 (1949): 1403–1406.

Ford, Malcolm J., and Barbara Glenn. "Undetected Diabetes among the Relatives of Diabetes: An Epidemiologic Note." *Southern Medical Journal* 44 (1951): 239–244.

Frazier, E. Franklin. *Black Bourgeoisie: The Rise of a New Middle Class in the United States*. New York: Free Press, 1957.

Frear, George W. "Diabetes." *Parents' Magazine* 8 (1933): 32, 76.

Freimer, Nelson, Dean Echenberg, and Norman Kretchmer. "Cross-Cultural Medicine: Cultural Variation-Nutritional and Clinical Implications." *Western Journal of Medicine* 193 (1983): 928–933.

Fujimoto, W. Y., K. Hershon, J. Kinyoun, W. Stolov, C. Weinberg, K. Ishiwata, H. Kajinuma, Y. Kanazawa, and N. Kuzuya. "Type II Diabetes Mellitus in Seattle and Tokyo." Supplement, *Tohoku Journal of Experimental Medicine* 141 (1983): 133–139.

Fulghum, J. E. "Diabetes as a Health Problem in Florida." *Journal of the Florida Medical Association* 50 (1963): 284–285.

Furdell, Elizabeth Lane. *Fatal Thirst: Diabetes in Britain until Insulin*. Leiden: Brill, 2009.

Futcher, Thomas B. "The Frequency and Aetiology of Diabetes Mellitus." *New York Medical Journal* 66 (1897): 753–757.

Gabaccia, Donna R. *We Are What We Eat: Ethnic Food and the Making of Americans*. Cambridge, MA: Harvard University Press, 1998.

Gadson, Sandra L. "Health Equality: The New Civil Rights Frontier." *Journal of the National Medical Association* 98, no. 3 (2006): 324–329.

Gains, Kevin. *Uplifting the Race: Black Leadership, Politics, and Culture in the Twentieth Century*. Chapel Hill: University of North Carolina Press, 1996.

Gamble, Vanessa Northington. *Making A Place for Ourselves: The Black Hospital Movement, 1920–1945*. New York: Oxford University Press, 1995.

Gamble, Vanessa Northington, and Deborah Stone. "U.S. Policy on Health Inequities: The Interplay of Politics and Research." *Journal of Health Politics, Policy and
Law* 31, no. 1 (2006): 93–126.

Gardner, L. I., Jr., M. P. Stern, S. M. Haffner, S. P. Gaskill, H. P. Hazuda, J. H. Rele-
thford, and C. W. Eifler. "Prevalence of Diabetes in Mexican Americans: Relationship to Percent of Gene Pool Derived from Native American Sources," *Diabetes* 33,
no. 1 (1984): 86–92.

Garvin, Charles H. "Negro Health." *Opportunity: Journal of Negro Life* 2, no. 13 (1924):
341–342.

"Garvin, Charles H.," *Encyclopedia of Cleveland History.* Case Western Reserve University, https://case.edu/ech/articles/g/garvin-charles-h, accessed May 26, 2019.

Gebel, Erika. "Problem of Pounds: The Parallel Paths of Obesity and Type 2 Diabetes." *Diabetes Forecast* 64, no. 9 (September 2011): 35–36.

Gerstle, Gary. *American Crucible: Race and Nation in the Twentieth Century.* Princeton,
NJ: Princeton University Press, 2001.

Gieryn, Thomas. "Boundary-Work and the Demarcation of Science from Non-
Science: Strains and Interests in Professional Ideologies of Scientists." *American
Sociological Review* 48 (December 1983): 781–795.

Gilman, Sander L. "Fat as Disability: The Case of the Jews." *Literature and Medicine*
23, no. 1 (2004): 46–60.

Ginzburg, Gershon. "Frequency of Diabetes among Jews: Pathogenesis and Prevention," *Harofé Haivri* 1 (1941): 191–193.

Gohdes, D. M. "Diabetes in American Indians: A Growing Problem." *Diabetes Care*
9, no. 6 (1986): 609–613.

Golden, Janet. *Message in a Bottle: The Making of Fetal Alcohol Syndrome.* Cambridge,
MA: Harvard University Press, 2005.

Goldstein, Eric L. "Contesting the Categories: Jews and Government Racial Classification in the United States." *Jewish History* 19 (2005): 79–107.

———. *The Price of Whiteness.* Princeton, NJ: Princeton University Press, 2006.

———. "The Unstable Other: Locating the Jew in Progressive-Era Racial Discourse."
American Jewish History 89 (2001): 383–409.

Goldstein, Hyman I. "Diabetes in the Negro. With Report of Eight Cases." *American
Journal of Clinical Medicine* 29 (1922): 905–909.

Goldstein, Jan. "The Wandering Jews and the Problem of Psychiatric Anti-Semitism
in Fin-de- Siècle France." *Journal of Contemporary History* 20, no. 4 (1985): 521–552.

Goldstein, Marcus S. "Longevity and Health Status of the Negro American." *Journal
of Negro Education* 32, no. 4 (1953): 337–348.

———. "Longevity and Health Status of Whites and Non-Whites in the United
States." *Journal of the National Medical Association* 46 (March 1954): 83–104.

Goren, Arthur A. "Jews." Pp. 571–598 in *Harvard Encyclopedia of American Ethnic
Groups*, ed. Stephan Thernstrom, Ann Orlov, and Oscar Handlin. Cambridge, MA:
Belknap, 1980.

Gottheil, Richard. "Israel among the Nations." *Review of Reviews: An International
Magazine* 13 (January–June 1896): 52–58.

Gottlieb, K., and W. J. Kimberling. "Admixture Estimates for the Gene Pool of Mexican-Americans in Colorado." *American Journal of Physical Anthropology* 50, no. 3 (1979): 444–448.

Gover, Mary. *Mortality among Negroes in the United States: Public Health Bulletin No. 174*. Washington, DC: Government Printing Office, 1927.

———. "Trend of Mortality among Southern Negroes since 1920." *Journal of Negro Education* 6, no. 3 (1937): 276–288.

Graham, George. *The Pathology and Treatment of Diabetes Mellitus*. London: Henry Frowde and Hodder & Stoughton, 1923.

Grahm, Lawrence Otis. *Our Kind of People: Inside America's Black Upper Class*. New York: Harper Collins, 1999.

Greene, Jeremy A. *Prescribing by Numbers: Drugs and the Definition of Disease*. Baltimore: Johns Hopkins University Press, 2007.

Grey, Michael R. *New Deal Medicine: The Rural Health Programs of the Farm Security Administration*. Baltimore: Johns Hopkins University Press, 1999.

Grissom, Robert J., and Robert C. Rosenlof. "The Management of the New Adult Diabetic." *Nebraska Medical Journal* 39 (1954): 461–465.

Grove, Robert D., and Alice M. Hetzel. *Vital Statistics Rates in the United States, 1940–1960*. Washington, DC: U.S. Department of Health, Education, and Welfare, 1968.

Gunby, Phil. "San Antonio Heart Study Compares Ethnic Groups." *Journal of the American Medical Association* 244, no. 3 (1980): 225.

Guthrie, M. C. "The Health of the American Indian." *Public Health Reports (1896–1970)* 44, no. 16 (1929): 945–957.

Guthrie, Nobel, John W. Runyan, Glenn Clark, and Oscar Marvin. "The Clinical Nursing Conference: A Preliminary Report." *New England Journal of Medicine* 270, no. 26 (1964): 1411–1413.

Guttmacher, Alan. "Hereditary Counseling: Diabetes, Pregnancy and Medicine." *Eugenics Quarterly* 1, no. 3 (1954): 191–192.

Haller, John S. *Outcasts from Evolution: Scientific Attitudes of Racial Inferiority, 1859–1900*. New York: McGraw-Hill, 1971.

Hamilton, Gloria. "Williams, Wilberforce A." Pp. 698–700 in *Notable Black American Men, Book II*, ed. Jessie Carney Smith. Detroit: Gale, 2007.

Hamlin, H. "A Health Survey of the Seminole Indians." *Yale Journal of Biology and Medicine* 6 (1933): 157–177.

Hammonds, Evelynn, and Rebecca Herzig, eds., *The Nature of Difference: Sciences of Race in the United States from Jefferson to Genomics*. Cambridge, MA: MIT Press, 2009.

Hancock, J. C. "Diseases among the Indians." *Southwestern Medicine* 17 (1933): 126–129.

Hanis, Craig L., Robert E. Ferrell, Sara A. Barton, Lydia Aguilar, Ana Garzaibarra, Brian R. Tulloch, Charles A. Garcia, and William J. Schull. "Diabetes among Mexican Americans in Starr County, Texas." *American Journal of Epidemiology* 118, no. 5 (1983): 659–672.

Harmon, Amy. "Why White Supremacists Are Chugging Milk (and Why Geneticists Are Alarmed)." *New York Times,* October 17, 2018.

Harmon, Katherine. "County-Level 'Diabetes Belt' Carves a Swath through U.S. South." *Scientific American,* March 8, 2011, https://www.scientificamerican.com/article/diabetes-belt, accessed May 28, 2019.

Hart, Mitchell B. "Racial Science, Social Science, and the Politics of Jewish Assimilation." *Isis* 90 (1999): 268–297.

———. *Social Science and the Politics of Modern Jewish Identity.* Stanford, CA: Stanford University Press, 2000.

———, ed. *Jews and Race: Writings on Identity and Difference, 1880–1940.* Waltham, MA: Brandeis University Press, 2011.

Hatch, Anthony Ryan. *Blood Sugar: Racial Pharmacology and Food Justice in Black America.* Minneapolis: University of Minnesota Press, 2016.

Hay, Travis. "Commentary: The Invention of Aboriginal Diabetes: The Role of the Thrifty Gene Hypothesis in Canadian Health Care Provision." *Ethnicity & Disease* 28, no. S1 (2018): 247–252.

Haynes, M. Alfred. "The Gap in Health Status between Black and White Americans." P. 1–30 in *Textbook of Black-Related Diseases,* ed. Richard Allen Williams. New York: McGraw-Hill, 1975.

"Health Director Warns against High T.B. Rate." *Afro-American,* April 8, 1933, 4.

Heat-Moon, William Least. "A Stark Reminder of How the U.S. Forced American Indians into a New Way of Life," *Smithsonian* (November 2013).

Henry, R. E., T. A. Burch, P. H. Bennett, and Max Miller. "Diabetes in the Cocopah Indians." *Diabetes* 18, no. 1 (1969): 33–37.

Henry, Walter Lester, Jr. "Endocrine Diseases." Pp. 317–330 in *Textbook of Black-Related Diseases,* ed. Richard Allen Williams. New York: McGraw-Hill, 1975.

"Heredity and Diabetes—A Medical View." *Journal of Heredity* 23 (January 1932): 30.

Herskovits, Melville J. *The American Negro: A Study in Racial Crossing.* New York: A. A. Knopf, 1928.

Hill, Jacqueline, Marcia Nielsen, and Michael H. Fox. "Understanding the Social Factors That Contribute to Diabetes: A Means to Informing Health Care and Social Policies for the Chronically Ill." *Permanente Journal* 17, no. 2 (2013): 67–72.

Hine, Darlene Clark. *Black Women in White: Racial Conflict and Cooperation in the Nursing Profession, 1890–1950.* Bloomington: Indiana University Press, 1989.

Hirschman, Charles. "Immigration to the United States: Recent Trends and Future Prospects." *Malaysian Journal of Economic Studies* 51, no. 1 (2014): 69–85.

Hirschmann, Nancy J., and Beth Linker. "Disability, Citizenship, and Belonging: A Critical Introduction." Pp. 1–21 in *Civil Disabilities: Citizenship, Membership, and Belonging,* ed. Nancy J. Hirschmann and Beth Linker. Philadelphia: University of Pennsylvania Press, 2015.

———, eds. *Civil Disabilities: Citizenship, Membership, and Belonging.* Philadelphia: University of Pennsylvania Press, 2015.

Hoffman, Frederick L. "Diabetes Record of 1931." *American Journal of Public Health* 23 (1933): 152.

—————. "Race Traits and Tendencies of the American Negro." *Publications of the American Economic Association* 11 (1896): 1–329.

Hollinger, David. "Amalgamation and Hypodescent: The Question of Ethnoracial Mixture in the History of the United States." *American Historical Review* 108, no. 5 (2003): 1363–1390.

Hopkins, James A. "Letter to the Editor: Increase of Diabetes." *Journal of the American Medical Association* 29 (1897): 450–451.

Howell, Ron. "Diabetes: Black Women Are Its No. 1 Victim." *Ebony* 34 (March 1979): 64–66, 68, 71.

Hrdlička, Aleš. *Physiological and Medical Observations among the Indians of the Southwestern United States and Northern Mexico.* Bulletin 24. Washington, DC: Smithsonian Institute, 1908.

Humphreys, Margaret. *Intensely Human: The Health of the Black Soldier in the American Civil War.* Baltimore: Johns Hopkins University Press, 2008.

—————. *Malaria: Poverty, Race, and Public Health in the United States.* Baltimore: Johns Hopkins University Press, 2001.

Humphreys, Margaret, Philip Costanzo, Kerry L. Haynie, Truls Østbye, Idrissa Boly, Daniel Belsky, and Frank Sloan. "Racial Disparities in Diabetes a Century Ago: Evidence from the Pension Files of US Civil War Veterans." *Social Science & Medicine* 64 (2007): 1766–1775.

Igo, Sarah E. *The Averaged American; Surveys, Citizens, and the Making of a Mass Public.* Cambridge, MA: Harvard University Press, 2007.

—————. *The Known Citizen: A History of Privacy in Modern America.* Cambridge, MA: Harvard University Press, 2018.

"Improved Health Habits Aimed at Black Community." *Baltimore Afro-American,* September 8, 1984, 12.

"Incidence of Diabetes Mellitus." *Journal of the American Medical Association* 149, no. 9 (1952): 886.

"Indian Health Act Is 'Dying' in Congress." *Navajo Times,* September 25, 1975, A10.

"Industrial Health of Nation Surveyed." *New York Times,* August 14, 1928.

"Is the Negro Dying Out? (A Symposium)." *Colored American Magazine* 15, no. 1 (January 1909): 659–679.

"Is Race 'Real?'" Web forum organized by the Social Science Research Council, http://raceandgenomics.ssrc.org, accessed May 26, 2019.

Iverson, Margot Lynn. "Blood Types: A History of Genetic Studies of Native Americans, 1920-1955." PhD diss., University of Minnesota, 2007.

Jablons, Benjamin. "Diabetes, a Controllable Disease." *Hygeia* 10 (1932): 423–425.

Jackson, William Peter Uprichard. "Diabetes Mellitus in Different Countries and Different Races: Prevalence and Major Features." *Acta Diabetologica* 7 (1970): 361–401.

Jacobs, Joseph, and Maurice Fishberg. "Diabetes Mellitus," *JewishEncyclopedia.com,* http://www.jewishencyclopedia.com/articles/5161-diabetes-mellitus, accessed October 5, 2019.

—————. "Nervous Diseases." *JewishEncyclopedia.com,* http://www.jewishencyclopedia.com/articles/11446-nervous-diseases, accessed May 26, 2019.

Jacobson, Matthew Frye. *Whiteness of a Different Color: European Immigrants and the Alchemy of Race*. Cambridge, MA: Harvard University Press, 1999.

Jennings, H. S. "Health Progress and Race Progress: Are They Incompatible?" *Journal of Heredity* 18 (1927): 271–276.

Jernigan, Valarie Blue Bird, Elizabeth J D'Amico, Bonnie Duran, and Dedra Buchwald. "Multilevel and Community-Level Interventions with Native Americans: Challenges and Opportunities." *Prevention Science* (June 2018): 1–9, doi:10.1007/s11121-018-0916-3.

Joe, Jennie R., and Robert S. Young, eds. *Diabetes as a Disease of Civilisation: The Impact of Culture Change on Indigenous Peoples*. Berlin: Mouton de Gruyter, 1994.

Johnson, John E., and C. Wallace McNutt. "Diabetes Mellitus in an American Indian Population Isolate." *Texas Reports on Biology and Medicine* 22 (1964): 110–125.

Jolly, F. *Handbuch der practischen Medicine*. Stuttgart: Ebstein and Schwalbe, 1900.

Jones, David S. *Rationalizing Epidemics: Meanings and Uses of American Indian Mortality since 1600*. Cambridge, MA: Harvard University Press, 2004.

———. "Virgin Soils Revisited." *William and Mary Quarterly* 60, no. 4 (October 2003): 703–742.

Jones, Edith Irby. "President's Column: Closing the Health Status Gap for Blacks and Other Minorities." *Journal of the National Medical Association* 78, no. 6 (1986): 485–488.

Jones, James. *Bad Blood: The Tuskegee Syphilis Experiment*. Rev. ed.; New York: Free Press, 1993.

Joslin, Elliott P. "The Changing Diabetic Clientele." *Transactions of the Association of American Physicians* 39 (1924): 304–307.

———. "Diabetes among Jews." *Harofé Haivri* 1 (1941): 220–222.

———. *A Diabetic Manual for the Mutual Use of Doctor and Patient*. Philadelphia: Lea & Febiger, 1918.

———. "The Diabetic Problem of Today." *Journal of the American Medical Association* 83, no. 10 (1924): 727–729.

———. "The Prevention of Diabetes Mellitus." *Journal of the American Medical Association* 76, no. 2 (1921): 79–84.

———. "The Shattuck Lecture: The Treatment of Diabetes Mellitus." *Boston Medical and Surgical Journal* 186 (1922): 833–852.

———. "Social and Medical Aspects of the Problem of Heredity in Diabetes." *Medical Clinics of North America* 18 (1935): 1033–1040.

———. *The Treatment of Diabetes Mellitus*. Philadelphia: Lea & Febiger, 1916.

———. *The Treatment of Diabetes Mellitus*, 2nd ed. Philadelphia: Lea & Febiger, 1917.

———. *The Treatment of Diabetes Mellitus*, 6th ed. Philadelphia: Lea & Febiger, 1937.

———. *The Treatment of Diabetes Mellitus*, 8th ed. Philadelphia: Lea & Febiger, 1946.

———. "The Universality of Diabetes: A Survey of Diabetic Mortality in Arizona. The Billings Lecture." *Journal of the American Medical Association* 115, no. 24 (1940): 2033–2038.

———. "The Unknown Diabetic." *Postgraduate Medicine* 4 (October 1948): 302–306.

Joslin, Elliott P., Louis I. Dublin, and Herbert H. Marks. "Studies in Diabetes Mellitus I: Characteristics and Trends of Diabetes Mortality throughout the World." *American Journal of the Medical Sciences* 6 (1933): 753–773.

———. "Studies in Diabetes Mellitus II: Its Incidence and the Factors Underlying Its Variations." *American Journal of the Medical Sciences* 184, no. 4 (1934): 433–457.

Jou, Chin. *Supersizing Urban America: How Inner Cities Got Fast Food with Government Help.* Chicago: University of Chicago Press, 2017.

Joyner, John E. "President's Inaugural Address: Future of Health Care in America: What Is the NMA's Role?" *Journal of the National Medical Association* 79, no. 11 (1987): 1129–1133.

Justice, James. "The History of Diabetes Mellitus in the Desert People." Pp. 69–127 in *Diabetes as a Disease of Civilisation: The Impact of Culture Change on Indigenous Peoples,* ed. Jennie R. Joe and Robert S. Young. Berlin: Mouton de Gruyter, 1994.

Kahn, Jonathan. *Race in a Bottle: The Story of BiDil and Racialized Medicine in a Post-Genomic Age.* New York: Columbia University Press, 2014.

Kalmar, Ivan Davidson, and Derek J. Penslar, eds. *Orientalism and the Jews.* Waltham, MA: Brandeis University Press, 2005.

Kandimalla, Ramesh, V. Thirumala, and P. H. Reddy. "Review: Is Alzheimer's Disease a Type 3 Diabetes? A Critical Appraisal." *Biochimica et Biophysica Acta (BBA)— Molecular Basis of Disease* 1863, no. 5 (2017): 1078–1089.

Karter, Andrew John. "Race and Ethnicity: Vital Constructs for Diabetes Research (Commentary)." *Diabetes Care* 26, no. 7 (July 2003): 2189.

Katz, Michael B. *In the Shadow of the Poorhouse: A Social History of Welfare in America.* New York: Basic Books, 1986.

Kawate, Ryoso, Michio Yamakido, Yukio Nishimoto, Peter H. Bennett, Richard F. Hamman, and William C. Knowler. "Diabetes Mellitus and Its Vascular Complications in Japanese Migrants on the Island of Hawaii." *Diabetes Care* 2, no. 2 (1979): 161–170.

Kemp, Tage. "Danish Experiences in Negative Eugenics, 1929–45." *Eugenics Review* 38, no. 4 (1947): 181–186.

Kevles, Daniel J. *In the Name of Eugenics: Genetics and the Uses of Human Heredity.* 2nd ed. Cambridge, MA: Harvard University Press, 1995.

Kimball, Chase Patterson. "The Patient and Diabetes: Impressions from Dialogues." *Journal of the American Medical Association* 219, no. 1 (1972): 83–85.

King, Desmond. *In the Name of Illiberalism: Illiberal Social Policy in the USA and Britain.* New York: Oxford University Press, 1999.

King, Richard H. *Race, Culture, and the Intellectuals, 1940–1970.* Washington, DC: Woodrow Wilson Center Press, 2004.

Kirchhof, Mark, Nooreen Popat, and Janet Malowany. "A Historical Perspective of the Diagnosis of Diabetes." *University of Western Ontario Medical Journal* 78, no. 1 (2008): 7–11.

Kitagawa, Evelyn M., and Philip M. Hauser. "Trends in Differential Fertility and Mortality in a Metropolis—Chicago." Pp. 59–85 in *Research Contributions to Urban*

Sociology, ed. Ernest W. Burgess and Donald J. Bogue. Chicago: University of Chicago Press, 1964.

Kleen, Emil. *On Diabetes Mellitus and Glycosuria*. Philadelphia: P. Blakiston's Son & Co., 1900.

Kline, Wendy. *Building a Better Race: Gender, Sexuality, and Eugenics from the Turn of the Century to the Baby Boom*. Berkeley: University of California Press, 2001.

Klingle, Matthew. "Inescapable Paradoxes: Diabetes, Progress, and Ecologies of Inequality." Part of the special issue "Forum: Technology, Ecology, and Human Health since 1850." *Environmental History* 20 (October 2015): 736–750.

Klunker, Ilse. "Genügen unsere heutigen Kenntnisse über den Diabetes mellitus zu dessen Einreihung unter die Erbkrankheiten im Sinne des Gesetzes vom 14. Juli 1933?" Diss. Med. Muenchen, 1936.

Knadler, Stephen. "Unsanitized Domestic Allegories: Biomedical Politics, Racial Uplift, and the African American Woman's Risk Narrative." *American Literature* 85, no. 1 (2013): 93–119.

Knowler, William C., David J. Pettitt, Peter H. Bennett, and Robert C. Williams. "Diabetes Mellitus in the Pima Indians: Genetic and Evolutionary Considerations." *American Journal of Physical Anthropology* 62, no. 1 (1983): 107–114.

Knowler, William C., David J. Pettitt, Mohammed F. Saad, and Peter H. Bennett. "Diabetes Mellitus in the Pima Indians: Incidence, Risk Factors and Pathogenesis," *Diabetes/Metabolism Reviews* 6, no. 1 (1990): 1–27.

Knowler, William C., David J. Pettitt, Peter J. Savage, and Peter H. Bennett. "Diabetes Incidence in Pima Indians: Contributions of Obesity and Parental Diabetes." *American Journal of Epidemiology* 113, no. 2 (1981): 144–156.

Kohler, Robert E. *Lords of the Fly. Drosophila Genetics and the Experimental Life*. Chicago: University of Chicago Press, 1994.

Kraus, Bertram S. *Indian Health in Arizona: A Study of Health Conditions among Central and Southern Arizona Indians*. Second Annual Report of the Bureau of Ethnic Research. Tucson: University of Arizona, 1954.

Kraut, Alan M. *Silent Travelers. Germs, Genes, and the Immigrant Menace*. Baltimore: Johns Hopkins University Press, 1995.

Krieger, Nancy. *Epidemiology and the People's Health. Theory and Context*. Oxford, UK: Oxford University Press, 2014. Pp. 249–261.

———. "If 'Race' Is the Answer, What Is the Question?—On 'Race,' Racism, and Health: A Social Epidemiologist's Perspective." In "Is Race 'Real?,'" web forum organized by the Social Science Research Council, http://raceandgenomics.ssrc .org/Krieger, accessed May 26, 2019.

———. "Stormy Weather: Race, Gene Expression, and the Science of Health Disparities." *American Journal of Public Health* 95 (2005): 2155–2160.

Krikler, Dennis M. "Diseases of Jews." *Postgraduate Medical Journal* 46 (1970): 687–697.

Krout, Maurice H. "Race and Culture: A Study in Mobility, Segregation, and Selection." *American Journal of Sociology* 37, no. 2 (1931): 175–189.

Ladd-Taylor, Molly. *Fixing the Poor: Eugenic Sterilization and Child Welfare in the Twentieth Century*. Baltimore: Johns Hopkins University Press, 2017.

Lang, Gretchen Chesley. "'In Their Tellings': Dakota Narratives about History and the Body." Pp. 53–71 in *Indigenous Peoples and Diabetes: Community Empowerment and Wellness*, ed. Mariana Leal Ferreira and Gretchen Chesley Lang. Durham, NC: Carolina Academic Press, 2006.

————. "Talking about a New Illness with the Dakota: Reflections on Diabetes, Foods, and Culture." Pp. 203–230 in *Indigenous Peoples and Diabetes: Community Empowerment and Wellness*, ed. Mariana Leal Ferreira and Gretchen Chesley Lang. Durham, NC: Carolina Academic Press, 2006.

Largent, Mark A. *Breeding Contempt: The History of Coerced Sterilization in the United States*. New Brunswick, NJ: Rutgers University Press, 2008.

Larkin-Gilmore, Juliet C. "Native Health on the Move: Public Health and Assimilation on the Lower Colorado River, 1890-1934." PhD diss., Vanderbilt University, 2019.

Laughlin, Harry H. "The Scope of the Committee's Work." *Eugenics Record Office* 10A (1913): 5–65.

Lawrence, "Framing Obesity: The Evolution of News Discourse on a Public Health Issue." *Press/Politics* 9, no. 3 (2004): 45–75.

Lawson, Nadya J. "Mary Fitzbutler Waring." Pp. 680–683 in *Notable Black American Women Book II*, ed. Jessie Carney Smith. New York: Gale Research, 1996.

Leach, William. *Land of Desire: Merchants, Power, and the Rise of a New American Culture*. New York: Vintage, 1993.

Lees, Hannah. "Two Million Tightrope Walkers." *Collier's*, May 16, 1936, 18, 34, 36, 38, available in the UnzReview: An Alternative Media Selection, http://www.unz .com/print/Colliers-1936may16-00018, accessed October 5, 2019.

Lefkowitz, Bonnie. *Community Health Centers: A Movement and the People Who Made It Happen*. New Brunswick, NJ: Rutgers University Press, 2007.

Lemann, Isaac Ivan. "Diabetes Mellitus among the Negroes." *New Orleans Medical and Surgical Journal* 63 (1911): 461–467.

————. "Diabetes Mellitus in the Negro Race." *Southern Medical Journal* 14, no. 7 (1921): 522–525.

Leonard, Ione. "A Diabetic's Disposition." *Hygeia* 17 (April 1939): 308–310.

Leopold, Eugene J. "Diabetes in the Negro Race." *Annals of Internal Medicine* 5 (1931): 285–293.

Levine, Philippa, and Alison Bashford. "Introduction: Eugenics and the Modern World." Pp. 3–24 in *The Oxford Handbook of the History of Eugenics*, ed. Alison Bashford and Philippa Levine. Oxford, UK: Oxford University Press, 2010.

Lewis, Julian Herman. *The Biology of the Negro*. Chicago: University of Chicago Press, 1942.

Lindee, Susan. "James Van Gundia Neel (1915–2000)." *American Anthropologist* 103, no. 2 (June 2001): 502–505.

Linder, Forrest E., and Robert D. Grove. *Vital Statistics Rates in the United States, 1900–1940*. Washington, DC: U.S. Government Printing Office, 1947.

Link, Bruce G., and Jo Phelan. "Social Conditions as Fundamental Causes of Disease." In the special issue "Forty Years of Medical Sociology: The State of the Art and Directions for the Future," *Journal of Health and Social Behavior* (1995): 80–94.

Linker, Beth. *War's Waste: Rehabilitation in World War I America*. Chicago: Chicago University Press, 2014.

Lyon, Ernst. *Diabetes Mellitus and the Jewish Race*. Jerusalem: Ludwig Mayer, 1940.

Lyons, Richard D. "Hunger and Sickness Afflict Mississippi Negro Children." *New York Times*, March 25, 1968.

MacDonald, Peter. "Hunger a Reality on Navajo Reservation." *Navajo Times*, April 2, 1970, 19–20.

"MacDonald Challenges Health Leaders to Develop New Medical Care Strategies." *Navajo Times*, November 5, 1987, 4, 10–11.

Macmillan, Amanda. "Researchers Identify Five Different Types of Diabetes, Not Just Type 1 and Type 2." *Time*, March 2, 2018.

Mancall, Peter. *Deadly Medicine: Indians and Alcohol in Early America*. Ithaca, NY: Cornell University Press, 1995.

Markel, Howard. *Quarantine!: East European Jewish Immigrants and the New York City Epidemics of 1892*. Baltimore: Johns Hopkins University Press, 1997.

Marks, Harry M. "Epidemiologists Explain Pellagra: Gender, Race and Political Economy in the Work of Edgar Sydenstricker." *Journal of the History of Medicine and Allied Sciences* 58, no. 1 (2003): 34–55.

——. *The Progress of Experiment: Science and Therapeutic Reform in the United States, 1900–1990*. New York: Cambridge University Press, 1997.

Marks, Herbert H. "Recent Statistics on Diabetes and Diabetics." *Medical Clinics of North America* 31, no. 2 (1947): 369–386.

Marquis, James. *The Metropolitan Life: A Study in Business Growth*. New York: Viking, 1947.

Martensen, Robert L., and David S. Jones. "Diabetes Mellitus as a 'Disease of Civilization.'" *Journal of the American Medical Association* 278, no. 4 (1997): 345.

Maty, Siobhan C., Sherman A. James, and George A. Kaplan. "Life-Course Socioeconomic Position and Incidence of Diabetes Mellitus among Blacks and Whites: The Alameda County Study, 1965–1999." *AJPH* 100, no. 1 (2010): 137–145.

Mauck, Aaron Pascal. "Managing Care: The History of Diabetes Management in Twentieth Century America." PhD diss., Harvard University, 2010.

McBride, David. *From TB to AIDS: Epidemics among Urban Blacks since 1900*. Albany, NY: State University of New York Press, 1991.

"McCann's Warning." *Time*, September 24, 1923.

McDermott, Robyn. "Ethics, Epidemiology and the Thrifty Gene: Biological Determinism as a Health Hazard." *Social Science and Medicine* 47, no. 9 (1998): 1189–1195.

McKusick, Victor A., John A. Hostetler, and Janice A. Egeland. "Genetic Studies of the Amish: Background and Potentialities." *Bulletin of the Johns Hopkins Hospital* 115 (1964): 203–222.

McLoughlin, Christopher. "Diabetes Detection in Georgia." *Journal of the Medical Association of Georgia* 40 (1951): 285–286.

McMillen, Christian W. *Discovering Tuberculosis: A Global History, 1900 to Present.* New Haven: Yale University Press, 2015.

———. "'The Red Man and the White Plague': Rethinking Race, Tuberculosis, and American Indians, ca. 1890–1950." *Bulletin of the History of Medicine* 82, no. 3 (2008): 608–645.

"Medic Says Two Million, Now Well, Will Get Diabetes." *Chicago Defender,* December 21, 1946.

Meldrum, Marcia. "David Rimoin Interview." UCLA Oral History of Human Genetics Project, http://ohhgp.pendari.com, accessed May 27, 2019.

Melillo, Wendy. "Why Are the Pima Indians Sick?" *Washington Post,* March 30, 1993, 7.

Mendosa, David. "Jewish Diabetes." *Mendosa.com* (updated January 14, 2002), http://www.mendosa.com/jewish.htm, accessed May 26, 2019.

Metzl, Jonathan M. *The Protest Psychosis: How Schizophrenia Became a Black Disease.* Boston: Beacon Press, 2009.

Mihesuah, Devon A., and Elizabeth Hoover, eds. *Indigenous Food Sovereignty in the United States: Restoring Cultural Knowledge, Protecting Environments, and Regaining Health.* Norman: University of Oklahoma Press, 2019.

"Mike Myers—Excerpts from an Interview." *Akwesasne Notes* 12, no. 4 (September 1980): 23.

Miller, Kelly. *A Review of "Hoffman's Race Traits and Tendencies of the American Negro."* American Negro Academy, Occasional Papers 1, 1897, Library of Congress, https://www.loc.gov/item/09024191, accessed December 6, 2019.

Miller, Max, Thomas A. Burch, Peter H. Bennett, and Arthur G. Steinberg. "Prevalence of Diabetes Mellitus in the American Indians: Results of Glucose Tolerance Tests in the Pima Indians of Arizona." Abstracts of Presented and by Title Papers of the 25th Annual Meeting of the ADA. *Diabetes* 14, no. 7 (1965): 439–440.

Miller, Max, Peter H. Bennett, and Thomas A Burch. "Hyperglycemia in Pima Indians: A Preliminary Appraisal of Its Significance." Pp. 89–103 in *Biomedical Challenges Presented by the American Indian.* Washington, DC: Pan American Health Organization, 1968.

Misra, A., and O. P. Ganda. "Migration and Its Impact on Adiposity and Type 2 Diabetes." *Nutrition* 23, no. 9 (2007): 696–708.

"The Missing Million." *Time,* October 17, 1949.

Molina, Natalia. *Fit to Be Citizens? Public Health and Race in Los Angeles, 1879–1939.* Berkeley: University of California Press, 2006.

Montagu, Ashley. "A Consideration of the Concept of Race." *Cold Spring Harbor Symposium on Quantitative Biology* 15 (1950): 315–336.

Montoya, Michael J. *Making the Mexican Diabetic: Race, Science, and the Genetics of Inequality.* Berkeley: University of California Press, 2011.

Mooney, Graham. "The Material Consumptive: Domesticating the Tuberculosis Patient in Edwardian England." *Journal of Historical Geography* 42 (2013): 152–166.

Moore, Amanda. "Tracking Down Martin Luther King, Jr.'s Words on Health Care." *Huffington Post,* January 18, 2013 (last updated March 20, 2013), http://www

.huffingtonpost.com/amanda-moore/martin-luther-king-health-care_b_2506393 .html, accessed May 27, 2019.

Moore, Martin D. *Managing Diabetes, Managing Medicine: Chronic Disease and Clinical Bureaucracy in Post-War Britain.* Manchester, UK: Manchester University Press, 2019.

Morrison, H. "A Statistical Study of the Mortality from Diabetes Mellitus in Boston from 1895 to 1913, with Special Reference to Its Occurrence among Jews." *Boston Medical and Surgical Journal* 175 (1916): 54–57.

"Mortality from Diabetes." *Journal of the American Medical Association* 92, no. 1 (1924): 42.

Mouratoff, George J., Nicholas V. Carroll, and Edward M. Scott. "Diabetes Mellitus in Athabaskan Indians in Alaska." *Diabetes* 18, no. 1 (1969): 29–32.

"Mrs. Clement Loses Limb." *Afro-American* (Baltimore), December 9, 1950, 10.

Mulligan, Jessica. "Biological Citizenship." In *Oxford Bibliographies in Anthropology* (2017), https://dx.doi.org/10.1093/obo/9780199766567-0164, accessed December 6, 2019.

Nasaw, David. *Going Out: The Rise and Fall of Public Amusements.* Cambridge, MA: Harvard University Press, 1993.

National Commission on Diabetes. *Report of the National Commission on Diabetes to the Congress of the United States,* vol. 1: *The Long-Range Plan to Combat Diabetes.* Bethesda: U.S. Department of Health, Education, and Welfare, 1976.

———. *Report of the National Commission on Diabetes to the Congress of the United States,* vol. 2: *Contributors to the Deliberations of the Commission. Part I: Public Testimony (Public Hearings 1–5).* Bethesda: U.S. Department of Health, Education, and Welfare, 1976.

National Institute of Diabetes and Digestive and Kidney Diseases. "Diabetes Overview." https://www.niddk.nih.gov/health-information/diabetes/overview, accessed May 27, 2019.

———. "Diabetes Statistics." https://www.niddk.nih.gov/health-information/health -statistics/diabetes-statistics, accessed May 28, 2019.

———. "Risk Factors for Type 2 Diabetes." https://www.niddk.nih.gov/health -information/diabetes/overview/risk-factors-type-2-diabetes, accessed May 27, 2019.

"Native People, Colonialism, and Food." *Akwesasne Notes* 13, no. 1 (March 1981): 24–25.

Navarro, Vicente. "Race or Class versus Race and Class: Mortality Differentials in the United States." *Lancet* 36 (1990): 1238–1240.

Neel, James V. "Diabetes Mellitus: A 'Thrifty' Gene Rendered Detrimental by 'Progress'?" *American Journal of Human Genetics* 14 (1962): 353–362.

———. "Editorial: Medicine's Genetic Horizons." *Annals of Internal Medicine* 49 (1958): 472–476.

———. "Heredity in the Prevention of Chronic Disease." *Eugenical News* 38, no. 2 (1953): 20–24.

———. "Opening Statement." *Biomedical Challenges Presented by the American Indians (Proceedings of the Special Session Held during the Seventh Meeting of the PAHO Advisory Committee on Medical Research, 25 June 1968)*, scientific publication no. 165. Washington, DC: Pan American Health Organization, 1968, 1.

———. *Physician to the Gene Pool.* New York: Wiley and Sons, 1994.

———. "The Study of Natural Selection in Primitive and Civilized Human Populations." *Human Biology* 30, no. 1 (1958): 43–72.

———. "The 'Thrifty Genotype' in 1998." *Nutrition Reviews* 57, no. 5 (1999): S2–S9.

———. "The Thrifty Genotype Revisited." Pp. 283–293 in *The Genetics of Diabetes Mellitus*, ed. J. Köbberling and R. Tattersall. New York: Academic Press, 1982.

———. "Towards a Better Understanding of the Genetic Basis of Diabetes." Pp. 240–244 in *The Genetics of Diabetes Mellitus*, ed. W. Creutzfeldt, J. Köbberling, and J. V. Neel. Berlin: Springer-Verlag, 1976.

Nelson, Alondra. *Body and Soul: The Black Panther Party and the Fight against Medical Discrimination.* Minneapolis: University of Minnesota Press, 2013.

"New Health Set-Up Urged for Indians." *New York Times*, June 2, 1951.

"New Hope in Health Care for Native Americans." *Akwesasne Notes* 6, no. 1 (April 1974): 28.

Newkirk II, Vann R. "What the 'Crack Baby' Panic Reveals about the Opioid Epidemic." *The Atlantic*, July 16, 2017, https://www.theatlantic.com/politics/archive/2017/07/what-the-crack-baby-panic-reveals-about-the-opioid-epidemic/533763, accessed May 29, 2019.

Ngai, Mae. "The Architecture of Race in American Immigration Law: A Reexamination of the Immigration Act of 1924." *Journal of American History* 86, no. 1 (1999): 67–92.

———. *Impossible Subjects: Illegal Aliens and the Making of Modern America.* Princeton, NJ: Princeton University Press, 2014.

Niswander, J. D. "Discussion." Pp. 133–136 in *Biomedical Challenges Presented by the American Indian.* Washington, DC: Pan American Health Organization, 1968.

Nobles, Melissa. "History Counts: A Comparative Analysis of Racial/Color Categorization in U.S. and Brazilian Censuses." *American Journal of Public Health* 90 (2000): 1738–1745.

"No Scientific Basis for 'Aryan' Race Theory, Dr. Jablons Proves," *Jewish Telegraphic Agency* archive, June 25, 1934, https://www.jta.org/1934/06/25/archive/no-scientific-basis-for-aryan-race-theory-dr-jablons-proves, accessed May 26, 2019.

Nott, Josiah. "Physical History of the Jewish Race." *Southern Quarterly Review* 1, no. 2 (1850): 428–430.

O-Day, J. Christopher, "The Blurring of Diabetes." *Medical Record* 155 (1942): 315–316.

O'Dea, Suzanne. *From Suffrage to Senate.* Amenia, NY: Grey House, 2013.

Oliver, C. P. "Concluding Remarks of the Chairman." *Cold Spring Harbor Symposium on Quantitative Biology* 15 (1950): 243–245.

Olson, Brooke. "Meeting the Challenges of American Indian Diabetes: Anthropological Perspectives on Prevention and Treatment." Pp. 163–184 in *Medicine Ways:*

Disease, Health, and Survival among Native Americans, ed. Clifford E. Trafzer and Diane Weiner. Walnut Creek: Alta Mira Press, 2001.

Omi, Michael, and Howard Winant. *Racial Formation in the United States: From the 1960s to the 1990s*. 2nd ed. New York: Routledge & Kegan Paul, 1994.

Omran, Abdel R. "The Epidemiological Transition: A Theory of the Epidemiology of Population Change." *Milbank Memorial Fund Quarterly* 49, no. 4 (1971): 509–538.

Oppenheimer, Gerald M. "Becoming the Framingham Study, 1947–1950." *American Journal of Public Health* 95, no. 4 (2005): 602–610.

"The Origin and Evolution of Man (Cold Spring Harbor Symposium, 1950)." *Eugenics Quarterly* 1 (1954).

Osler, William. *The Principles and Practice of Medicine*. New York: D. Appleton, 1892.

———. *The Principles and Practice of Medicine*, 8th ed. New York: D. Appleton, 1913.

———. *The Principles and Practice of Medicine*, 16th ed. New York: D. Appleton, 1947.

Pachon, Harry P., and Joan W. Moore. "Mexican Americans." *Annals of the American Academy of Political and Social Science* 454 (1981): 111–124.

Pancoast, Dr. "Diabetes in the Negro." *Johns Hopkins Hospital Bulletin* 9, no. 83 (1898): 40–41.

Paradies, Yin C. , Michael J. Montoya, and Stephanie M. Fullerton. "Racialized Genetics and the Study of Complex Diseases: The Thrifty Genotype Revisited." *Perspectives in Biology and Medicine* 50, no. 2 (2007): 203–227.

Parks, J. H., and E. Waskow. "Diabetes among the Pima Indians of Arizona." *Arizona Medicine: Journal of the Arizona State Medical Association* 18 (1961): 99–107.

Pate, James E. "The Public Health." *Social Forces* 18, no. 4 (1940): 525–535.

Pattillo-McCoy, Mary. *Black Picket Fences: Privilege and Peril among the Black Middle Class*. Chicago: University of Chicago Press, 1999.

Paul, Diane. *Controlling Human Heredity: 1865 to the Present*. Amherst, NY: Humanity Books, 1995.

———. *The Politics of Heredity: Essays on Eugenics, Biomedicine, and the Nature-Nurture Debate*. Albany: State University of New York Press, 1998.

Peiss, Kathy. *Cheap Amusements*. Philadelphia: Temple University Press, 1986.

Pérez-Peña, Richard. "Beyond 'I'm a Diabetic,' Little Common Ground." *New York Times*, May 17, 2006.

"Periodicals." *Eugenics Review* 55, no. 2 (1963): 123.

Pernick, Martin S. "Eugenics and Public Health in American History." *American Journal of Public Health* 87, no. 11 (1997): 1767–1772.

Perrott, George St. J., and Dorothy F. Holland. "The Need for Adequate Data on Current Illness among Negroes." In "The Health Status and Health Education of Negroes in the United States," *Journal of Negro Education* 6, no. 3 (1937): 350–363.

Peterson, Iver. "Surge in Indians' Diabetes Linked to Their History." *New York Times*, February 18, 1986, A10.

Pettigrew, Ann Hallman, and Thomas F. Pettigrew. "Race, Disease and Desegregation: A New Look." *Phylon* 24, no. 4 (1963): 315–333.

Phelan, Jo C., and Bruce G. Link. "Is Racism a Fundamental Cause of Inequalities in Health?" *Annual Review of Sociology* 41 (2015): 311–330.

Pollock, Anne. *Medicating Race: Heart Disease and Durable Preoccupations with Differ-ence.* Durham, NC: Duke University Press, 2012.

Porter, Roy. "Diseases of Civilization." Chap. 27 in *Companion Encyclopedia of the History of Medicine,* ed. W. F. Bynum and Roy Porter. London: Routledge, 1993.

Poudrier, Jennifer. "The Geneticization of Aboriginal Diabetes and Obesity: Adding Another Scene to the Story of the Thrifty Gene." *Canadian Review of Sociology & Anthropology* 44, no. 2 (2007): 237–261.

Proceedings of the St. Louis Medical Society of Missouri. Saint Louis: J. H. Chambers, 1885.

Proctor, Robert N. *Racial Hygiene: Medicine under the Nazis.* Cambridge, MA: Harvard University Press, 1988.

"Protect Your Health." *Black Worker* 26, no. 10 (1955): 6.

Purdy, Charles. *Diabetes: Its Causes, Symptoms, and Treatment.* Philadelphia: F.A. Davis, 1890.

Quinn, Sandra Crouse, and Stephen B. Thomas. "The National Negro Health Week, 1915–1951." *Minority Health Today* 2, no. 3 (2001): 44–49.

Rasmussen, Nicolas. *Fat in the Fifties: America's First Obesity Crisis.* Baltimore: Johns Hopkins University Press, 2019.

Rawlins, E. Elliott. "Diabetes." *New York Amsterdam News,* February 1, 1928, 13.

———. "The Increasing Frequency of Diabetes." *New York Amsterdam News,* August 15, 1928, 16.

———. "Keep a Cool Head and Save Your Ductless Glands." *New York Amsterdam News,* October 5, 1927, 14.

———. "The Mind and Disease." *New York Amsterdam News,* July 27, 1927, 15.

Raymond, Chris Anne. "Diabetes in Mexican-Americans: Pressing Problem in a Growing Population." *Journal of the American Medical Association* 259, no. 12 (1988): 1772.

"Reaction of Negroes to Disease." *Journal of the American Medical Association* 98, no. 12 (1931): 857.

Reardon, Jenny. *Race to the Finish: Identity and Governance in an Age of Genomics.* Princeton, NJ: Princeton University Press, 2005.

Reed, T. E. "Ethnic Classification of Mexican Americans." *Science* 185 (July 19, 1974): 283.

Reilly, Philip R. *The Surgical Solution: A History of Involuntary Sterilization in the United States.* Baltimore: Johns Hopkins University Press, 1991.

"Report of the Expert Committee on the Diagnosis and Classification of Diabetes Mellitus." *Diabetes Care* 25, suppl. 1 (2002): s5–s20.

Reverby, Susan M. *Examining Tuskegee: The Infamous Syphilis Study and Its Legacy.* Chapel Hill: University of North Carolina Press, 2013.

Rhoades, Everett R., and Dorothy A. Rhoades. "The Public Health Foundation of Health Services for American Indians & Alaska Natives." *American Journal of Public Health* 104, S3 (2014): S278–S285.

"Richard Allen Williams, M.D., President-Elect." *National Medical Association,* n.d., https://www.nmanet.org/general/custom.asp?page=President Elect, accessed May 28, 2019.

Rieser, A. C. *The Chautauqua Movement: Protestants, Progressives, and the Culture of Modern Liberalism.* New York: Columbia University Press, 2003.

Rimoin, David L. "Ethnic Variability in Glucose Tolerance and Insulin Secretion." *Archives of Internal Medicine* 124, no. 6 (1969): 695–700.

———. "Genetics of Diabetes Mellitus." *Diabetes* 16, no. 5 (1967): 346–351.

Rimoin, David L., and John H. Saiki. "Diabetes Mellitus among the Navajo. II. Plasma Glucose and Insulin Responses." *Archives of Internal Medicine* 122 (July 1968): 6–9.

"Rip Van Winkles." January 1930. Metropolitan Life Archives, National Advertisements, 1922-Welfare—1932.

"Rising Diabetes Death Rate Laid to Easier Living." *New York Tribune,* July 28, 1929.

Roberts, Dorothy. *Killing the Black Body: Race, Reproduction, and the Meaning of Liberty.* Vintage, 1998.

Roberts, Samuel Kelton, Jr. *Infectious Fear: Politics, Disease, and the Health Effects of Segregation.* Chapel Hill: University of North Carolina Press, 2009.

Roberts, Steward R. "Nervous and Mental Influences in Angina Pectoris." *American Heart Journal* 7 (1931): 21–35.

Robinson, Eugene. *Disintegration: The Splintering of Black America.* New York: Doubleday, 2010.

Rock, Melanie. "Classifying Diabetes; or, Commensurating Bodies of Unequal Experience." *Public Culture* 17, no. 3 (2005): 467–486.

Rodriguez, Joseph. "Hispanic-Americans Suffer More Often from Diabetes Type." *Hartford Courant,* March 31, 1985.

Roemer, Milton I. "Resistance to Innovation: The Case of the Community Health Center." *American Journal of Public Health* 78, no. 9 (1988): 1234–1239.

Root, Howard F., and Alexander Marble. "Progress in Diabetes Mellitus." *New England Medical Journal* 218, no. 22 (1938): 918–933.

Rose, Nikolas. *The Politics of Life Itself: Biomedicine, Power, and Subjectivity in the Twenty-First Century.* Princeton, NJ: Princeton University Press, 2006.

Rose, Nikolas, and Carlos Novas. "Biological Citizenship." Pp.1–40 in *Blackwell Companion to Global Anthropology,* ed. A. Ong and S. Collier. Oxford, UK: Blackwell, 2004.

Rosenberg, Charles E. "Body and Mind in Nineteenth Century Medicine: Some Clinical Origins of the Neurosis Construct." *Bulletin of the History of Medicine* 63 (1989): 185–197.

———. *The Cholera Years: The United States in 1832, 1849, and 1866.* Chicago: University of Chicago Press, 1962.

———. "Pathologies of Progress: The Idea of Civilization as Risk." *Bulletin of the History of Medicine* 72, no. 4 (1998): 714–730.

Runyan, John W., Roger Vander Zwaag Jr., and Stephen T. Miller. "The Memphis Diabetes Continuing Care Program." *Diabetes Care* 3, no. 2 (1980): 382–386.

Rusk, Howard A. "A Point Four for U.S. Indians Urged to Better Their Health." *New York Times,* November 1, 1953.

Saguy, Abigail C., and Kevin W. Riley. "Weighing Both Sides: Morality, Mortality, and

Framing Contests over Obesity." *Journal of Health Politics, Policy and Law* 30, no. 5 (2005): 869–921.

Sahagun, Louis. "Genetic Link Traced: Diabetes. A Special Risk for Latinos." *Los Angeles Times*, April 20, 1983.

————. "Needed: Facts in Spanish for Those Most Vulnerable. Diabetes Data Misdirected, Latinos Say." *Los Angeles Times*, May 12, 1983.

Sahota, Puneet Chawla. "Genetic Histories: Native American's Accounts of Being at Risk for Diabetes." *Social Studies of Science* 42, no. 6 (2012): 821–842.

Saiki, John H., and David L. Rimoin. "Diabetes Mellitus among the Navajo. I. Clinical Features." *Archives of Internal Medicine* 122, no. 1 (1968): 1–5.

Salsbury, C. G. "Disease Incidence among the Navajos." *Southwestern Medicine* 21 (1937): 230–233.

Sardell, Alice. *The U.S. Experiment in Social Medicine: The Community Health Center Program, 1965–1986*. Pittsburgh: University of Pittsburgh Press, 1987.

Savitt, Todd. *Medicine and Slavery: The Diseases and Health Care of Blacks in Antebellum Virginia*. Urbana: University of Illinois Press, 1978.

————. *Race and Medicine in Nineteenth- and Early-Twentieth-Century America*. Kent State University Press, 2007.

Scheder, Jo C. "A Sickly-Sweet Harvest: Farmworker Diabetes and Social Equality." *Medical Anthropology*, n.s. 2, no. 3 (1988): 251–277.

Scheper-Hughes, Nancy. "Foreword: Diabetes and Genocide—Beyond the Thrifty Gene." Pp. xvii–xxi in *Indigenous Peoples and Diabetes: Community Empowerment and Wellness*, ed. Mariana Leal Ferreira and Gretchen Chesley Lang. Durham, NC: Carolina Academic Press, 2006.

Schultz, Adolph H. *Biographical Memoir of Aleš Hrdlička, 1869–1943*. Washington, DC: National Academy of Sciences, 1944.

Schwartz, Hillel. *Never Satisfied: A Cultural History of Diets, Fantasies and Fat*. New York: Free Press, 1986.

Schwartz, Jacob. "The Etiology of Diabetes Mellitus among Jews." *Medical Times and Long Island Medical Journal* 62 (1934): 107–109.

Schwartz, Marie Jenkins. *Birthing a Slave: Motherhood and Medicine in the Antebellum South*. Cambridge, MA: Harvard University Press, 2006.

Schwartz, Shuly Rubin. *The Emergence of Jewish Scholarship in America: The Publication of the 'Jewish Encyclopedia.'* Cincinnati: Monographs of the Hebrew Union College, 1991.

Scott, Daryl Michael. "The Rise and Fall of Race Psychology in the Study of African Americans. Pp. 722–744 in *The Oxford Handbook of African American Citizenship, 1865–Present*, ed. Henry Louis Gates. Oxford, UK: Oxford University Press, 2012.

Scott, E. M., and G. J. Mouratoff. "Diabetes Mellitus in Alaskan Eskimos and Indians." In *Diabetes Mellitus in Asia, 1970: Proceedings of a Symposium. Kobe, Japan, May 24, 1970*, ed. S. Tsuji and M. Wada. Amsterdam: Excerpta Medica, 1971.

Seegen, Josef. *Der Diabetes Mellitus auf Grundlage zahlreicher Beobachtung*, 3rd ed. (Berlin: August Hirschwald, 1893).

"Seventy-Five Per Cent of Diabetes Cases Occur in Jews, Magazine Declares." *Jewish Post*, October 31, 1941, https://newspapers.library.in.gov/?a=d&d=JPOST19411031-01.1.1&e=, accessed December 6, 2019.

"72% of 506 Diabetic Clinic Patients Previously Overweight." *Atlanta Daily World*, January 19, 1961.

Shah, Nyan. *Contagious Divides: Epidemics and Race in San Francisco's Chinatown*. Berkeley: University of California Press, 2001.

Shapiro, Laura. "Do Our Genes Determine Which Foods We Eat?" *Newsweek* 122, no. 6 (1993): 1.

Shattuck, Frederick C. "The General Management of Diabetes." *Albany Medical Annals* 25, no. 4 (1904): 367–375.

Sheridan, Clare. "'Another White Race': Mexican Americans and the Paradox of Whiteness in Jury Selection." *Law and History Review* 21, no. 1 (2003): 109–144.

Shihipar, Abdullah. "The Opioid Crisis Isn't White." *New York Times*, February 26, 2019.

Signorello, Lisa B., David G. Schlundt, Sarah S. Cohen, Mark D. Steinwandel, Maciej S. Buchowski, Joseph K. McLaughlin, Margaret K. Hargreaves, and William J. Blot. "Comparing Diabetes Prevalence between African Americans and Whites of Similar Socioeconomic Status." *American Journal of Public Health* 97 (2007): 1–8.

Singerman, Robert. "The Jew as Racial Alien: The Genetic Component of American Anti-Semitism." Pp. 103–129 in *Anti-Semitism in American History*, ed. David A. Gerber. Urbana: University of Illinois Press, 1986.

"600,000 Diabetics Are Health Asset to Nation." *Science News Letter* 35 (May 13, 1939): 297.

Skipper, Eric. "Diabetes Mellitus and Pregnancy: A Clinical and Analytical Study." *Quarterly Journal of Medicine*, n.s. 2 (1933): 353–380.

Slater, Eliot. "German Eugenics in Practice." *Eugenics Review* 27, no. 4 (1936): 287–295.

Sloan, Norman. "Ethnic Distribution of Diabetes Mellitus in Hawaii." *Journal of the American Medical Association* 183, no. 6 (1963): 419–424.

Smedley, Audrey, and Brian D. Smedley. "Race as Biology Is Fiction, Racism as Social Problem Is Real: Anthropological and Historical Perspectives on the Social Construction of Race." *American Psychologist* 60 (January 2005): 216–226.

Smith, Susan L. *Sick and Tired of Being Sick and Tired: Black Women's Health Activism in America, 1890–1950*. Philadelphia: University of Pennsylvania Press, 1995.

Smith, T. Lynn. "The Redistribution of the Negro Population of the United States, 1910–1960." *Journal of Negro History* 51, no. 3 (1966): 155–173.

Smith-Morris, Carolyn. *Diabetes among the Pima: Stories of Survival*. Tucson: University of Arizona Press, 2006.

Smits, David. "The Frontier Army and the Destruction of the Buffalo: 1865–1883." *Western Historical Quarterly* 25, no. 3 (Autumn 1994): 312–338.

Solomon, Rivers. "I Have Diabetes. Am I to Blame?" *New York Times*, October 12, 2016.

Speak, Allan H. *Black Chicago: The Making of a Negro Ghetto, 1890–1920.* Chicago: University of Chicago Press, 1967.

"Special Notice." *National Negro Health News* 18, no. 2 (1950).

Stallard, Karin, Barbara Ehrenreich, and Holly Sklar. *Poverty in the American Dream: Women & Children First.* Boston: South End Press, 1983.

Starr, Paul. *The Social Transformation of American Medicine.* New York: Basic Books, 1982.

Stearns, Peter N. *Fat History: Bodies and Beauty in the Modern West.* New York: New York University Press, 1997.

Stearns, Samuel. "Some Emotional Aspects of the Treatment of Diabetes Mellitus and the Role of the Physician." *New England Journal of Medicine* 249, no. 12 (1953): 471–476.

Stein, Jay H., Keey M. West, James M. Robey, Dean F. Tirador, and Glen W. McDonald. "The High Prevalence of Abnormal Glucose Tolerance in the Cherokee Indians of North Carolina." *Archives of Internal Medicine* 116, no. 6 (1965): 842–845.

Steinitz, H. "The Incidence of Diabetes in Israel." *Harefuah* 50, no. 1 (March 1956): 106–107.

Stepan, Nancy. *The Idea of Race in Science: Great Britain, 1800–1960.* New York: Macmillan, 1982.

Stepan, Nancy Leys, and Sander L. Gilman. "Appropriating the Idioms of Science: The Rejection of Scientific Racism." Pp. 170–195 in *The "Racial" Economy of Science: Toward a Democratic Future*, ed. Sandra Harding. Bloomington: Indiana University Press, 1993.

Stern, Alexandra. *Eugenic Nation: Faults and Frontiers of Better Breeding in Modern America.* Berkeley: University of California Press, 2005.

———. *Telling Genes: The Story of Genetic Counseling in America.* Baltimore: Johns Hopkins University Press, 2012.

Stern, Heinrich. "The Mortality from Diabetes Mellitus in the City of New York (Manhattan and the Bronx) in 1899." *Medical Record* 58 (1900): 766–774.

Stern, Michael P., Sharon Parten Gaskill, Clarence R. Allen Jr., Virginia Garza, José L. Gonzales, and Reuel H. Waldrop. "Cardiovascular Risk Factors in Mexican Americans in Laredo, Texas. I: Prevalence of Overweight and Diabetes and Distributions of Serum Lipids." *American Journal of Epidemiology* 113, no. 5 (1981): 546–555.

Stern, Michael P., Sharon Parten Gaskill, and Steven M. Haffner. "Does Obesity Explain Excess Prevalence of Diabetes among Mexican Americans? Results of the San Antonio Heart Study." *Diabetologia* 24 (1983): 272–277.

Stern, Michael, Jacqueline A. Pugh, Sharon Parten Gaskill, and Helen P. Hazuda. "Knowledge, Attitudes, and Behavior Related to Obesity and Dieting in Mexican Americans and Anglos: The San Antonio Heart Study." *American Journal of Epidemiology* 115 (1982): 917–928.

Stocking, George W., Jr. *Race, Culture and Evolution: Essays in the History of Anthropology.* Chicago: University of Chicago Press, 1997.

———. "The Turn-of-the-Century Concept of Race." *Modernism/Modernity* 1, no. 1 (1994): 4–16.

Stoddard, Lothrop. "The Pedigree of Judah." *Forum* (March 1926): 326.

Stratford, Mary. "H.D. Doctor's Study Raises Hope for Diabetics." *Afro-American*, November 16, 1957, 20.

Striker, C. "American Diabetes Association." *Hygeia* 23 (1945): 522, 532, 534.

Stunkard, A. J. "Presidential Address—1974: From Explanation to Action in Psychosomatic Medicine: The Case of Obesity." *Psychosomatic Medicine* 37, no. 3 (1975): 195–236.

Swan, John. *The Works of Thomas Sydenham*. Vol. 1. London: G.G.J. and J. Robinson, 1788.

"Symposium on Diabetes," *Journal of the American Medical Association* 82, no. 23 (1924): 1887–1888.

Tallbear, Kim. *Native American DNA: Tribal Belonging and the False Promise of Genetic Science*. Minneapolis: University of Minnesota Press, 2013.

Tattersall, Robert. *Diabetes: The Biography*. New York: Oxford University Press, 2009.

———. "Maturity Onset Diabetes of the Young: A Clinical History." *Diabetic Medicine* 15, no. 1 (1998): 11–14.

Taylor, Carol M. "W. E. B. Du Bois's Challenge to Scientific Racism." *Journal of Black Studies* 11, no. 4 (1981): 449–460.

Tessaro, Irene, Shannon L. Smith, and Sheila Rye. "Knowledge and Perceptions of Diabetes in an Appalachian Population." *Preventing Chronic Disease: Public Health Research, Practice, and Policy* 2, no. 2 (2005): 1–9.

Thomas, David Hurst. *Skull Wars: Kennewick Man, Archaeology, and the Battle for Native American Identity*. New York: Basic Books, 2000.

"Thomas E. Malone, Ph.D." National Institutes of Health. Last modified August 7, 2015. https://www.nih.gov/about-nih/what-we-do/nih-almanac/thomas-e-malone -phd, accessed December 6, 2019.

Thomas, W. H. "Medical Treatment of Diabetes." *Albany Medical Annals* (April 1904), abstracted in the *Journal of the American Medical Association* 42 (May 28 1904): 1451.

Tomasson, Richard F. "Patterns in Negro-White Differential Mortality, 1930–1957." *The Milbank Memorial Fund Quarterly* 38, no. 4 (October 1960): 362–386.

Tomes, Nancy. *Remaking the American Patient: How Madison Avenue and Modern Medicine Turned Patients into Consumers*. Chapel Hill: University of North Carolina Press, 2016.

Tom-Orme, Lillian. "Traditional Beliefs and Attitudes about Diabetes among Navajos and Utes." Pp. 271–291 in *Diabetes as a Disease of Civilisation: The Impact of Culture Change on Indigenous Peoples*, ed. Jennie R. Joe and Robert S. Young. Berlin: Mouton de Gruyter, 1994.

Toon, Elizabeth. "Managing the Conduct of the Individual Life: Public Health Education and American Public Health, 1910–1940." PhD diss., University of Pennsylvania, 1998.

Trafzer, Clifford E., and Jean A. Keller. *Boarding School Blues: Revisiting Indian Educational Experiences*. Lincoln: University of Nebraska Press, 2006.

Trennert, Robert A. *The Phoenix Indian School: Forced Assimilation in Arizona, 1891–1935*. Norman: University of Oklahoma Press, 1988.

Treuting, T. F. "The Role of Emotional Factors in the Etiology and Course of Diabetes Mellitus." *American Journal of Medical Science* 244 (1962): 93–110.

Tuchman, Arleen Marcia. "Biometrics and Citizenship: Measuring Diabetes in the United States in the Interwar Years." *History of Science* special issue: *Measurement, Self-Tracking and the History of Science* (forthcoming, 2020), doi: 10.1177/00732753/19869762.

———."Diabetes and 'Defective' Genes in the Twentieth-Century United States." *Journal of the History of Medicine and Allied Sciences* 70, no. 1 (2013): 1–33.

———."Diabetes and Race: A Historical Perspective." *American Journal of Public Health* 101, no. 1 (2011): 24–33.

Tuomi, T., N. Santoro, S. Caprio, M. Cai, J. Weng, and L. Groop. "The Many Faces of Diabetes: A Disease with Increasing Heterogeneity." *Lancet* 383, no. 9922 (2014): 1084–1090.

Turner, Patricia A. *Ceramic Uncles & Celluloid Mammies: Black Images and Their Influence on Culture*. New York: Anchor Books, 1994.

"Two Important Cures Announced." *New York Times*, December 6, 1922.

Unger, Jeff. "Editorials: Latent Autoimmune Diabetes in Adults." *American Family Physician* 81, no. 7 (2010): 843–847.

Urquhart, Brian. *Ralph Bunche: An American Odyssey*. New York: W.W. Norton, 1998.

U.S. Bureau of the Census. "History. Through the Decades. Index of Questions. 1930." https://www.census.gov/history/www/through_the_decades/index_of_questions/1930_1.html, accessed May 28, 2019.

———. *A Report of the Seventeenth Decennial Census of the United States*. Vol. 2, part 21: Massachusetts. Washington, DC: U.S. Government Printing Office, 1953.

U.S. Congress. *Dictionary of Races or Peoples: Reports of the Immigration Commission, Document No. 662*. Washington, DC: U.S. Government Printing Office, 1911.

———. *Statements and Recommendations Submitted by Societies and Organizations Interested in Immigration: Document No. 764*. Washington, DC: U.S. Government Printing Office, 1911.

U.S. Department of Health, Education, and Welfare. *Diabetes Mellitus Mortality in the United States, 1950–67*. Washington, DC: Government Printing Office, 1971.

———. *Diabetes Source Book. PHS Publication no. 1168*, rev. Washington, DC: U.S. Government Printing Office, 1968.

U.S. Department of Health and Human Services. *Report of the Secretary's Task Force on Black & Minority Health*. (Heckler Report.) Washington, DC: U.S. Government Printing Office, 1985.

U.S. Interdepartmental Committee to Coordinate Health and Welfare Activities. *National Health Conference, July 18–20, 1938*. Washington, DC, 1938.

U.S. President's Research Committee on Social Trends. *Recent Social Trends in the United States: Report of the President's Research Committee on Social Trends, with a Foreword by Herbert Hoover*. New York: McGraw-Hill, 1933, https://archive.org/

stream/recentsocialtren0runitrich/recentsocialtren0runitrich_djvu.txt, accessed May 27, 2019.

U.S. Public Health Service. *Preliminary Reports, Bulletin 6: The Magnitude of the Chronic Disease Problem in the United States.* Washington, DC: United States Public Health Service, 1938 [rev. 1939]. HathiTrust, http://hdl.handle.net/2027/mdp .39015007748299, accessed October 5, 2019.

———. *Preliminary Reports, Bulletin 9: Disability from Special Causes in Relation to Economic Status.* Washington, DC: National Health Survey, 1938 (rev. 1939).

"U.S. Studies Latino Health in Alhambra." *Los Angeles Times,* August 14, 1983.

Vantrease, Dana. "Commod Bods and Frybread Power: Government Food Aid in American Indian Culture." *Journal of American Folklore* 126, no. 499 (2013): 55–69.

Wailoo, Keith. *Dying in the City of Blues: Sickle Cell Anemia and the Politics of Race and Health.* Chapel Hill: University of North Carolina Press, 2001.

———. *How Cancer Crossed the Color Line.* New York: Oxford University Press, 2011.

Wailoo, Keith, and Stephen Pemberton. *The Troubled Dream of Genetic Medicine: Ethnicity and Innovation in Tay-Sachs, Cystic Fibrosis, and Sickle Cell Disease.* Baltimore: Johns Hopkins University Press, 2006.

Walker-Barnes, Chanequa. *Too Heavy a Yoke: Black Women and the Burden of Strength.* Eugene, OR: Cascade, 2014.

Wang, Alexandra. "The Changing Face of Diabetes: How Diabetes Came to Be an Issue in African Americans." Undergraduate honors thesis, Wesleyan University, 2012.

"War on Diabetes." *Time,* April 21, 1923.

Ward, Thomas J., Jr. *Black Physicians in the Jim Crow South.* Fayetteville: University of Arkansas Press, 2003.

Waring, Mary Fitzbutler. "Degenerative Diseases." *National Notes* 30, no. 8 (1928): 6.

———. "Sanitation." *National Association Notes* (April–May 1917): 8–9.

Weindling, Paul. "German Eugenics and the Wider World: Beyond the Racial State." Pp. 315–331 in *The Oxford Handbook of the History of Eugenics,* ed. Alison Bashford and Philippa Levine. Oxford, UK: Oxford University Press, 2010.

Weiner, Diane. "Interpreting Ideas about Diabetes, Genetics, and Inheritance." Pp. 108–135 in *Medicine Ways: Disease, Health, and Survival among Native Americans,* ed. Clifford E. Trafzer and Diane Weiner. Walnut Creek, CA: Alta Mira, 2001.

Weisz, George. *Chronic Disease in the Twentieth Century: A History.* Baltimore: Johns Hopkins University Press, 2014.

———. "Epidemiology and Health Care Reform: The National Health Survey of 1935–1936." *American Journal of Public Health* 101, no. 3 (2011): 438–447.

West, Kelly M. "Diabetes in American Indians and Other Native Populations of the New World." *Diabetes* 23, no. 10 (1974): 841–855.

———. *Epidemiology of Diabetes and Its Vascular Lesions.* New York: Elsevier, 1978.

White, Deborah Gray. *Too Heavy a Load: Black Women in Defense of Themselves, 1894–1994.* New York: W. W. Norton, 1999.

White, Priscilla, "Diabetes in Childhood." Pp. 587–617 in *Treatment of Diabetes Mellitus,* ed. Elliott P. Joslin, 6th ed. Philadelphia: Lea & Febiger, 1937.

————. "Pregnancy Complicating Diabetes." Pp. 618–637 in *Treatment of Diabetes Mellitus*, ed. Elliott P. Joslin, 6th ed. Philadelphia: Lea & Febiger, 1937.

Whitney, L. Baynard. "Harlem Mourns Passing of Beloved Pioneer Physician: Final Rites Held over Remains of E. Elliott Rawlins." *New York Amsterdam News*, September 19, 1928, 1–2.

Wiebe, Robert H. *The Search for Order*. New York: Hill and Wang, 1967.

Wiley, H. W. "The League for Longer Life." *Good Housekeeping* 72 (1921): 30, 186–190.

Wilkerson, Hugh. "Problems of an Aging Population." *American Journal of Public Health* 37 (1947): 177–188.

Wilkerson, Hugh, and Leo P. Krall. "Diabetes in a New England Town." *Journal of the American Medical Association* 135, no. 4 (1947): 209–216.

Wilkerson, Isabel. *The Warmth of Other Suns: The Epic Story of America's Great Migration*. New York: Random House, 2010.

Williams, A. Wilberforce. "Defender Health Editor Looks Back." *Chicago Defender*, May 4, 1935, 24.

————. "Diabetes." Talks on Preventive Measures, First Aid Remedies, Hygienics and Sanitation. *Chicago Defender*, August 23, 1924, 24.

————. "Diabetes." Talks on Preventive Measures, First Aid Remedies, Hygienics and Sanitation. *Chicago Defender*, January 31, 1925, 24.

————. "Diabetes." Talks on Preventive Measures, First Aid Remedies, Hygienics and Sanitation. *Chicago Defender*, June 18, 1927, A2.

————. "The Way to Health: Diabetes Management." Talks on Preventive Measures, First Aid Remedies, Hygienics and Sanitation. *Chicago Defender*, December 22, 1934, 12.

————. "What to Do for Diabetes." Talks on Preventive Measures, First Aid Remedies, Hygienics and Sanitation. *Chicago Defender*, June 25, 1927, A2.

Williams, Daniel H., M.D., "Is the Negro Dying Out?" *Colored American Magazine* 15, no. 1 (January 1909): 662.

Williams, David R. "Race and Health: Basic Questions, Emerging Directions." *Annals of Epidemiology* 5 (1997): 322–333.

Williams, John R. "An Evaluation of the Allen Method of Treatment of Diabetes Mellitus." *American Journal of the Medical Sciences* 162 (1921): 62–72.

————. "A Study of the Significance of Heredity and Infection in Diabetes Mellitus." *American Journal of the Medical Sciences* 154, no. 3 (1917): 396–406.

Williams, Richard Allen. "Introduction." Pp. xv–xvi in *Textbook of Black-Related Diseases*, ed. Richard Allen Williams. New York: McGraw-Hill, 1975.

————. "An Introduction to the New NMA President, by Himself." *Journal of the National Medical Association* 108, no. 3 (2016): 138–139.

————, ed. *Textbook of Black-Related Diseases*. New York: McGraw-Hill, 1975.

Williams, R. C., W. C. Knowler, W. J. Butler, D. J. Pettitt, J. R. Lisse, P. H. Bennett, D. L. Mann, A. H. Johnson, and P. I. Teraski. "HLA-A2 and Type 2 (Insulin Independent) Diabetes Mellitus in Pima Indians: An Association of Allele Frequency with Age." *Diabetologia* 21 (1981): 460–463.

Williamson, R. T. "Increased Death Rate from Diabetes, and the Possibility of Preventing the Disease, or of Postponing Its Onset." *The Practitioners (London)* (April 1909): 455–467.

Willrich, Michael. *Pox: An American History.* New York: Penguin, 2012.

Wilson, J. G. "The Crossing of the Races." *Popular Science Monthly* 79 (July–December 1911): 486–495.

———. "Increase in the Death Rate from Diabetes—A Possible Explanation." *Medical Record* 82 (1912): 662–663.

———. "A Study in Jewish Psychopathology." *Popular Science Monthly* (1913): 264–271.

Wise, P. H., F. J. Edwards, R. J. Craig, B. Evans, J. B. Murchland, B. Sutherland, and D. W. Thomas. "Diabetes and Associated Variables in the South Australian Aboriginal." *Australian and New Zealand Journal of Medicine* 6 (1976): 191–196.

Wohl, Michael G. "Diabetes: A Public Health Problem." *Hygeia* 12 (1934): 409–411.

Wolfe, B. "Racial Integrity Laws (1924–1930)." In *Encyclopedia Virginia.* Last modified November 4, 2015, available at http://www.EncyclopediaVirginia.org/Racial_Integrity_Laws_of_the_1920s, accessed May 29, 2019.

Wood, Bertha M. *Foods of the Foreign-Born: In Relation to Health.* Boston: Whitcomb & Barrows, 1922.

Wright, Greg. "Rising Diabetes Rates in Appalachia Shock Health Officials." *Gannett News Service,* September 13, 2003.

Wright, Lawrence. "One Drop of Blood." *New Yorker,* July 25, 1994, 46–55.

Zaccardi, Francesco, et al. "Pathophysiology of Type 1 and Type 2 Diabetes Mellitus: A 90-Year Perspective." *Postgraduate Medical Journal* 92 (2016): 63–69.

Zackondik, Teresa. "Fixing the Color Line: The Mulatto, Southern Courts, and Racial Identity." *American Quarterly* 53 (September 2001): 420–451.

Zimmet, Paul. "Epidemiology of Diabetes and Its Macrovascular Manifestations in Pacific Populations: The Medical Effects of Social Progress." *Diabetes Care* 2, no. 2 (1979): 144–153.

Zisserman, Louis. "Diabetes Mellitus: A Survey of 155 Deaths in Diabetic Patients." *Journal of Clinical Endocrinology & Metabolism* 1, no. 4 (1941): 314–315.

ACKNOWLEDGMENTS

The time has come to thank everyone who has helped me to bring this book to frui-tion. Without the assistance, support, and encouragement of family, friends, col-leagues, students, librarians, and archivists, the journey would have been far more tumultuous and the days to completion even longer. It is with considerable pleasure that I now acknowledge them all.

Several undergraduate students who helped me in the early stages of this project are now well into their own careers in medicine, law, development, and city planning. Others, who helped me recently, are still carving out a path for themselves. I wish to thank Michael Ahillen, Stacy Clark, Miriam Goldstein, Laura Grove, and Brett Sklaw for their assistance over the life of this book. I also want to acknowledge the help of the archivists and librarians at the following institutions: Columbia University Health Sciences Library; Francis A. Countway Library of Medicine; Joslin Diabetes Center; Metropolitan Life Insurance Company Archives; National Library of Medicine; and the New York Academy of Medicine.

The weeks I spent doing research at the Joslin Diabetes Center came with the added pleasure of getting to know Dr. Donald M. Barnett and Dr. Donna Younger, both of whom had begun working at the Joslin Clinic when Dr. Elliott P. Joslin was still alive. I appreciate their generosity, their love of history, and their guidance when I encountered bumps in the road. I owe a special debt to Christopher Ryland and James Thweatt in Special Collections at the Eskind Biomedical Library, as well as to the wonderful staff in the Interlibrary Loan Office at Vanderbilt University, for their ongoing help and support.

Several funding institutions made it possible for me to carry out my research. I wish to thank the American Council of Learned Societies, the National Institutes of Health (G13LM012252–01), and Vanderbilt University's Office of the Provost (Re-search Scholars Grant Program) for their generous financial support of my work. I particularly appreciate the year I spent as a fellow at Vanderbilt's Robert Penn Warren

Center for the Humanities in 2013–2014. The wide-ranging and provocative discussions with members of the "Seminar on Diagnosis in Context" led to new friendships, new understandings, and, I believe, a more sharply focused book.

Over the years, I have had countless conversations with colleagues whose insights have simply become part of how I think about history. Much scholarly writing takes place in solitude, but the ideas we express are only partly our own. I appreciate the conversations and email exchanges I have had with Missy Foy, Matt Klingle, Aaron Mauck, Richard Mizelle, and Robert Tattersall about our shared interest in the history of diabetes. Special thanks to those who read parts of this book and gave me valuable feedback: Dave Aftlandian, Lisa Bob, Brandon Byrd, Michell Chresfield, David S. Jones, Beth Linker, Matt Klingle, Sarah Rose, Dan Usner, and Jackie Wolf. I am especially indebted to friends and colleagues who read the entire manuscript and helped me to hone my argument: Len Braitman, Kate Daniels, Mona Frederick, Janet Golden, Jeremy Greene, Margaret Humphreys, Robert Kauffman, Marilyn Place, and Dave Zolensky. Thanks also to Janet Golden, Sue Lederer, and Naomi Rogers, who sent materials about diabetes to me that they came across while doing their own research. I also want to acknowledge the excellent editorial staff at Yale University Press. Jean Thomson Black has been an ideal editor, finding the perfect balance between patience and pressure as I completed this book. And Julie Carlson is the copyeditor every author wants. Her ability to cut through my verbiage and sharpen my prose has improved this manuscript tremendously.

Portions of Chapters 1 and 2 appeared in Arleen Marcia Tuchman, "Diabetes and Race: A Historical Perspective," *American Journal of Public Health* 101, no. 1 (2011): 24–33, published by the Sheridan Press, and Tuchman, "Diabetes and 'Defective' Genes in the Twentieth-Century United States," *Journal of the History of Medicine and Allied Sciences* 70, no. 1 (2013): 1–33, published by Oxford University Press. I want to thank both presses for granting me permission to use portions of my previously published work.

I want to give a particular shout-out to Sarah Igo and Ruth Rogaski, who have been my writing buddies since the spring of 2015. Not only did they read the entire manuscript as it came together, asking tough questions while expressing enthusiasm for my work, but they also kept me accountable. There was something steadying and comforting about our weekly meetings during the craziness of the semester, when, whatever else might be going on, we would get together, give each other a brief update on our work, and then just write.

In the years I spent working on this book I leaned especially heavily on friends. With those who lived far away, texts and phone calls were my lifeline. With those close to home, our long walks around Sevier Park, Radnor Lake, and through the streets of the neighborhood sustained and nurtured me. Thank you to Kate, Marilyn, Mona, Pat, and Vanessa for being there, whether I needed to talk about scholarship, teaching, children, blended families, aging parents, or anything else life threw my way. You reminded me of what is important in life, and kept me balanced.

My greatest debt goes to my family. I want to thank my sister, Shendl, for her love and wisdom; my stepdaughter, Rachel, for modeling what a life committed to social justice can look like; my stepson, Peter, and his wife, Heather, for making sure that our ever-growing family remains closely knit; my grandchildren, Sam and Lena, who keep my heart filled with joy; and my son, Andrew, who somehow, overnight, has changed from an adorable child into a remarkable young man, filled with passion for life, learning, and the mysteries of the mind. Finally, my deepest thanks go to my husband, Dave, who has lost count of the number of drafts he has read of this manuscript. I am grateful for his unconditional support of my work and his unconditional love for me.

My father passed away in 2013, two weeks after Andrew became a Bar Mitzvah. He was never an easy man to be around, but in the last decade of his life we grew close, for which I am deeply grateful. Through him, I got to see what it could mean to live with diabetes. This book is dedicated to him.

INDEX

Page numbers in *italics* indicate illustrations and figures.